Paediatric Anaesthesia and Critical Care in the District Hospital

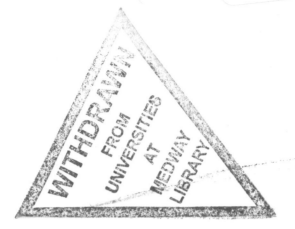

Commissioning Editor: Paul Fam
Project Development Manager: Claire Whittaker
Project Manager: Susan Skinner
Illustration Manager: Mick Ruddy
Design Direction: Andy Chapman

Paediatric Anaesthesia and Critical Care in the District Hospital

Neil S Morton MBChB FRCA FRCPCH
Consultant in Paediatric Anaesthesia
Intensive Care and Pain Management
Department of Anaesthesia
Royal Hospital for Sick Children
Yorkhill NHS Trust
Glasgow
UK

and

Jane M Peutrell MBBS FRCP FRCA
Consultant in Paediatric Anaesthesia
Department of Anaesthesia
Royal Hospital for Sick Children
Yorkhill NHS Trust
Glasgow
UK

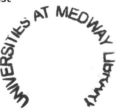

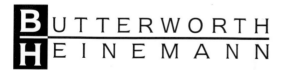

BUTTERWORTH
HEINEMANN

An imprint of Elsevier Science

EDINBURGH • LONDON • NEW YORK • OXFORD • PHILADELPHIA • ST LOUIS • SYDNEY • TORONTO   2003

BUTTERWORTH-HEINEMANN
An imprint of Elsevier Limited

First published 2003
  Reprinted 2004

ISBN 0 7506 4302 1

British Library Cataloguing in Publication Data
A catalogue record for this book is available from the British Library

Library of Congress Cataloging in Publication Data
A catalog record for this book is available from the Library of Congress

Note
Medical knowledge is constantly changing. Standard safety precautions must be followed,
but as new research and clinical experience broaden our knowledge, changes in treatment and
drug therapy may become necessary or appropriate. Readers are advised to check the most
current product information provided by the manufacturer of each drug to be administered to
verify the recommended dose, the method and duration of administration, and
contraindications. It is the responsibility of the practitioner, relying on experience and
knowledge of the patient, to determine dosages and the best treatment for each individual
patient. Neither the Publisher nor the editors assumes any liability for any injury and/or
damage to persons or property arising from this publication.

The Publisher

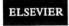
your source for books,
journals and multimedia
in the health sciences
www.elsevierhealth.com

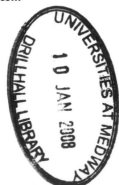

The
publisher's
policy is to use
**paper manufactured
from sustainable forests**

Printed in China
C/02

Contents

Preface

The practice of paediatric anaesthesia and critical care in district hospitals has been influenced in the last fifteen years by a trend towards centralisation of paediatric services in regional or tertiary hospitals. This was driven by clinical governance aspects of anaesthesia which came to the fore after the NCEPOD report of 1989 and subsequent recommendations about case-load and case-mix requirements to maintain skills. Recently the pendulum has swung back somewhat because it is clear that the tertiary centres cannot cope with the total volume of paediatric work, the public wish to have some services provided locally and the old recommendations are too proscriptive and many district hospitals are able to provide a very high standard of care for the majority of children who are, in the main, healthy with only one problem to fix. In addition, the old recommendations did not address difficulties imposed by geography and the particular needs of remote and rural parts of the UK.

A more rational approach has now developed for the provision of paediatric anaesthesia and critical care and the aim of this book is to draw together the myriad of guidelines and recommendations to enable district hospitals to design and then set the limits of their local service. The book also gives advice on when to refer cases on to regional and tertiary facilities. As recently emphasised by the Royal College of Anaesthetists, district hospitals who receive children must always be able to resuscitate and stabilise the critically ill child pending transfer and detailed guidance is given on these important aspects of care.

We hope that the information in this book will be helpful to and supportive of colleagues working in district hospitals and will encourage comprehensive provision of paediatric anaesthetic and critical care services for all children in the UK wherever and whenever they present.

Neil S. Morton & Jane M. Peutrell

Contributors

Alison Carr MBBS, BSc, DA, DCH, FRCA
Consultant Paediatric Anaesthetist, Department Directorate of Anaesthesia, and Director of Phase 2, Peninsula Medical School Derriford Hospital, Plymouth NHS Trust, Plymouth

Pauline M Cullen MBCHB, FFARCSI
Consultant in Paediatric Anaesthesia & Intensive Care, Department of Anaesthesia, Royal Hospital for Sick Children, Yorkhill NHS Trust, Glasgow

Ann Harvey MBCHB, FRCA, DCH
Consultant Anaesthetist, Royal Cornwall Hospital (Treliske), Truro

Roddie McNicol MBCHB, FRCA
Consultant in Paediatric Anaesthesia, Department of Anaesthesia, Royal Hospital for Sick Children, Yorkhill NHS Trust, Glasgow

Neil S Morton FBCHB, FRCA, FRCPCH
Consultant in Paediatric Anaesthesia, Intensive Care & Pain Management, Department of Anaesthesia, Royal Hospital for Sick Children, Yorkhill NHS Trust, Glasgow

Jane M Peutrell MBBS, FRCP, FRCA
Consultant in Paediatric Anaesthesia, Department of Anaesthesia, Royal Hospital for Sick Children, Yorkhill NHS Trust, Glasgow

Anna-Maria Rollin MBBS, MRCS, LRCP, FRCA
Consultant Anaesthetist, Department of Anaesthesia, Epsom General Hospital, Epsom and St Helier NHS Trust, Epsom

Bruce L Taylor BSC, MBCHB, FFARCS, FANZCA, FFICANZCA
Consultant in Critical Care and Anaesthesia, Queen Alexandra Hospital, Portsmouth Hospitals NHS Trust, Portsmouth

Kathy Wilkinson MBBS, FRCA, MRCP, DCH
Consultant Paediatric Anaesthetist, Norfolk and Norwich Health Care Trust, Norwich

Acknowledgements

We also gratefully acknowledge contributions submitted by:

Dr Judith Dunnet, Frenchay Hospital, Bristol

Dr Jo Eastwood, King's Mill Centre, Sutton-in-Ashfield

Dr Ian Gauntlett, Musgrove Park, Taunton

Dr Dave Higgins, Southend Hospital, Trust

Dr Anna Johnson, Derriford Hospital, Plymouth

Dr Jerry Luntley, Barnsley District General Hospital

Dr Mike Mowbray, King's Mill Centre, Sutton-in-Ashfield

Dr John Pook, The Children's Hospital, Lewisham

Dr Anna Maria Rollin, Epsom General Hospital

Dr John Rutherford, Dumfries & Galloway Royal Infirmary

Dr Mike Tremlett, South Tees Acute Hospitals NHS Trust

Dr Jill White, Northampton General Hospital NHS Trust

Dr Kathy Wilkinson, Norfolk and Norwich Healthcare Trust

Cover illustration by Lauren McLaughlan

CHAPTER 1

Development of current practice

Roddie McNicol, Anna-Maria Rollin

Resistance to change	Networking
Achieving agreement	Monitoring the system
Standards	**Conclusion**
Resources	**References**
Recognition of limitations	

SECTION 1: Organisational framework

HISTORICAL BACKGROUND

In 1948 the new National Health Service (NHS) was established to offer a comprehensive health and rehabilitation service involving local authorities, hospitals and other medical and welfare services. As the NHS developed, hospital treatment was made available to many more sick children and the differences in the way children were cared for at home compared with hospital became more obvious. It became apparent that hospitals had to cater as much for the emotional needs of children as for their medical ones. This was summed up by one of the major campaigners for change, James Robertson, who stated in 1958 that 'the greatest single cause of distress for the young child in hospital is not illness or pain but separation from mother'.[1]

The Platt report: *The Welfare of Children in Hospital* (1959)[2]

By the 1950s, some progress had been made. For example, a few hospitals did allow mothers to stay with their children, but this practice was rare. In 1956, a wide range of professional and voluntary bodies lobbied the Central Health Services Council to take action and a special committee was set up under the chairmanship of Sir Harry Platt, President of the Royal College of Surgeons. This committee produced its report, *The Welfare of Children in Hospital*, in 1959.[2] Platt's remit was to make a special study of the arrangements in hospital for the emotional welfare of ill children (as distinct from their medical or nursing treatment) and make suggestions for improvement.

It is interesting to examine aspects of the Platt Report and their subsequent development because, although reports may change policy or lead to further reports, they are often ignored through differences of opinion or lack of financial resources and do not always produce legislative changes.

The 1955–59 Conservative government immediately accepted the recommendations of the Platt committee and the Ministry of Health issued a series of circulars endorsing them (particularly those calling for an end to caring for children in adult wards, or urging unrestricted visiting of children in hospital).[3] Since 1959 numerous official circulars have been issued pressing for a more widespread implementation of the recommendations. *Visiting of Children in Hospital*, published in 1966,[4] urged hospitals immediately to abolish routine restrictions for visiting children, to provide accommodation for mothers to stay with their children in hospital and to produce explanatory leaflets for parents on visiting arrangements. *Accommodation of Children in Hospital in Children's Departments* (1969)[5] urged hospital authorities to end the practice of admitting children to adult wards by 1971. In 1971, the authors of a comprehensive paper, *Hospital Facilities for Children*,[6] examined the essential requirements of a hospital service for children. Hospital boards were asked 'to review existing provision and secure further improvements at an early stage'. The Department of Health and Social Security (DHSS) revised and reissued this circular in 1977.[7] They noted that, although the principles of the Platt report were widely accepted, they were not universally practised and 'serious mistakes have been made when specially trained paediatric medical and nursing staff have not been involved in the care of a young child'.

National Association for the Welfare of Children in Hospital/Action for Children in Hospital

In 1961 the National Association for the Welfare of Children in Hospital (NAWCH) was formed to press for implementation of the principles of the Platt report and to advise parents about becoming more involved in their child's experience in hospital. Many changes in the care of children in hospital are due to the persistence of this association, now known as Action for Children in Hospital (ACH).

NAWCH/ACH has also undertaken surveys, some of which challenge official government figures. For instance a Health Ministry census, published in 1967,[8] claimed that 85% of hospitals allowed 'unrestricted visiting'. NAWCH/ACH, however, showed that only 57% of hospitals in one region allowed this practice, with over 25% forbidding morning visits. In their survey, NAWCH/ACH found that 55% of hospitals had no accommodation for mothers wishing to stay with their children.[9]

The Court committee: *Fit for the Future* (1976)[10]

In 1976, the Court committee published its report, *Fit for the Future*. It criticised the poor attempts by the health service to improve paediatric services, particularly the failure to implement the recommendations of the Platt committee,[2] which, it thought, could have been done with little or no additional expense. The Court committee reaffirmed the principles of the Platt report,[2] considered the existing structure of health care for children and called for integration of health services. In paragraph 12.20, p. 183, the authors stated:

> the development of (district general) hospitals has been one of the most significant contributions by the NHS to the care of children. Their intended structure and function in relation to children have been expressed with clarity and conviction in the Department of Health's memorandum [HM (71)22] and its explanatory annex 'Hospital Facilities for Children'. We are in essential agreement with these recommendations and wish to see them fully implemented. The central conclusion of the circular was this: to make the most efficient and economic use of resources, the district services for acutely ill children should be centralized in one department, in one part of the main hospital, accommodating all children and providing paediatric and specialty services. This also implies, for example, that in urban areas where closely adjacent district hospitals may each maintain a children's department, every effort must be made, without ignoring all the complex geographical, human and other factors, to concentrate the paediatric services in one hospital only. In this way alone can duplication of staff, accommodation and equipment be avoided, and families seem on the whole prepared to recognize that greater inconvenience for some may be the price that has to be paid to ensure better care for all.

The Consumers' Association survey: *Children in Hospital* (1980)[11]

In 1980, the Consumers' Association published the results of a national survey in its report *Children in Hospital*.[11] One of its aims was to assess how far the recommendations of the Platt committee[2] had been implemented. In all, 58 hospitals and 300 parents took part. The main findings are given in Box 1.1. The Consumers' Association found that, despite consistent support from successive governments for the principles of the Platt committee, progress towards full implementation had been slow.

CURRENT RECOMMENDATIONS

NHS Management Executive: *Welfare of Children and Young People in Hospital* (1991)[12]

Welfare of Children and Young People in Hospital, issued by the NHS Management Executive, is the most recent report aimed at improving health services for children. The

3

Box 1.1 Consumers' Association survey *Children in Hospital*: principal findings[11]

- Few hospitals had separate facilities for children in outpatients. Paediatric nurses were commonly not on duty in the outpatients' department
- 15% of children were admitted to adult wards. This practice was particularly common for children having ear, nose and throat surgery. The main reasons cited were lack of resources, conflict between paediatricians and other specialists or administrative anomalies
- Although all hospitals surveyed employed one or more consultant paediatrician, these individuals were not always responsible for all the children admitted to the hospital
- Although most sisters in charge of children's wards were registered children's nurses, there was little attempt to train staff lower down the hierarchy in paediatric nursing

Executive recommended it should form the basis of all health-service contracts for the provision of children's services and was therefore designed to assist purchasers to identify the standards of service they should seek and help providers to achieve these. The authors based their paper on the afore-mentioned Platt report[2] and the recommendations following its publication, not all of which had been implemented by every hospital. They also incorporated some of the findings and recommendations of the National Confidential Enquiry into Perioperative Deaths (NCEPOD) 1989 (see below).[13]

The NHS Management Executive advocated admitting children only as a last resort (i.e. if day treatment was not possible) and treating them only in hospitals with paediatric wards. They advised that the care of all children admitted to hospital should be supervised by a paediatric physician or surgeon and an adequate 'safety net' of paediatric cover should be provided. Any department in which children were treated should also have at least two registered sick children's nurses (RSCNs) on duty at all times. In support of NCEPOD,[13] the authors stated that anaesthetists and surgeons should not undertake 'occasional prac-

Box 1.2 Principal recommendations of the NHS Management Executive issued in *Welfare of Children and Young People in Hospital*[12]

- Children should only be treated as inpatients if day care is not possible
- Facilities should be available to ensure that children are separated from adult patients
- There should be open visiting for parents and siblings
- There should be facilities for parents to be resident a maximum distance of 'a dressing gown journey' away
- There should be facilities for play, ideally in the presence of a play leader
- There should be a designated paediatrician or surgeon to supervise the care of children with appropriate cover during periods of absence
- Adolescents should be able to choose whether they are admitted to a children's or adult's ward
- Two registered sick children's nurses (or nurses who have completed the child branch of Project 2000) should be on ward duty for every 24-h period
- There should be a registered sick children's nurse available 24 h a day to advise on the nursing of children in other departments, e.g. the intensive care unit, the casualty department and outpatients
- All anaesthetic and surgical staff should be experienced at dealing with children, as should be members of other medical specialities, such as radiology and laboratory medicine and members of the professions allied to medicine
- Staff rosters should provide for adequate safety-net cover in both the children's department and other departments where paediatric support is required

tice' in children, and adequate cover should be provided for designated anaesthetists during their absence.

The principal recommendations of the NHS Management Executive are summarised in Box 1.2.

It is important to note that the authors of the *Welfare of Children and Young People in Hospital*[12] state that there are specific instances when they must provide more than simple advice and be prescriptive because of legal obligations or the requirements of statutory and professional bodies responsible for clinical standards or key principles of government policy. Under these circumstances, they have used the word 'should'. It is interesting to see from Box 1.2 how frequently this word appears in the recommendations and guidelines.

The Audit Commission report: *Children First: A Study of Hospital Services* (1993)[14]

In 1993 the Audit Commission published a report *Children First: A Study of Hospital Services*.[14] The Commission first analysed data for the treatment of children in hospital to put paediatric surgery in a national context. It then assessed the quality of service provided and made recommendations for improvement.

Data for the treatment of children in hospital

There are about 14 million children and young people aged 18 and younger in England and Wales (28% of the population). About one in 11 children are admitted to hospital each year, amounting to about 16% of all inpatient admissions. Forty-two per cent of children or young people are admitted to hospital under the care of paediatric physicians. Forty-four per cent of the remaining are admitted to one of eight surgical specialities, usually ear, nose and throat (ENT), general surgery or trauma and orthopaedics. A large proportion of children admitted to medical paediatrics are younger than 1 year. In contrast, the ages of children admitted to surgical specialities are more evenly spread (although there is a peak at 5 years because of admissions for ENT surgery). Almost all admissions to medical paediatrics are emergencies, compared with about two-thirds of children admitted for surgery. These findings are summarised in Figure 1.1. Most surgeons operating on children also operate on adults. Only a small proportion of children (usually very young babies) are operated on by surgeons actually specialising in paediatric surgery.

Quality of service and recommendations for improvement

In the summary of their report, the Audit Commission stated that, although the principles for the care of children in hospital had been established by the Platt report as long ago as 1959,[2] they were sometimes not implemented. The main aims of the Audit Commission's study were to investigate why the various recommendations had not been met and to suggest ways of implementing them. In addition, it established six principles for the care of sick children (Box 1.3).

The root problem identified by the Audit Commission was that clinicians, managers and other staff gave insufficient attention to the needs of children and their families. This was manifest in a lack of written policies, management focus and poor communication between staff and parents. The authors state that the aims of the Platt report[2] could only be implemented if there was a major change in the attitudes of managers, doctors, nurses and other staff involved in running the service. However, attitudes cannot be changed overnight. Like the authors of the Court report,[10] the Commission claimed much could be achieved with little or no additional cost. They recommended that the management team of a hospital should include a consultant with overall responsibility for the policies for all services for children; a children's nurse (more senior than a ward sister) to provide the focus for implementing consistent policies throughout the

42% of child inpatients are admitted to paediatrics and 44% to eight surgical specialties

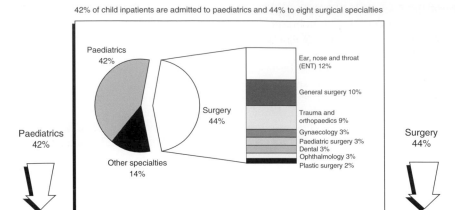

whereas...

42% of children admitted to paediatrics are aged <1 year

The incidence of surgery peaks at age 5, mainly due to ENT

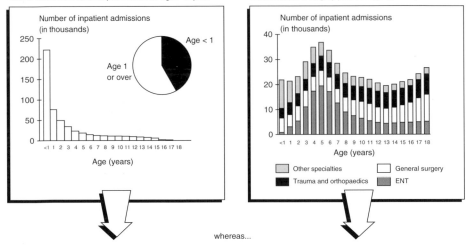

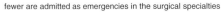

whereas...

Most admissions are emergencies in paediatrics

fewer are admitted as emergencies in the surgical specialties

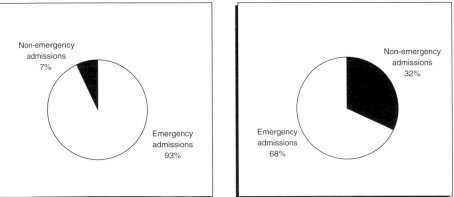

Fig. 1.1 Child inpatients aged 0–18, by specialty, in England and Wales 1990–1991. With permission from the Audit Commission.

Box 1.3 The six principles for services for sick children from the Audit Commission's report *Children First: A Study of Hospital Services*[14]

- Child- and family-centred care
- Specially skilled staff
- Separate facilities
- Effective treatments
- Appropriate hospitalisation
- Strategic commissioning

hospital; and appropriate managerial and financial support. A summary of the conclusions and recommendations of the Audit Commission is given in Box 1.4.

The Commission was clear that much could be done to improve communication between hospital staff and families and gave three key areas for change:

1. greater involvement of parents;
2. a more widespread use of named nurses;
3. more written information.

GREATER INVOLVEMENT OF PARENTS

The Commission thought staff needed to recognise the importance of parents in the care of their children in hospital. Staff should encourage parents to be with their children at all times (including in the accident and emergency or outpatients' departments, wards, anaesthetic or recovery rooms and X-ray facilities) and recognise the knowledge and skills of parents of children with chronic illnesses. Parents (and siblings) should also be encouraged to care for and support the child as they would at home and obtain the knowledge and confidence to do more for the child themselves. Many families will need support (both in hospital and at home) to help them cope with the long-term consequences of illness and advice from staff specially skilled to deal with the particular condition.

Box 1.4 *Children First: A Study of Hospital Services*: summary of the conclusions and recommendations of the Audit Commission[14]

- Children have special health-care needs because they are physically and emotionally different from adults and need the constant care and support of their parents. The principles of care for sick children (Box 1.3) are often not implemented because many clinicians, managers and other staff pay insufficient attention to their needs and those of their families
- Senior managers in every hospital should make services for children a priority to ensure the special needs of children and families are recognised. Written standards and indicators to monitor these standards are needed
- Children should receive care from specially skilled staff in facilities designed to meet their needs
- For some groups (e.g. neonates or children with cancer) outcome can be improved at lower cost in large tertiary or regional centres compared with smaller general hospitals
- The outcomes of many treatments used in children are not routinely monitored. Guidelines for monitoring outcomes should be implemented in all hospitals
- There is a lack of clear guidance on when an admission is appropriate and a failure to consider alternatives. Children are sometimes kept in hospital unnecessarily because of administrative delays, organising discharge or a lack of services for care at home
- Health authorities set the broad strategy for services providing an important catalyst for change

WIDESPREAD USE OF NAMED NURSES

Nurses have a major role to communicate with parents and children. All hospitals now allocate a named nurse to each child who has overall responsibility for his or her care and provides a link with other staff involved in his or her management. This named nurse should also ensure the child and parents obtain all the information they need.

MORE WRITTEN INFORMATION

Finally, the authors of the Audit Commission report claimed good personal communication and written information were equally important. Families need constant reassurance, time to take in and review information and opportunities to ask questions. The report referred to practice in North America where good-quality information is a central part of the responsibilities of management. The Commission advocated giving parents information leaflets containing the main elements of hospital policy and child care when they came with their children to hospital. In addition, all hospital departments dealing with children should provide a range of leaflets covering their specific policies, facilities and services; details about the management of individual medical conditions; and procedures for more information (including contact names and telephone numbers). An example of a suitable leaflet is given in Figure 1.2.

The Audit Commission report is one of a few to incorporate the recommendations of the NCEPOD (see below).[13] The commission advised district hospitals to appoint a designated consultant anaesthetist with responsibility for paediatric anaesthesia (including

---

....

was operated on today for repair of .... hernia.

- The stitches will dissolve.

- He/she may be uncomfortable to begin with but this can be eased by giving pain relief tablets/syrup, e.g. paracetamol.

- There may be some swelling and bruising which will settle.

- Light diet on day of operation, normal diet thereafter.

- If you are concerned in any way, please contact:

    a   **Day Surgery Unit – 0141 • 201 • 0108/9**
          from 7.30 a.m. - 7.00 p.m., Monday   Friday.

    b   **Receiving Surgical Registrar – A&E Dept**
          0141 • 201 • 0078

- ....should wear loose clothing for the first few days after the operation

- His/her first bath should be on the day after the operation.

- He/she should return to school/playgroup as soon as he/she feels comfortable.

- Your child should refrain from strenuous exercise or activities likely to cause knocks or bumps, e.g. football, cycling or PE for 10 days.

Fig. 1.2 Aftercare guidelines for hernia repair. Patient information for parents produced by the Day Surgery Unit, Yorkhill NHS Trust.

training). The NHS Management Executive, in its document *Welfare of Children and Young People in Hospital*, published in 1991,[12] made it clear that this individual could not be expected to take on this responsibility on his/her own and colleagues with paediatric experience should provide cover during his or her absence. The Audit Commission went further and stated that if an adequate 'safety net' of cover was not available, children should be transferred to another hospital where appropriate care was available.

If the physical environment in which children should be treated is well defined, the same cannot be said for whom should be treating them. As a direct result of the publication in 1990 of the NCEPOD,[13] the surgical treatment of children in district general hospitals has been hotly debated. This publication has had such a profound effect that it deserves to be described in some detail.

Enquiries into perioperative deaths

Confidential Enquiry into Perioperative Deaths (1987)

In 1987, the report of a Confidential Enquiry into Perioperative Deaths (CEPOD) was published.[15] This was a milestone in the quest for quality assurance in surgery and anaesthesia. CEPOD was initiated in 1982 as a joint venture between the Association of Anaesthetists of Great Britain and Ireland and the Association of Surgeons, and was supported financially by the Nuffield Provincial Hospital's Trust and the King Edward's Hospital Fund for London. The enquiry reviewed surgical and anaesthetic practice over 1 year in three NHS regions and was deemed of sufficient importance to be funded by the government for a review of anaesthetic and surgical care throughout England and Wales. This enquiry became NCEPOD.

National Confidential Enquiry into Perioperative Deaths (1989)

The aims of the 1989 enquiry[13] were to investigate the clinical practices of anaesthesia and surgery and identify remedial factors. Because of criticisms of the methods used for CEPOD 1987 (which were based on peer review), an early decision was made to adopt a more conventional, and potentially rigid, approach for the national enquiry. Good practice would be identified by comparing patients who died with a random sample of those surviving similar operations. In order to test the new system, children aged 10 years or younger dying within 30 days of surgery were chosen for full investigation. This was a small and easily defined group. From the results of CEPOD 1987, it was calculated that approximately 400 children aged 10 years or younger died each year after surgery. This was thought to be a reasonable sample size for the first year of the enquiry.

However, it proved extremely difficult to match each death with a survivor and after the assessment of only 62 survivors' cases, the authors reverted to peer review of deaths (as in CEPOD 1987[15]). This method had been heavily criticised, especially by consultants in district general hospitals, because they thought those reviewing cases expected an unattainably high standard of care. However, in the national enquiry the authors used index cases for comparison. These were patients preselected at random having similar operations to those who died. This allowed the reviewers to compare management of the dead children with what might be assumed to be normal practice.

Deaths occurring in 417 children were reviewed. The authors of the report divided these into 262 children having cardiac operations and 141 who had other surgery. They based their report on a review of non-cardiac deaths because they reasoned that many of the deaths associated with heart surgery could be expected as the children were all critically ill. The authors' general conclusions are given in Box 1.5.

It is interesting to note that, in general, the authors reported an excellent overall standard for the surgical and anaesthetic care of children. However, they also found potential for improvement and made several recommendations, summarized in Box 1.6. It is the implications of these that have caused concern in some quarters, and an ongoing debate in general.

> **Box 1.5** Conclusions of the National Confidential Enquiry into Perioperative Deaths (1989)[13]
>
> - The overall surgical and anaesthetic care of children as revealed to this enquiry is excellent
> - Few children die following surgery. Those who do die have multiple congenital anomalies often not compatible with life, or malignant tumours, or suffer severe multiple trauma
> - Much surgery and anaesthesia for children is given by clinicians with a regular paediatric practice. However, this is not always so
> - While most children's surgery and anaesthesia is undertaken by, or under the direct supervision of, consultants, on some occasions this supervision was lacking
> - The clinical competence of some locum appointees to care for the special needs of children must be questioned
> - The needs of children in single surgical specialty units are not always fully met. Whilst the natural dominance of surgical requirements (neurosurgery and burns in particular) is paramount, an absence of facilities in intensive care for children and a lack of skilled paediatric anaesthetists, paediatricians and paediatric nurses were found in some units
> - Local audit meetings to review the management of children occurs in 83% of cases. This is a considerable improvement on the situation reported in the Report of the Confidential Enquiry into Perioperative Deaths[15]

Although the authors of NCEPOD[13] stated it was pleasing that children were generally managed by consultant staff with appropriate training and current experience, this was not always the case in every hospital, especially district general hospitals (having to manage, for example, an infant with multiple injuries) or specialist quaternary referral centres (e.g. neurosurgical or orthopaedic hospitals). The staff from both types of hospital, although experts in their own field, were not necessarily expert with small children.

The interpretation of the relatively broad recommendations and conclusions from the NCEPOD[13] is obviously a matter of professional opinion but it is clear that since its publication opinion has hardened. Most now believe paediatric anaesthesia should be the province of a relatively small group of anaesthetists with a sufficiently large practice to maintain their skills.

LUNN'S CRITERIA

Lunn was one of the authors of the NCEPOD[13] and in 1992 wrote about its implications.[16] He thought it important to distinguish a 'paediatric anaesthetist' (a specialist anaesthetist for children) from a 'children's anaesthetist' (anaesthetists with a commitment to paediatric anaesthesia during part of their working week). He pointed out that, at the time, the

> **Box 1.6** Principal recommendations of the National Confidential Enquiry into Perioperative Deaths (1989)[13]
>
> - The National Confidential Enquiry into Perioperative Deaths should continue
> - Information systems should be improved to provide accurate and timely information for audit and quality assurance. All consultants should assist in achieving this improvement
> - Local audit meetings are essential to good clinical practice. All consultants should participate
> - Surgeons and anaesthetists should not undertake occasional paediatric practice. The outcome of surgery and anaesthesia in children is related to the experience of the clinicians involved
> - Consultants who take responsibility for the care of children (particularly in district general or single-speciality hospitals) must keep up-to-date and competent in the management of children
> - Consultant supervision of trainees needs to be kept under scrutiny. No trainee should undertake any anaesthetic or surgical operation on a child of any age without consultation with his or her consultant

Association of Paediatric Anaesthetists of Great Britain and Ireland expected their members to spend in excess of 50% of their clinical time anaesthetising children of all ages suffering a wide range of complicated conditions. Using data from the NCEPOD[13] 2294 were asked how many children they anaesthetised annually. Of the 92% who replied, 62% thought they anaesthetised between 10 and 49 children aged 6 months and 3 years; 39% (22% of the total number of anaesthetists involved in the report) thought that they anaesthetised the same number of babies less than 6 months of age.

It was clear that a large number of children were managed by anaesthetists not given the accolade 'paediatric anaesthetist'. Such anaesthetists may reasonably be termed 'children's anaesthetists'. However it was apparent that the vast majority of children's anaesthetists only anaesthetised a child occasionally. They had achieved consultant status and most worked in district general or single-surgical specialty hospitals. On the basis of figures derived in 1984 from data of 1975, they were believed to supervise 70% of anaesthesia for children aged less than 3 years in the UK.[17] More recent data[13, 16] would suggest that this figure is now less than 60%.

The current situation is interesting. As part of an ongoing review by the NCEPOD, Ingram & Sherry[18] commented, in 1998, on data showing that in 1 week in hospitals in Northern Ireland, England and Wales there were 841 emergency operations on children of 10 years and under. They made allowance for the small number of hospitals not taking part and some under-reporting, and thought it not unreasonable to suggest that about 1000 emergency operations occur in children aged 10 years or less each week. Considering the number of hospitals admitting emergencies, this probably equates to about three children a week for each hospital. Many operations will be relatively minor and will occur during normal working hours when it is probably easier to provide more senior clinicians. Therefore, these data make it clear that major emergency surgery in children occurring out of hours is relatively uncommon and most children's anaesthetists and surgeons must be obtaining experience only occasionally.

These authors used this argument to make a case for recommending that emergency operations in children should be concentrated in far fewer hospitals where appropriate consultant cover could be provided. This reiterated the recommendations made by the Court Committee in 1976[10] and the Audit Commission in 1993.[14] In a review in 1992 of the provision of safe surgery for children, Atwell & Spargo[19] calculated that 2000 children less than 3 years of age were anaesthetised each year in their own unit (2900 children under 5 years of age). This equated to only one or two children per week for each consultant.

One of the recommendations of the authors of NCEPOD[13] was that 'surgeons and anaesthetists should not undertake occasional practice', but what is 'occasional practice'? Using data from the NCEPOD and his own experience, Lunn's personal conclusion was that adequate practice meant not less than one full operating session (one half-day) per week. However, he thought case mix should also be taken into consideration. He recommended that a 'children's anaesthetist' should anaesthetise 12 babies younger than 6 months per year (one each month); 50 babies or children aged 6 months to 3 years per year (one each week); and approximately 300 children aged between 3 and 10 years per year (one each day). These recommendations are summarised in Box 1.7.

Results of a postal survey of consultants in the UK suggest that fewer than 20% of those anaesthetising children fulfil the criteria for a 'children's anaesthetist', although 41% of respondents had a regular paediatric practice equivalent to at least one operating session per week.[20] These results are consistent with Lunn's calculations[16] derived from NCEPOD.[13]

Report of the National Confidential Enquiry into Perioperative Deaths (1999): Extremes of Age[21]

NCEPOD reconsidered perioperative deaths in children 10 years after the first enquiry in the report *Extremes of Age*.[21] Deaths occurring in children aged less than 16 not associated with congenital heart disease were included. The changes that have occurred since the first NCEPOD make interesting reading and are summarised in Box 1.8.

> **Box 1.7** Lunn's recommendations for minimum case load for a children's anaesthetist[9]
>
> | Babies younger than 6 months | 1 per month (12 per year) |
> | Children and babies < 3 years | 1 per week (50 per year) |
> | Children < 10 years | 1 per day (300 per year) |

> **Box 1.8** Summary of the findings of the National Confidential Enquiry into Perioperative Deaths (1999): *Extremes of Age*[21]
>
> - The proportion of anaesthetists who do not anaesthetise infants less than 6 months of age has increased from 16 to 58%
> - A significant number of anaesthetic consultants giving anaesthesia to children still do a small number of cases each year
> - There has been a considerable shift in practice (with more specialisation in children's surgery) within some specialties, for example orthopaedic surgery, whereas in other areas there has been little change when compared with data from 10 years ago
> - Very occasional practice in emergency situations persists within surgery on children

The recommendations proposed by Hoile & Ingram,[21] two members of the editorial team who compiled the report, are given in Box 1.9.

It is plain that, although fewer units are indulging in occasional practice, there is still room for improving surgical services for children. Indeed, even in twenty-first-century medicine there are still echoes of Platt and Court.

EVIDENCE AGAINST OCCASIONAL PRACTICE

If, as it appears, occasional paediatric practice occurs in district general hospitals, is it associated with an increased morbidity? There are no data on anaesthetic morbidity in district general hospitals compared with regional paediatric units, although there are a number of

> **Box 1.9** Recommendations for children's surgical services from the authors of *Extremes of Age* (National Confidential Enquiry into Perioperative Deaths 1999)[21]
>
> - Concentrating children's surgical services would increase expertise and further reduce 'occasional practice'
> - A review of staff planning is required to enable anaesthetists and surgeons to train in the management of small children
> - There is a need for a system to assess the severity of surgical illness in children to gather meaningful information about outcomes
> - Anaesthetic and surgical trainees need to know when to inform their consultants and national guidelines are required
> - A regional organisational perspective, led by (specialist) paediatric units, is required in the management of acute surgical conditions in children, including transfer of patients
> - All trusts should address the requirements of the framework document on intensive care[22]
> - The death of any child occurring within 30 days of anaesthesia or surgery should be subject to peer review
> - The events surrounding the perioperative death of any child should be the subject of multidisciplinary clinical audit
> - There should be central guidance to ensure uniformity of data collection

large surveys of perioperative complications in children, notably from the UK, France and Canada. In the light of the results of these surveys and the infrequent experience of most anaesthetists with children, some authors have argued that services could be improved if small or sick children were sent to central specialist paediatric units.[19]

Incidence of perioperative complications in babies and children

Anaesthetic problems occur most frequently in children younger than 3 years,[23] while the incidence in older children is similar to adults. Several large studies have confirmed the high incidence of perioperative anaesthetic complications in neonates and older babies. Tiret and colleagues reported the incidence of major complications in a prospective survey of anaesthesia for children in France.[24] A major complication was defined as: 'a fatal or life threatening accident or any incident producing severe sequelae, which occurred during, or within 24 hours of, anaesthesia'. The authors reported 27 major complications amongst 40 240 anaesthetics in children younger than 15 years, including 2103 younger than 12 months (5% of the total). This gave an overall incidence of major complications of 0.7 per 1000 anaesthetics. The risk of complications was significantly higher ($P < 0.001$) in babies (4.3 per 1000) than older children (0.5 per 1000). Nine of the complications occurred in babies, seven of which were primary respiratory problems (including mismanagement of the airway, complications of intubation, aspiration or postoperative respiratory depression) and four of which were associated with cardiac arrest. The authors concluded that most complications were probably avoidable.

Cohen and colleagues, in a study from Canada, confirmed these findings.[25] Of 29 220 patients younger than 16 years, neonates had the highest rate of adverse events, both intra-operatively and during recovery. Babies aged 1–12 months had the next highest incidence (8 per 10 000 anaesthetics). Adverse events included respiratory, cardiovascular or surgical problems or death. Death within 3 days of operation occurred in 5 per 10 000 babies, again the highest in any age group apart from neonates. The authors commented that the majority of children had been healthy and 70% had no preoperative medical conditions.

The transport of infants and children for surgery

It is not possible to discuss the problems of 'occasional' paediatric anaesthesia in isolation as it is, of necessity, associated with 'occasional' paediatric surgery. Atwell & Spargo[19] reviewed the provision of safe surgery for children and gave their arguments for transferring small or sick children to specialist paediatric centres. They pointed out that there was a tendency for neonatologists to refer sick neonates to local surgeons rather than transfer them to an appropriate specialised unit. They argued, firstly, that most major neonatal disorders could be diagnosed antenatally and the mother transferred to specialised unit for delivery, and, secondly, that transferring sick children was common with virtually all major paediatric centres running a retrieval service.

The authors then examined the perioperative management of babies, using congenital pyloric stenosis and intussusception as models for comparison and obtaining data from a variety of reports. For pyloric stenosis, they found an incidence of surgical complications greater than 20% for the 'occasional' paediatric surgeon compared with less than 1% for a specialist paediatric surgeon. Of the 33 children dying after intussusception in England and Wales between 1984 and 1989, only one had been under the care of a specialist paediatric surgeon, and this child had been transferred from a district general hospital after inappropriate surgery. The principal causes of death were delay in diagnosis (either at home or shortly after arrival in hospital), inadequate resuscitation or inappropriate surgery.

Atwell & Spargo[19] pointed out that, in children younger than 5 years, the outcomes of surgery for inguinal hernia, undescended testis or appendicitis depended on the paediatric experience of the surgeon. For example, testicular atrophy occurred less frequently after orchidopexy by a specialist compared with an 'occasional' surgeon. The authors also recommended that all children younger than 5 years with appendicitis should be treated by surgeons specialising in the care of children because the mortality rate was significantly higher than in older children.

Although data are available showing clear differences in the standard of surgery between general hospitals and specialist paediatric centres, there are none for anaesthesia. This has been put forward as a reason for maintaining paediatric anaesthesia on an 'occasional' basis.[26] However, it is clear that if a surgical complication occurs because of 'occasional' paediatric surgery, the anaesthetist, undertaking anaesthesia knowing the limitations of his surgical colleague, must be prepared to accept some responsibility.

In 1993 a joint report *The Transfer of Infants and Children for Surgery* was published under the auspices of the British Paediatric Association.[27] The authors also included representatives of the Royal College of Anaesthetists and the Association of Anaesthetists of Great Britain and Ireland. The authors reiterated that most anaesthetic and surgical morbidity occurred in children younger than 3 years of age. They recommended that all children younger than 3 years requiring emergency surgery should be treated in specialised paediatric units, unless physicians with appropriate skills were available and the services provided by the district general hospital were consistent with the standards laid down by the NHS Management Executive in its report *Welfare of Children and Young People in Hospital*.[12]

Ideally, the authors of *The Transfer of Infants and Children for Surgery*[27] would have liked to see the recommendations broadened to include all children less than 5 years old, but recognised the logistical difficulties, and so compromised with the under–3-years age group. They added that anaesthetists and surgeons with paediatric practice equivalent to one full operating list per week, working in district general hospitals, should be capable of dealing with all children aged 5 years or older having uncomplicated surgery. This is consistent with the opinion of Lunn.[16]

More recent recommendations are, interestingly, less prescriptive. Rather than using absolute criteria, the Royal College of Anaesthetists seems to advocate critically reviewing local provision. Anaesthetists must always 'recognise and work within the limits of their professional competence' and 'if there is doubt about training, skills, facilities, or ongoing experience, the child should be transferred'. However, the College has stated that ' there is no absolute lower age limit for treatment in a district general hospital as management of common surgical problems in healthy children should be within the competence of designated consultant surgeons and anaesthetists' although neonates, children with significant comorbidity (e.g. ex-premature babies) or children having complex surgery (e.g. for serious trauma) should be treated in specialist paediatric units.[28]

STAFF TRAINING AND CONTINUING EXPERIENCE

Anaesthetists

Training for all anaesthetists

The competent authority in the UK responsible for medical training is the Specialist Training Authority (STA) created by the European Specialist Medical Qualifications Order. The STA delegates authority to the Royal Colleges and Faculties to organise and oversee training programmes. Paediatric anaesthesia is a core subject of the curriculum for both parts of the examination for the diploma of Fellowship of the Royal College of Anaesthetists. All specialist registrars must also undertake 3 months' clinical training in paediatric anaesthesia.

Training for specialist paediatric anaesthetists or consultants with an interest in paediatric anaesthesia

Early in 1999 the STA approved a change to the training programme for specialist registrars in anaesthesia, extending it from 4 to 5 years on condition it was based on competency. The

Royal College of Anaesthetists is currently reformulating the programme. It is now hoped that those wishing to work in district general hospitals as consultants with significant paediatric workloads, or as full-time paediatric anaesthetists, will be able to take part in training programmes which are more rigidly defined than at present.

The regulations for training in paediatric anaesthesia are confusing. The Association of Paediatric Anaesthetists has advised the Royal College of Anaesthetists that:

1. for appointment as a consultant with a significant paediatric workload in a district general hospital, individuals would be advised to obtain an extra 6 months' training in a recognised paediatric centre;
2. for appointment as consultant in a specialist children's hospital, an extra 12 months would be essential.

The Royal College of Anaesthetists now states that 'consultants with a substantial commitment to paediatric anaesthesia, including full-time paediatric anaesthetists ... should have obtained at least one year of equivalent full-time specialist training in paediatric anaesthesia in a specialist paediatric unit ... (started in years 3–5 of the specialist registrar training programme)'. The College also recommends that consultants appointed to posts with a designated subspecialty interest in paediatric anaesthesia should have obtained at least 6 months' similar experience in a specialist unit.[28]

Hopefully these recommendations will be incorporated into the new competency-based training programme (see section 2).

Box 1.10 A position statement published in 1997 by the UK Central Council for Nursing, Midwifery and Health Visiting[29]

- The Council's position on the matter is declared by *The Scope of Professional Practice*. It is accepted that those qualified before Project 2000 might have gained knowledge and competence in a different speciality to their registered speciality through the course of their career, and that some of their knowledge and competence obtained as registered nurses will be transferable. On this basis, all registered nurses will make accountable decisions about their ability to practise in a safe and appropriate manner in a care area outside their registration status, acknowledging limitations in knowledge and competence in accordance with clause 4 of the *Code of Professional Conduct*
- Project 2000-registered nurses will have experience and knowledge of a range of skills relevant to all branches by virtue of the Common Foundation Programme, although they will only be registered in one field of nursing. The individual registered nurse will be accountable for acknowledging limitations in his/her knowledge and competence[†]
- The nursing care provided by any registered nurse working outside the registration status should be conducted with support of, and supervised by, a first-level registered nurse with the appropriate knowledge and qualifications for that area of care. For example, a registered sick children's nurse working in an Accident and Emergency unit could act as a supervisor and primary nurse for children requiring treatment in the Accident and Emergency unit, and also act as a caregiver within the limitations of his/her knowledge and competence, under the supervision of a suitably qualified nurse for the whole range of patients admitted to the unit
- When working in a care area outside that of registration, the registered nurse cannot take on the registration of the new areas, but remains as registered in the area that he/she has qualified in. It is unacceptable for a registered nurse to give the impression that he/she holds a qualification that he/she does not

---

[†]Registered sick children's nurses (RSCNs) are being replaced by nurses who have completed Project 2000, a fundamental reform of preregistration training. All student nurses undergo a common foundation programme for the first half of their training and then specialise in their own specialist interest.

Nurses

Nursing requirements are important issues. The UK Central Council for Nursing, Midwifery and Health Visiting (UKCC) acknowledges that, although only nurses with specific registered qualifications can hold posts which make use of these qualifications, there are occasions when nurses may be employed in posts not related to their registration status. Part of a position statement published by the council in 1997 is given in Box 1.10.[29]

The position statement is relevant to operating departments in children's and district general hospitals. If a nurse not registered as a qualified children's nurse is prepared to accept his/her limitations and is supervised by a registered children's nurse then he/she may be employed in a position outwith his/her registered qualifications. Therefore, nurses trained in adult hospitals in theatre techniques can transfer their skills to a paediatric environment if they are constantly supervised by trained children's nurses and have regular experience working with children. This includes nurses assisting either surgeons or anaesthetists, or caring for children in recovery.

Nurses working outside their registered qualifications must accept the limitations of their training. The UKCC would take a very dim view of any nurse who undertook paediatric practice (particularly outwith a paediatric environment) who did not have regular experience working with children or who was not directly supervised by a registered children's nurse.

SECTION 2: Implementing the recommendations

As demonstrated in the first section of this chapter, there is no shortage of guidance for the organisation of surgical and anaesthetic services for children. However, as any clinician practising in the resource-limited, and somewhat conservative, environment of the NHS knows, change can be difficult to implement. This is especially true when the change involves many different departments, each with its own priorities and agenda.

When considering how to effect change, it can be helpful to identify the factors driving the change, so the individuals involved understand the reasons for altering practice. It is also helpful for them to agree minimum standards of practice, usually by adopting national guidelines (if available) modified to suit local circumstances. If the absolute standards are clearly unattainable within a realistic time scale or available resources, intermediate targets should be set and a plan agreed for attaining the absolute standards later.

Implementing change is almost never easy, but understanding clearly the reasons for, and benefits of, altering established practice can make agreement easier. In this section, I will examine some of these drivers of change. I will then discuss how the recommendations from the various professional and government bodies described in section 1 can be implemented in district or major acute general hospitals to provide a safe and satisfactory surgical service for children.

DRIVERS OF CHANGE

The roles of doctors and all other health-care professionals and their relationships with patients have altered radically in the last few years. There are a number of reasons for this.

Expectations of patients and/or parents

The rise in consumerism has inevitably affected medicine. Patients are better informed than ever before. Knowledge, once available only in specialist libraries, now appears in the mass media and on the internet. That not all of it is correct unfortunately only complicates the situation.

Political pressure

Anxieties over the variations in standards of practice between different hospitals or practitioners has led to increasing calls for 'transparency' and accountability. There is no doubt that institutions and individual doctors in the future will have to demonstrate that they are maintaining acceptable standards of competence. League tables of performance, for all their dubious value, are a powerful political tool.

Purchasers

Purchasers, when placing contracts, should take account of clinical standards. The Royal College of Anaesthetists published in 1994[30] the standards purchasers could reasonably demand of departments of anaesthesia in their document *Guidance for Purchasers*. This was revised in 1999, as *Guidance on the Provision of Paediatric Anaesthetic Services*[31], and again in July 2001.[28] A summary is given in Box 1.11.

Audit

Doctors now have a professional obligation to audit quality of care. Audit has shown that surgical services for children in many hospitals are less than ideal, although clear evidence of detriment is difficult to find.[13, 19] However, since the publication of the report of the NCEPOD,[13] opinion has swung to support the recommendations of the authors (Box 1.6),[18] and it is no longer considered acceptable to provide surgical services for children in a haphazard fashion.

Risk management

Until 1996, hospitals were covered by Crown indemnity. Since then, however, trusts have been responsible for their own risks. Each chief executive now has overall responsibility for risk management within his or her trust. In response to these developments and the demands of the Clinical Negligence Scheme for Trusts (CNST), hospitals have implemented formal policies for risk management requiring services to be organised and run to nationally approved standards.

Clinical governance

It is uncertain how clinical governance will work, but it is clear that individual doctors will be subject to revalidation and it will no longer be acceptable for them to practise outside their recognised fields of clinical competence.

Box 1.11 Guidelines from the Royal College of Anaesthetists for the provision of anaesthetic services for children[28]

- Anaesthesia for children requires specially trained medical and nursing staff and special facilities
- Parents (or carers) should be involved in all aspects of the care and decisions regarding the care of their children
- The service should be led at all times by consultants anaesthetising children regularly
- Adequate assistance for the anaesthetist by staff with paediatric training and skills must be available
- Paediatric anaesthetic equipment must be available where children are treated
- Staff must receive regular retraining in paediatric life support
- There should be a properly staffed and funded acute pain service covering the needs of children

Technical developments

Technical developments requiring expensive equipment, and the general move to hospitals serving populations of 400 000–500 000, are leading to the closure of some small institutions and merger of others. These changes will inevitably alter patterns of work.

Doctors' perceptions

Doctors' perceptions of their role are changing in response to the changing expectations of society. Some doctors see the new demand for accountability as a threat to their position. More constructively, however, it is possible to use it to improve communication with patients or parents, allowing them to act as educated participants in making clinical decisions.

National guidelines versus clinical judgement

The imposition of guidelines agreed nationally (e.g. the Scottish Intercollegiate Guidelines Network) and the emerging roles of the National Institute of Clinical Excellence in England and the Scottish Health Technology Assessment Centre are seen by some as threats to clinical freedom. Although the indiscriminate use of guidelines is not necessarily in the interest of individual patients, good guidelines do represent a consensus on which to base policies that can be adapted for local conditions.

STANDARDS AND TARGETS

Several government and professional bodies have established minimum standards for the provision of anaesthetic and surgical services for children[12, 13, 16, 27, 28, 32, 33–36] (see section 1). Although the recommendations vary in detail, there is consensus on many requirements for the provision of a 'competent' service.

Named consultants

Any hospital admitting children for surgery should have named consultants in anaesthesia and the relevant surgical specialities, who are responsible for leading children's services.[13, 27] The Royal College of Anaesthetists now requires that any department of anaesthesia recognised for training should have such a named (or designated) consultant.[28, 34] Typically, a designated consultant will anaesthetise the equivalent of at least one children's list each week and organise and oversee all the anaesthetic services for children, including resuscitation and pain control.[28] A summary of the possible responsibilities of the designated consultant's is given in Box 1.12.

Although the designated consultant will be in charge of anaesthesia for children, there has never been any intention that all anaesthetics for children will be administered by a single specialist. This would be clearly impossible and highly undesirable. Several authors have expressed valid anxieties that reorganising children's services will deskill many consultants in district general hospitals;[26, 35] it is argued that as many consultants as possible should retain paediatric skills to be able to resuscitate a child in an emergency. The number who can remain 'competent' to anaesthetise children largely depends on the total workload for paediatric surgery within the hospital. This work should be shared as widely as possible, provided each anaesthetist meets the minimum recommended criteria. This will ensure that as many as possible retain the skills to resuscitate and stabilise critically ill babies and children, at least until more specialist help arrives, and to provide cover for emergency surgery out of hours.

Guidelines for trainees

All children should be anaesthetised by a consultant or other career-grade anaesthetist with regular relevant paediatric practice, or a trainee supervised by such a person.[28] The

Box 1.12 Possible responsibilities of the designated consultant for paediatric anaesthesia in a district hospital

- To ensure that the competencies of those working in the service are maintained, e.g. consultant colleagues, operating department personnel, nurses
- To ensure that the standards of the facilities are adequate (e.g. suitable equipment, separate wards from adults, child-friendly environment)
- To act as the department's liaison with colleagues in other specialities and disciplines, including surgeons, paediatricians, intensivists, staff working on the children's wards or in the operating theatre, pharmacists, staff in the radiology or Accident and Emergency departments, physiotherapists, porters
- To function as a central coordinator for all queries about general aspects of the anaesthetic service for children, so standards are maintained and colleagues do not 'shop around' until they obtain the advice they wish to hear
- To provide general clinical advice to colleagues about children's anaesthesia (although individual anaesthetists should retain full clinical responsibility for all children they anaesthetise)
- To produce departmental guidelines and protocols in consultation with colleagues, e.g. the supervision of trainees, duration of preoperative fast, or management of postoperative pain, nausea or vomiting
- To produce information leaflets for parents and children, e.g. for consent, preoperative procedures, the induction of anaesthesia, postoperative analgesia (including the use of suppositories), regional blocks or other invasive procedures

consultants in each department must, therefore, establish guidelines for trainees on the levels of supervision required for children of different ages and for different operations. These guidelines will vary from department to department, depending on the type of work and the seniority of the trainees.[28] As a general principle, children under 5 years of age should normally be anaesthetised by, or under the close supervision of, consultants with appropriate training and continuing experience.[16, 36]

Adequate training

The Royal College of Anaesthetists has made recommendations for training in paediatric anaesthesia. These are given in section 1, above. The details are still under discussion, but it is likely that they will become more stringent with the introduction of the 5-year training programme for specialist registrars. However, the College insists that all anaesthetists must be able to provide life-saving care to a child of any age in an emergency. To this end, paediatric anaesthesia is a core subject for the curriculum of both parts of the examination for the diploma for Fellowship of the Royal College of Anaesthetists. Competency-based training and assessment (introduced in February 2001) will, in the future, require a senior house officer to demonstrate an understanding of the implications of childhood in the perioperative period (for children > 5 years), and acquire the clinical skills necessary for simple anaesthesia in this age group.[37] In addition, a trainee must spend a minimum of 3 months as a specialist registrar (SpR) in clinical paediatric anaesthesia. Additional specialist training is required for anyone intending appointment as a consultant with a special interest in children in district general or specialist children's hospitals. However, there is consensus[27] that all trained anaesthetists should be able to manage anaesthesia for all commonly occurring operations in children over 5 years of age.

Many consultants practising now will have trained before the introduction of structured training, and in a more haphazard fashion than is now regarded as appropriate. Nevertheless, it does not seem sensible to suggest that those who have maintained adequate ongoing experience after standard training for their day should be excluded from anaesthetising children. Apart from anything else, the work needs to be done by those capable of doing it, until more formalised systems are introduced.

Continuing education

For all anaesthetists, but especially the more senior, continuing medical education (CME) and continuing professional development (CPD) are increasingly important. The individual doctor has a responsibility to ensure he or she stays, in the words of the authors of the NCEPOD[13] report, 'up to date and competent' in the management of children.[13] This can be achieved in a number of ways, and a combination of methods might be best. Since the introduction of compulsory CME, the number of formal courses has grown apace. Almost all the central and regional bodies involved with training and education in anaesthesia run courses, seminars and workshops from time to time. In addition, the Royal College of Anaesthetists now recognises visits to other centres as legitimate CME and suggests establishing formal links with the specialist unit for continuing education, professional development and refresher training.[28] This may encourage consultants to spend time in other centres, perhaps learning new techniques in specialist centres, or using the opportunity to gain new perspectives on old problems. The College is particularly supportive of this approach for consultants with no regular paediatric commitment but who may have to provide emergency cover out of hours.[28]

Individuals must be responsible for their own continuing education and standards of competence. However, the designated consultant for paediatric anaesthesia is probably best able to coordinate the educational requirements of individuals with the needs of the department and hospital. For example, resuscitation courses, such as Paediatric Advanced Life Support (PALS) or Advanced Paediatric Life Support (APLS) should be available to all those working with children.

The Association of Paediatric Anaesthetists of Great Britain and Ireland exists to further clinical care and research in the subspeciality. Membership is now open to any consultant with an interest in paediatric anaesthesia, and is not dependent on the type of hospital in which they practise or the number of children's list in their weekly programme.

Ongoing experience

In 1990, the authors of the NCEPOD[13] stated 'Surgeons and anaesthetists should not undertake occasional practice and stated that the outcome of surgery and anaesthesia in children is related to the experience of the clinicians involved'.[13] Although this statement aroused some controversy at the time it was published, it is now accepted as an axiomatic truth. However, there is still dissent about what constitutes 'occasional practice' or 'adequate ongoing experience'. Lunn's recommendations (or Lunn's criteria), published in 1992,[16] have not been formally superseded (Box 1.7). His suggestion of a minimum of one operating list per week was generally accepted as reasonable and realistic. However, he further recommended a minimum case load per year of 12 babies younger than 6 months, 50 babies and children under 3 years of age and 300 children under the age of 10. It is more difficult to accept this latter recommendation without qualification. One could argue that anaesthetising one small baby each month is insufficient to maintain competence, since these are the most challenging cases. Conversely, it should not be necessary to anaesthetise one large child per day to be able to do this competently. It may also be more realistic and appropriate to examine the local case load, and ensure that those anaesthetising children have sufficient practice in the sort of work they actually do, rather than trying to achieve a national standard with no local relevance. However, all anaesthetists must recognise and work within the limits of their professional competence.[28]

Paediatricians

The Department of Health recommended in 1991 in their document *Welfare of Children and Young People in Hospital*[12] that all children admitted to hospital as inpatients should be under the care of a children's physician or surgeon (Box 1.2). For this to be possible, the paediatric department must be staffed 24 hours a day to the standards published in 1996 by the British Paediatric Association.[33] These standards include the minimum on-call of one consultant paediatrician and a resident doctor with at least 12 months' experience in paediatrics (see Ch. 2).

In practice, most children having surgery in district general hospitals are admitted under the care of surgeons with a special interest in paediatrics, rather than specialist paediatric surgeons. It is to the benefit of all children admitted for surgery in district hospitals to come automatically under the joint care of the paediatricians (perhaps most conveniently the team on call at the time of admission) and the surgical consultant. Once this principle is established, the paediatricians can become involved in the management and progress of any child when appropriate, without waiting for elaborate (and often slow) referral mechanisms. Paediatricians are also the doctors spending the most time on children's wards and the clinicians to whom the nurses will usually turn for help and advice. In addition, the routine involvement of paediatricians should be educational for trainees in anaesthesia and surgery.

Paediatric nurses

There should be at least two RSCNs on duty at all times in any unit to which children are admitted for surgery.[12] This includes day-surgery units. Nurses with appropriate experience but without paediatric registration may assist in the care of children, provided they remain within their area of competence and under the supervision of a registered children's nurse. The implications of these requirements are discussed in detail in section 1, above. However, the current shortage of RSCNs is seriously limiting the development of children's surgery within district general hospitals.

Other staff

There is a consensus that children should be treated, whenever possible, by staff with a special interest and ongoing experience in paediatrics. Most district hospitals, for example, will have a radiologist with a paediatric interest, and radiographers experienced at dealing with children.

The Royal College of Paediatrics and Child Health advises that all accident and emergency departments accepting children should have special facilities and staff.[36] The key recommendations of a multidisciplinary working party on accident and emergency services for children are summarised in Box 1.13.

Theatre and recovery nurses will need appropriate training, specialised skills and ongoing experience. Nurses without paediatric registration may work outside their area of

---

Box 1.13 Key recommendations for the provision of accident and emergency services for children[41]

- There must be audiovisual separation of children from adult patients
- Inpatient facilities for children should be available on the same hospital site
- There must be a registered sick children's nurse on duty
- There must be a consultant who has undertaken a recognised training programme in paediatric accident and emergency medicine
- There must be liaison between a designated paediatrician and the consultant in accident and emergency
- Practitioners in accident and emergency medicine, primary care and paediatrics must collaborate in planning services for the management of acute illness and injury in children

registration under the supervision of an RSCN (Box 1.10). Operating department assistants (ODAs) and operating department practitioners (ODPs) are not currently registered and therefore not subject to statutory regulation. The Association of Operating Department Practitioners (AODP, formerly the British Association of Operating Department Assistants) operates a voluntary register. An executive letter, dated 20 March 2000, stipulated that employment within the NHS should be limited to those whose names appear on this register.[38] Despite the lack of formal registration, the ODA or ODP is a vital member of the anaesthetic team and it is important that an appropriate number are trained as a district hospital develops its children's surgical services to a competent standard.

Dedicated operating lists

Although nearly half of all admissions to hospital during childhood are for surgery,[36] the absolute numbers for each speciality in a district hospital tend to be rather small, with the otorhinolaryngologists taking the lion's share. Most surgical specialist societies advocate nominating one consultant in each speciality in the hospital as a lead clinician for children and recommend that clinicians should not undertake 'occasional practice'.[36] Although not all the societies stipulate a minimum workload to maintain skills, where it is laid down one full list a week (i.e. half a day) seems to be the consensus.

If the advice from individual societies is followed, children should not appear on adult surgical lists. Although this was normal before the publication of the report from the NCEPOD 1989,[13] it now seems utterly inappropriate.

All children should have surgery on dedicated children's operating lists (wherever possible), managed by individuals with special skills. Fortunately, anaesthetists, nurses, ODAs and ODPs can work across surgical specialities. Once a group of trained people has been established, it should be possible to cover for regular personnel who are absent. The authors of the report of the NCEPOD 1989[13] expressed anxiety about the qualifications and experience of locums. It is preferable to cancel lists if suitable staff are unavailable rather than to put children at risk.

Dedicated wards

The Royal College of Paediatrics and Child Health firmly recommend 'children should be treated, both as in-patients and day cases, in facilities appropriate to their age, which meet the standards laid down in the Department of Health document Welfare of Children and Young People in Hospital, and in particular should not be admitted to adult wards'.[36]

Any district general hospital with a workload sufficient to run a surgical service for children should be able to provide dedicated ward facilities. Ideally, medical and surgical facilities should be separated, since children with medical illnesses are often much sicker than those admitted for (often minor) surgery. Nursing the two groups together can cause distress to both groups of children and parents, and the nurses may find they concentrate their attention on the 'medical' children who seem to need them more. However, this counsel of perfection may be difficult to achieve because of the current shortage of trained children's nurses and of resources generally.

Anaesthetic and recovery rooms

The Royal College of Anaesthetists recommends that 'theatre design and temperature control, appearance and working practices should reflect the emotional and physical needs of children'.[28] In larger district hospitals, with a substantial paediatric workload, it may be possible to set aside an operating theatre and adjoining anaesthetic room solely for the use of children. This is clearly ideal, since appropriate equipment can be gathered in one place, and the room made as child-friendly as possible.

However, many general hospitals have insufficient work for 10 sessions of children's surgery each week. As more hospitals merge to serve larger populations, this may change. Additionally, many specialities, including orthopaedics and ENT, require special equipment and facilities for both adults and children. Their needs are best met by concentrating all relevant equipment in one purpose-built theatre. The appropriate solution lies in the best available compromise, which must be negotiated locally.

It is, nevertheless, possible to make any anaesthetic room suitable for children by, for example, keeping appropriate anaesthetic equipment on a mobile trolley, or improving the decor and physical surroundings. With a small investment in money and a larger investment of time and imagination, the room can be made welcoming. It may be possible to involve local schools or colleges in such a project. Few adults will object to being anaesthetised in a room which is obviously designed for use by children. A few may welcome it.

Recovery facilities should cater to the special needs of children. Children should be segregated from adults, either by providing a separate facility or using screens.[28] All necessary equipment must be available, and care should be provided by nursing staff with appropriate training and experience, to the standard laid down in *Welfare of Children and Young People in Hospital*.[12] Parents should be allowed to join their children in recovery at an appropriate time whenever possible.[14, 28]

Equipment

Any hospital wanting to provide a 'competent' anaesthetic service for children must have the full range of equipment needed to make those services safe. This includes properly serviced and maintained anaesthetic, monitoring and resuscitation equipment appropriate to the ages of the children and the nature of the surgery.

Monitoring throughout anaesthesia and recovery must be to the standards published in the *Recommendations for Standards of Monitoring During Anaesthesia and Recovery* by the Association of Anaesthetists of Great Britain and Ireland.[39]

Accommodation for parents

Accommodation should be provided for parents whenever children are admitted overnight.[28]

ACHIEVING CHANGE

The will to change

It is always difficult to change established practice in an organisation as complex as a hospital. When change requires the cooperation of staff working in many departments, it is inevitably slow and must be taken at a steady pace. Usually, there are one or two individuals who see the need to alter the pattern of work, and who have the drive and energy to make it happen. It is important they identify those of their colleagues who will be crucial to the new development, and bring them on board. This will take time and powers of persuasion. It will also need hard facts, and a grasp of the evidence.

An assessment of the current workload is usually the first step. This should include total workload, and a breakdown by age, speciality and type of admission (routine or emergency). The types of operations within each speciality, the time they occur, and the seniority and experience of the clinicians involved should also be identified. Only when this information is available can rational discussion commence.

Resistance to change

Until the publication of the report of the NCEPOD,[13] the special needs of children having surgery received scant attention in many hospitals. Minor children's surgery was regarded as easy, and many operating lists with small children were left for the trainees (both

23

anaesthetic and surgical). The NCEPOD[13] report changed all that. Given that the very first of its general conclusions was that 'the overall surgical and anaesthetic care of children as revealed to this Enquiry is excellent',[13] it is interesting that it set in train a change in attitudes revolutionising the provision of surgical services for children throughout the UK.

It did not, of course, change all attitudes. Certainly, the evidence in the report was anecdotal, and there has been considerable resistance to some of the suggested changes in practice. This was predictable, and understandable. Surgeons and anaesthetists who for decades undertook 'occasional paediatric practice' without apparent morbidity or mortality were unlikely to respond positively when told they were no longer permitted to do what they had always done. Many doctors find the management of children interesting, enjoyable and satisfying and are understandably reluctant to give it up. When it is suggested that the whole system needs reorganising, the first response is often resistance and a suggestion that 'if it ain't broke, don't fix it!' It is here that an audit of the workload can be valuable. Even in larger district hospitals, where all the surgeons operate on children, the personal workload of each surgeon is likely to be very small. This is especially true when considering children under the age of 6 months, or emergencies in the very young.

Regrettably, even when confronted with the inadequacy of a system which has been in place for many years, it often takes the threat of action by an outside body (for example, loss of recognition for training by a Royal College) to concentrate minds.

Achieving agreement

It is important that all interested parties are involved at the beginning of any reorganisation. A multidisciplinary working group including surgeons, anaesthetists, paediatricians, ward nurses, theatre staff, the professions allied to medicine and managers may seem cumbersome, but these are the people who will be required to agree and implement change and they should be represented. It is much easier for a multidisciplinary group, with all the interested parties involved in the debate and decision-making, to progress towards an agreed goal, than for any single-interest group to impose its needs or wishes on the service. The Royal College of Anaesthetists suggests including a paediatrician, anaesthetist, surgeon, pharmacist and registered children's nurse,[28] although membership may be broader. The membership of the group established at the Epsom and St Helier NHS Trust is given in Box 1.14.

Any working party should have a clear remit, and a defined task, to prevent it becoming simply a 'talking shop'. For the same reason, it should have executive and advisory powers. The Royal College of Anaesthetists advocates that these groups should be responsible for the overall management, improvement, integration and audit of services for children.[28]

Standards

The multidisciplinary group will need to review the nationally published guidelines in the light of local circumstances. Armed with workload figures, they should assess local demand and clinical priorities, and attempt to match these with the facilities and clinical expertise available. The members of the group should also agree standards of practice. The list of requirements for a competent children's surgical service can function as a template against which to assess the current provision of services.

Resources

Many requirements for a competent service for children can be achieved by reorganising and redeploying existing resources. Any hospital admitting children for surgery should have consultant anaesthetists and surgeons who can take on the role of designated consultants for children, as described above. The workload of a department should be redistributed to ensure consultants working with children have adequate continuing experience. It is, however, important to ensure as many people as possible retain their competence and the service must not be so dependent on one or two people that it grinds to a halt in their absence.

Box 1.14 The multidisciplinary working party for children's surgical services, Epsom and St Helier NHS Trust

Two anaesthetists
- Lead consultant for paediatric anaesthesia
- Consultant with an interest in paediatric anaesthesia

Three local surgical consultants with paediatric interests in:
- Ear, nose and throat
- Urology
- Orthopaedics

Visiting specialist paediatric surgeon

Consultant paediatrician

Paediatric nurse manager

Two other managers
- Inpatient theatre manager
- Day-surgery theatre manager

Three senior sisters/charge nurses
- From the children's medical ward
- From the children's day surgery ward
- With responsibilities for paediatric high-dependency unit

Pharmacist

The routine involvement of paediatricians in the care of children having surgery should simply be a matter of local agreement. The additional workload is unlikely to be heavy, but the 'safety net' is invaluable.

The provision of dedicated children's operating lists is, again, a matter of reorganisation. Since the work is already being done, it should be feasible to schedule it within existing resources.

Providing dedicated children's wards for inpatient and day-case surgery in hospitals where they do not already exist is expensive. Involving a senior manager at every stage of planning can be enormously helpful in achieving this major objective. Managers and committees, understandably, tend to concentrate on the financial resources required, to the detriment of other resources. A major change in organisational culture of the sort we are discussing requires both good will and time.

It is unlikely any clinician or manager will disagree, in theory, with the requirement for nursing and other staff with specialised training and experience. This does, however, have substantial implications for resources, since it usually means employing additional skilled staff. Even with money available, it can be difficult, given the current shortages, to recruit trained personnel in sufficient numbers.

It is not easy to change the practice of a professional lifetime or the way a large organisation functions. It is unrealistic to expect everybody in the organisation to be enthusiastic about change. All proposed changes should have a realistic time scale, so change can be gradual and evolutionary. This is not the same as a statement of good intentions, followed by aimless drift, but does mean accepting that systems need time to turn around. It may even be necessary to allow some senior consultants a little more flexibility (within the limits of safety) until they retire, on the firm understanding that their replacements will work in the agreed manner.

Recognition of limitations

The fact that a district general hospital can admit children for surgery does not mean that it can undertake *all* children's surgery. Put at its simplest, a hospital may be perfectly competent to do an elective tonsillectomy on a 5-year-old child in the middle of the morning, but not have skilled staff available to do a laparotomy on the same child in the middle of the night.

It is essential that the multidisciplinary working party establishes the limits of competence of the service, taking into account the available infrastructure, the facilities for postoperative high-dependency or intensive care, the skill mix of the staff and the available clinical expertise. These decisions should never be made by individual clinicians on the spur of the moment, but as a group around a committee table with adequate information available (e.g. the audit data for workload). All consultants whose practice is likely to be affected by the limitations established for the hospital's competence should have the opportunity to participate in the discussions.

In most small and medium-sized district general hospitals with insufficient trained and experienced staff to run a separate rota for children, the competence of the hospital will vary from time to time. The system should be flexible enough to take account of this.

The working party should also establish guidelines for managing emergencies. The British Paediatric Association believes all consultant anaesthetists working in general hospitals should be competent to manage most common surgical emergencies in children older than 5 years of age. Surgical emergencies in very young children are uncommon, and it is these patients who most require an expert team with full supporting infrastructure.[27] In the absence of staff with the appropriate training and skills, these children should be transferred to a specialist paediatric hospital.

Networking

There are some hospitals so isolated that it is impossible to establish close links with a specialist paediatric unit easily. Most district general hospitals, however, especially in urban areas, already have close clinical and academic links with a neighbouring teaching or specialist centre. These links can be very valuable in establishing a competent children's surgical service.

Specialist departments of paediatric surgery are increasingly willing to send their consultants into the district hospitals to conduct outpatient clinics and, often, to operate. This provides valuable training opportunities for staff of all disciplines, who can then increase the range of work they are able to undertake. Once relationships have been established, it is relatively easy to organise the occasional visit to the teaching centre, as part of CPD.

Guidelines on the transfer from district general to specialist hospitals of children needing elective or emergency surgery should be agreed by surgeons and anaesthetists from both hospitals. It is far simpler and safer to decide in principle on what should be transferred than to negotiate case-by-case in an emergency. However, the guidelines should not be so rigid as to preclude clinical judgement in individual cases.

Monitoring the system

The NCEPOD revisited perioperative deaths in children 10 years after its initial report.[21] The main recommendations are summarised in Box 1.8. The authors identified a number of changes in anaesthetic practice, the most important of which was that 58% of anaesthetists do not anaesthetise babies younger than 6 months, compared with only 16% 10 years ago. Comparing the data, they concluded that 'the process and structure for the provision of anaesthesia and surgery for children have changed for the better'.

Paediatric surgery (as with all services) also needs to be reviewed regularly locally. Performance should be assessed perhaps annually, and it may be useful to assess it formally against the standards set by the multidisciplinary working party. Indeed, this group may be empowered to do the assessment, and also to take action on any lapses which become apparent.

Box 1.15 Paediatric 'audit recipes' from the Royal College of Anaesthetists[40]

- Preoperative parent and patient information
- Consent for paediatric surgery
- Staffing for paediatric anaesthetic services
- Ongoing consultant education in paediatric anaesthesia
- Preoperative fasting
- Premedication in children of school age
- Use of local and regional blocks
- Temperature control
- Pain management
- Parent satisfaction for the arrangements for them to accompany their child for induction of anaesthesia

Audits of clinically relevant topics (e.g. duration of preoperative fasting, quality of post-operative analgesia, the incidence of transfers for emergency surgery or surgery occurring out-of-hours) can highlight problems and suggest solutions. The Royal College of Anaesthetists recently published a book of 'audit recipes'.[40] The paediatric section provides a number of templates that can be modified for local use (Box 1.15). The authors include guidance on standards of best practice, suggested indicators for audit and the data that should be collected. Many projects involve the participation of nurses, theatre staff and pharmacists, as well as patients and parents, and are suitable for multidisciplinary audit. In addition, critical incidents and morbidity and mortality should be reported routinely and discussed.

CONCLUSION

In conclusion, paediatric anaesthesia should only be undertaken in district general hospitals whose standards of provision are consistent with the recommendations of the various government and professional bodies. Anaesthetists should not undertake occasional practice and should keep themselves abreast of current developments in paediatric anaesthesia. Anaesthetists play an important role in the running of hospitals in general, and can be instrumental in effecting improvements in the running and organisation of paediatric services. Many changes in attitude which have improved surgical services for children have been driven by anaesthetists. As 'perioperative physicians' they are often the specialists with the best overview of the problems of treating children in general hospitals.

REFERENCES

1. Robertson J. Young children in hospital. Tavistock Publications;1958.
2. Platt H. The welfare of children in hospital. 1959.
3. Visits to children in hospital. 1959; Department of Health circular HM (59) 19 1959.
4. Visiting of children in hospital. 1966; Department of Health circular HM (66) 18 1966.
5. Accommodation of children in hospital in children's departments. 1969; Department of Health circular HM (69) 4 1969.
6. Hospital facilities for children. 1971; Department of Health Circular HM (71) 22 1971.
7. Hospital facilities for children. 1977; Department of Health and Social Security HC (77) 30 1977.
8. Health Ministry census. 1967.
9. Rogers R. Crowther to Warnock. How 14 reports tried to change children's lives. London: Heinemann Educational; 1983.
10. The Court Committee: Fit for the future 1976. Cmnd 6684 1976.
11. Consumers' Association survey. Children in hospital 1980.
12. Department of Health. Welfare of Children and young people in hospital. London: HMSO; 1991.

13. Campling EA, Devlin HB, Lunn JN. The report of the National Confidential Enquiry into Perioperative Deaths (1989). London: NCEPOD; 1990.
14. The Audit Commission report: Children first: a study of hospital services. London: HMSO; 1993.
15. Buck N, Devlin HB, Lunn JN. The report of the National Confidential Enquiry into Perioperative Deaths (1987). London: NCEPOD; 1987.
16. Lunn JN. Implications of the National Enquiry into Perioperative Deaths for paediatric anaesthesia. Paediatr Anaesth 1992; 2:69–72.
17. Hatch DJ. Anaesthesia for children. Anaesthesia 1984; 39:405–406.
18. Ingram S, Sherry K. Paediatric anaesthesia – who should do it? Anaesthesia 1998; 53:604–605.
19. Atwell JD, Spargo PM. The provision of safe surgery for children. Arch Dis Child 1992; 67:345–349.
20. Stoddart PA, Brennan L, Hatch DJ, et al. Postal survey of paediatric practice and training amongst consultant anaesthetists in the UK. Br J Anaesth 1994; 73:559–563.
21. Extremes of Age. The report of the National Confidential Enquiry into Perioperative Deaths (1997-98). London: NCEPOD; 1999.
22. NHS Executive. Paediatric intensive care. A framework for the future. UK: National co-ordinating group on Paediatric Intensive Care/NHS Executive; 1997.
23. Anonymous. Paediatric anaesthesia (editorial). Br Med J 1978; ii:717.
24. Tiret L, Nicoche Y, Hatton F et al. Complications related to anaesthesia in infants and children. Br J Anaesth 1988; 61:263–269.
25. Cohen NM, Cameron CB, Duncan PG. Anesth Analg 1990; 70:160–167.
26. Heneghan CM, Harrison C. Paediatric anaesthesia – who should do it? Anaesthesia 1998; 53:201–202.
27. The transfer of infants and children for surgery: report of the joint working group. London: British Paediatric Association; 1993.
28. Royal College of Anaesthetists. Guidance on the provision of paediatric anaesthetic services. London: Royal College of Anaesthetists Bulletin 2001; 8:355–359.
29. UK Central Council for Nursing, Midwifery and Health Visiting (UKCC) Position statement 1997.
30. Royal College of Anaesthetists. Guidance for purchasers. London: Royal College of Anaesthetists; 1994.
31. Royal College of Anaesthetists. Guidance for the provision of paediatric anaesthetic services. London: Royal College of Anaesthetists; 1999.
32. McNicol LR. Paediatric anaesthesia – who should do it? The specialist's view. Anaesthesia 1997; 51:513–515.
33. Future configuration of paediatric services. London: British Paediatric Association; 1996.
34. Guidelines for the provision of anaesthetic services. London: Royal College of Anaesthetists; 1997.
35. Rollin A-M. Paediatric anaesthesia – who should do it? The view from the district general hospital. Anaesthesia 1997; 52: 513–516.
36. Children's surgical services. Report of an ad-hoc multi-disciplinary children's surgical liaison group. London: Royal College of Paediatrics and Child Health; 1996.
37. Royal College of Anaesthetists. The CCST in anaesthesia II. Competency based senior house officer training and assessment. A manual for trainees' trainers. London: Royal College of Anaesthetists; 2000.
38. NHS Executive. The employment of operating department practitioners (ODPs) in the NHS. London: NHS Executive; 2000.
39. Association of Anaesthetists of Great Britain and Ireland. Recommendations for standards of monitoring during anaesthesia and recovery, edition 3. London: Association of Anaesthetists of Great Britain and Ireland; 2000.
40. Lack JA, White LM, Thoms GM, et al. Raising the standard – a compendium of audit recipes for continuous quality improvement in anaesthesia. London: Royal College of Anaesthetists; 2000.
41. Royal College of Paediatrics and Child Health. Accident and emergency services for children. Report of a multi-disciplinary working party. London: Royal College of Paediatrics and Child Health; 1999.

CHAPTER 2

Criteria for referring babies and children to specialist paediatric centres

Kathy Wilkinson

INTRODUCTION

In the last decade recommendations for the standards of surgical services for children have become increasingly specific. The National Confidential Enquiry into Perioperative Deaths (NCEPOD 1989[1]) revealed that many anaesthetists caring for babies and small children did so infrequently (see Box 1.5). Amongst deaths in children having non-cardiac surgery, half had been managed by anaesthetists caring for fewer than 12 babies younger than 6 months per year. In the summary of the report, the authors condemned 'occasional paediatric practice' (see Box 1.6) and suggested change was necessary in some district general (DGH) and single-speciality hospitals that had demonstrated difficulties maintaining the required skills. The interpretation of the data and the conclusions made within the NCEPOD (1989) report have been criticised. A particular problem was the paucity of available statistics and, especially, the lack of numerators, making it difficult to know the amount of paediatric surgery in the various centres and whether there was actually an excess of deaths in any particular type of institution. Most surgery was almost certainly taking place (as now) in district hospitals and the number of deaths reported in NCEPOD (1989) were relatively few. Nevertheless, it was the character of many of the deaths which provoked concern, making them worthy of close consideration. The reviews following the publication of this first NCEPOD report[2, 3] have been influential in shaping current service provision, planning and practice.

In particular, the British Paediatric Association (BPA), now the Royal College of Paediatrics and Child Health (RCPCH), produced clear recommendations for the organisation of surgical services for children in its report, *The Transfer of Infants and Children for Surgery* (Box 2.1).[4] Age is widely used throughout this document as the principal reason for referral and the authors advocate transferring all children younger than 3 years to a specialist centre unless the local provision is of an adequate standard.

However, other factors also need consideration, including:

1. the quality of local provision (e.g. appropriately trained and experienced staff);
2. the need for specialist facilities or care (e.g. paediatric intensive care unit (PICU), treatment for major burns, etc.);
3. the presence of concomitant disease (e.g. congenital heart disease (CHD));
4. the choice of the parent and child.

In this chapter, I will attempt to describe the pattern of surgical and anaesthetic practice for children in the UK. I will then discuss the criteria (particularly that of age) for referral to a specialist paediatric centre and examine in detail the evidence supporting the available recommendations. I will then consider some alternatives for delivering surgical care for babies and children.

THE PATTERN OF SURGICAL AND ANAESTHETIC PRACTICE FOR CHILDREN

Statistics

Surgery accounts for almost half of all inpatient admissions of children in the UK.[5] Recent statistics from the Department of Health suggest that only one-third of children younger than 16 years having surgery are cared for in specialist centres (i.e. children's hospitals, university or single-speciality hospitals).[6] The majority of children's surgery occurs in non-specialist units (i.e. DGH or other major acute hospitals), generally without a large range of paediatric services on site. Although it is impossible to identify the percentage of operations that are of a specialist nature, most tertiary centres provide a mixed service, i.e. specialist surgery, routine surgery for children with complex problems and some non-specialist surgery for the local population. For the first two categories of care, children are often referred from a wide geographical area.

Box 2.1 The British Paediatric Association's main recommendation for *The Transfer of Infants and Children for Surgery* (1994)[4]

RECOMMENDATION 3

Children aged 0–3 years requiring emergency surgery should be transferred from a district hospital to a specialist surgical unit unless consultant surgical and anaesthetic staff experienced in emergency surgery for infants and young children are available in the district hospital, and the service is able to meet the standards set in *The Welfare of Children and Young People in Hospital*

Which surgeons operate on children?

According to the Health Episode Statistics in England from 1994 to 1995, 48 992 children requiring general surgery were managed by specialist paediatric surgeons and 84 377 by general surgeons.[7] Of children managed by general surgeons, 25 826 (31%) were aged 4 years or younger.

Data from 1997–98 is presented in Figure 2.1. This would tend to suggest that there has been a further reduction of children's surgery undertaken by general surgeons with primarily adult workloads. For children less than 4 years, only 13 089 cases were cared for by general surgeons, with 24 542 by specialist paediatric surgeons.

Both these reports show the considerable change since 1989–90 when the BPA noted that as many children younger than 4 years were cared for by general (i.e. 'adult') surgeons as by specialist paediatric surgeons.[4]

Statistics differ across the UK. In Scotland, with a population of approximately 5.5 million, it was estimated in 1998 that 15 paediatric surgeons provide about 80% of the general surgical care of children.[9] In 1993 the BPA commented[4] that children requiring surgery in Scotland were twice as likely to be under the care of a paediatric surgeon (as opposed to a general surgeon whose primary responsibilities was for adults). In England at the same time, the opposite was the case.

The pattern of work for other surgical subspecialties is somewhat different. Throughout childhood, ear, nose and throat surgery accounts for the largest percentage of elective surgical admissions,[5] with most children admitted to non-specialist units. The surgeons involved in their care will usually have a mixed (i.e. adult and paediatric) practice, as will be the case for many other specialist surgical specialities.

	Operations by 'adult' general surgeons	Operations by specialist paediatric general surgeons
All ages	1 353 477	51 349
<1 day–27 days	134 (**0.17**)	2 441 (**4.9**)
28 days to < 6 months	1 466 (**1.83**)	5 784 (**11.6**)
6 months to < 1 year	1 046 (**1.3**)	3 042 (**6.1**)
1–3 years	10 443 (**13.1**)	13 275 (**26.6**)
4–10 years	31 232 (**39**)	16 701 (**33.5**)
11–16 years	35 430 (**44**)	8 644 (**17.3**)
Total under 16 years	79 751	40 887
17 years and over	1 273 441	1 453
Not known	285	9

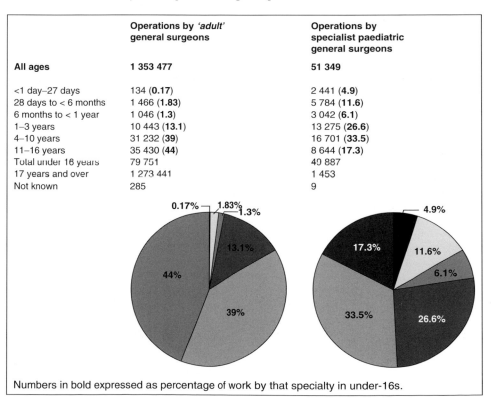

Numbers in bold expressed as percentage of work by that specialty in under-16s.

Fig. 2.1 Ordinary admissions and day cases combined for general surgery: completed episodes, NHS hospitals, England 1997–1998.[6]

Frequency of surgery at different ages

The frequency of all surgery related to age in England during 1997–98 is presented in Figure 2.2. Surgery for children aged 0–16 years accounts for 8.5% of the total surgery for all ages.

Twenty-six per cent of all surgery in childhood occurs in those younger than 4 years. Babies under 1 year account for more than a third of this work, which is probably explained by the number of serious congenital abnormalities requiring surgery soon after birth.

Geographical location

The delivery of surgical services for children in the UK may still depend to some extent on postcode. As already mentioned, a child under 4 years of age requiring general surgery is very much more likely to be operated on by a specialist paediatric surgeon than by an adult surgeon.[6] The RCPCH has reinforced, within its most recent report on children's surgical services,[8] that specialist paediatric surgical centres should provide a general surgical service for the local population and a specialist service to which children may be referred from the whole region. Such a centre would normally employ five specialist paediatric general surgeons and be based in a tertiary centre with a PICU. It suggests that general surgeons with a paediatric interest ought to provide non-specialist surgery for children living some distance from the paediatric surgical centre. However, if these recommendations were applied without exception, they might concentrate specialist paediatric surgical services into even fewer centres, possibly resulting in two standards of care (particularly for most non-specialist surgery) determined by geographical location – one provided by specialist paediatric surgeons and the other by ('adult') general surgeons with an interest in children's surgery. Obviously, this concern assumes that the paediatric surgeon provides a better standard of care, but whatever the standards, there is currently a marked shortage of general surgeons with a paediatric interest.[9] This may underlie the inequality of service between patients who live close to, compared with those who live more distant from, a paediatric surgical centre.

Indeed, hospital care in the UK continues to be concentrated primarily in large urban areas. Individuals living in more remote parts of the UK have relatively poor access to secondary and tertiary health-care services. This includes those living in much of rural Wales and Scotland, and the far west and east of England. At present, some children in these areas are

All ages (adults and children)	5,850,237		
			% of all operations in children aged 0–16 years
<1–27 days	16 758	3.4	(A)
28 days to < 6 months	15 030	3	(B)
6 months to < 1 year	12 315	2.5	(C)
1–3 years	85 187	17.2	(D)
4–10 years	211 216	42.7	(E)
11–16 years	154 616	31.2	(F)
Total 0–16 years	55 346 131		
17 years and over	8984		
Not known	495 122		

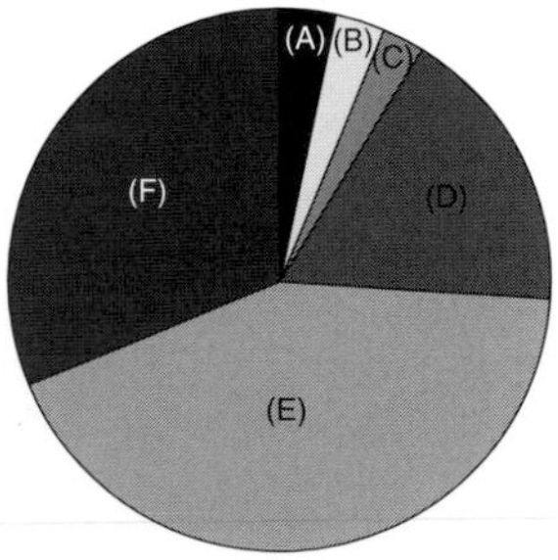

Fig. 2.2 Ordinary admissions and day cases combined (all surgery): completed episodes by primary operations. NHS hospitals, England, 1997–1998.[6]

served by large acute hospitals, some of which have established a paediatric surgical service with between one and three specialist paediatric surgeons. Such hospitals have limited subspecialty care on site, but do not generally provide PICUs. They are able to offer a more robust surgical service for children compared with the smaller DGHs, but fall short of complying with current recommendations for the model of paediatric surgery discussed above.

CRITERIA FOR REFERRAL

Age

The Royal College of Anaesthetists (RCA) has summarised many of the available recommendations for paediatric anaesthesia in its *Guidance to Purchasers* first published in 1994 and recently revised (see Box 1.11).[10] Within the introduction on paediatric anaesthetic services, the authors state: 'Treatment in a specialist paediatric unit will be required for neonates (less than 44 weeks' gestational age), children with significant co-morbidity ... and children with complex surgical conditions including major trauma'. What, however, is the evidence to support a recommendation to refer the very young child and/or those with comorbidity or complex surgical needs?

Transfer in utero

Prenatal diagnosis of congenital anomalies is increasingly common. The Royal College of Surgeons of England (RCSE) recommends transferring babies with suspected major congenital malformation for delivery in maternity units with ready access to appropriate surgical facilities (see Box 2.2).[11]

Evidence supporting in-utero transfer comes primarily from the study of two conditions – gastroschisis and diaphragmatic hernia.

The evidence for gastroschisis is inconclusive, but tends to show that those infants referred to a specialist paediatric hospital antenatally have a reduced period of ventilation and establish enteral feeding more quickly.[12, 13] For diaphragmatic hernia, at least one study showed good survival for babies diagnosed in utero and delivered at a site where paediatric

---

Box 2.2 Recommendations from the Royal College of Surgeons of England for *Surgical Services for the Newborn* (1999)[11]

- Surgical neonates should be concentrated within specialist paediatric surgical units with adequate numbers of appropriately trained medical and nursing staff and full facilities for the care of the infant and his/her family

- Neonatal surgical units should be adequately staffed by paediatric surgeons with access to a full range of supporting services. An ideal unit should be staffed by a minimum of four consultant paediatric surgeons and one paediatric urologist who provides adequate emergency cover and the development of subspecialties within centres

- The nursing care and support of newborns undergoing surgery should be undertaken by nurses with the appropriate knowledge and skills (normally a registered children's nurse with additional postregistration training). Their supportive and educational role in relation to parents and other family members must be recognised

- An integrated multidisciplinary approach to care is essential in the premature surgical neonate and in those with complex congenital malformations

- A fetus with a suspected major congenital malformation should ideally be delivered in a unit with ready access to paediatric surgical facilities. Close links between paediatric surgeons, neonatologists and fetal medicine specialists are essential. The prospective parents of such children should have access to expert prenatal counselling

surgery was available.[14] Although overall mortality was equivalent for these babies compared with those delivered elsewhere, the authors thought mortality should actually be increased in babies diagnosed early in utero (and therefore transferred for delivery) because the defect was usually larger. More controversial is whether early referral of babies with diaphragmatic hernias to centres providing very specialised methods of respiratory support improves outcome. A randomised controlled study showed extracorporeal membrane oxygenation (ECMO) was little better (in terms of mortality) than high-quality conventional treatment.[15] Nevertheless, ECMO may well have a place in the management of a small number of babies with diaphragmatic hernia and the UK now has five such centres adjacent to, or within, paediatric surgical units.

Neonates

During and immediately after the neonatal period the types of surgical problems which present are diverse and often complex, but the frequency of each condition is low. The neonate is physiologically fragile, particularly if born prematurely, and perioperative morbidity and mortality are increased.[16-18] Surgical problems are often associated with other congenital anomalies, especially CHD. Surgery and anaesthesia may be lengthy and neonates frequently need perioperative high-dependency or full intensive care. Few would argue, therefore, that highly specialised skills and ongoing experience are important to maintain a reliable standard of care. Several authors have recommended transferring neonates to a specialist paediatric surgical centre for surgery.[3, 17, 18] In the UK, such babies are almost exclusively dealt with in regional centres providing a minimum number of services on site. The 1999 RCSE report on surgical services for the newborn deals specifically with the requirements of this most vulnerable population.[11] The authors describe the current provision in the UK and recommend that neonatal surgery occurs only in large specialist centres providing a full range of paediatric services. They suggest that each of these centres should employ five specialist paediatric general surgeons (one with a major interest in urology) and serve a population of approximately two and a half million. This arrangement provides an adequate patient population to make the service economically viable and support training and academic research. It also allows clinicians to maintain and develop their expertise whilst having an acceptable on-call rota. Arul and Spicer have suggested that each specialist centre should care for a minimum of 60 neonates to maintain viability.[19]

Babies and preschool children

Most accept that neonates should be transferred to specialist paediatric hospitals for surgery. There may also be good reasons to refer all older babies for specialist care. They too have very different physiology, pathology and psychology compared with older children or adults. Certainly both perioperative morbidity and mortality in infants are generally believed to be higher. Morray's review of US paediatric closed malpractice claims from 1985 until early 1991 showed that the claims involving children 6 months of age or younger were the most numerous.[20] More recently, the Australian Incident Monitoring Scheme (AIMS) study of critical incidents during anaesthesia in children showed a very similar pattern of serious problems, most relating to the respiratory system and/or inadequate ventilation.[21] Given that babies have increased metabolic demands and rates of oxygen consumption, it is not surprising that critical incidents relating to the respiratory system lead rapidly to a poor outcome. In 1991, Keenan published a retrospective study of the incidence of cardiac arrests in babies managed by specialist paediatric anaesthetists compared with those managed by non-specialists working in the same university teaching hospital.[22] There were no arrests in the group cared for by paediatric anaesthetists compared with four in the non-specialist group. Holzman more recently reviewed the literature on the morbidity and mortality related to paediatric anaesthesia.[23] He concludes that:

no doubt should remain that children in the first year of life are at increased risk of anaesthetic related cardiac arrest ... there is some evidence that this risk may be decreased when anaesthetics are administered and supervised by experienced pediatric anesthesiologists.

What is the evidence to support transferring older children to specialist paediatric centres? In Morray's review of closed malpractice claims, 55% involved children 3 years or under.[20] Many young children are still cared for in non-specialist centres and it is important to know if anaesthetic morbidity or mortality is really greater in these hospitals. Although the literature is sparse, Morray judged that anaesthetic care was more likely to have been 'less than appropriate' in paediatric claims.[20] Of the first 2000 incidents reported to AIMS, 7% occurred in children aged 1–14 years (3% were in those < 1 year).[21] The majority of these children were American Society of Anesthesiology (ASA) 1 or 2. Holzman[23] has concluded that accidents beyond the infant age range are rare, but comments that healthy children continue to suffer injury and have greater rates of survival with more permanent damage.

There is a general belief that recommendations based on age have greatly influenced our paediatric anaesthetic practice in the UK over the last 10 years – but is there any objective evidence of this? In 1994, a questionnaire was sent to all Fellows of the RCA to try to find out if attitudes and practice had changed significantly since publication of the NCEPOD (1989) report.[24] Only those involved in anaesthesia for children aged under 3 were asked to participate. The majority of responding consultants' main paediatric practice was in district hospitals. Just under half stated that they had received the minimum period of specialist training in paediatric anaesthesia considered desirable. Although only 21% were caring for more than 12 infants under the age of 6 months per year, two-thirds of respondents managed infants for pyloromyotomy, with most caring for only one or two annually. In 1996, in a survey of the delegates attending the UK Association of Anaesthetists Linkman conference (more than two-thirds of whom represented DGHs),[25] 64.2% said that their hospital had no lower age limit for emergency work in childhood. In addition, 37% were unhappy to entrust the care of their own child to their DGH.

Both surveys indicate a lack of universal compliance with age-based guidelines. Nevertheless, in the last 10 years many trusts have undergone major reorganisation of theatre lists and on-call rotas in an attempt to improve the quality of anaesthetic care for children.

The most recent update of NCEPOD (covering paediatric deaths during 1997–98) perhaps demonstrates more convincingly the results of reorganisation.[26] Most deaths in this series were associated with congenital anomalies, necrotising enterocolitis, tumours or trauma. Very few children died following surgery in DGHs, with many more (compared with 1989) dying in specialist children's hospitals (Fig. 2.3).

Relatively few children who died were dealt with in a facility without a separate on-call rota for paediatric anaesthesia and the vast majority were anaesthetised by a consultant (83%, 71/85). In all but one case (1%, 1/93) consultant surgeons were aware and involved in the care of the children who died. The overall recommendations of the report are presented in Box 1.9.

The changes in paediatric anaesthetic and surgical provision made in the UK have to some extent been mirrored in North America where calls have been made for further subspecialisation.[27, 28] Moreover, in countries where subspecialisation has already been adopted, there is some evidence that mortality may have been reduced.[29]

If it is accepted that surgery in neonates and older babies is very different and that age alone may be sufficient reason to seek early transfer to a specialist surgical centre, what are the additional factors which come into play when deciding where to operate on children? Associated medical conditions and complexity of surgery undoubtedly matter. Complex surgery (which would include cardiac, neurosurgery, cancer and transplantation surgery or procedures with major blood loss) will not be discussed in detail here.

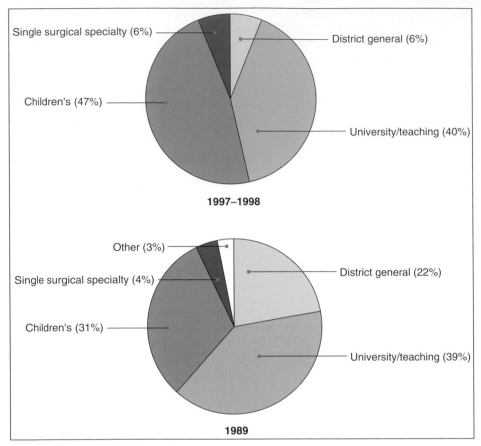

Fig. 2.3 Deaths after surgery in children: comparison of the types of hospitals in which surgery took place during 1997, 1998 and 1989 (percentage of total postoperative deaths). Note that these figures compare information collected from anaesthetic questionnaires on deaths in children in 1989, with the 1997–1998 data from both anaesthetic and surgical returns. Reproduced with permission from NCEPOD.[26]

Associated medical conditions

In reality, many children are referred to specialist centres because they have associated medical conditions. Some of the surgery they need will be minor and often within the capabilities of the local hospital. Which conditions in childhood generally preclude treatment in a DGH, even for minor surgery? A broad list is provided in Box 2.3.

Congenital heart disease

CHD is the single most common, and perhaps most significant, group of abnormalities. Although only a minority of children with heart murmurs require transfer to a tertiary centre for surgery, all will need to be assessed carefully before deciding to operate locally, using information gleaned from the history (in particular an assessment of exercise tolerance), a recent paediatric cardiology review and echocardiography. Infants and children with ventricular dysfunction or significant pulmonary hypertension should always be cared for in specialist hospitals. Moreover, anaesthetists and any others involved in the care of those with previous palliative procedures for CHD (e.g. the Mustard, Senning or Fontan proce-

---

Box 2.3 Associated medical conditions in which surgery should generally be avoided in the district general hospital

Complex or decompensated congenital heart disease (see text)

Syndromes in which difficult intubation and/or ventilation might be anticipated, e.g.
- Major craniofacial syndromes
- Mucopolysaccharidoses

Metabolic disease in which blood sugar/acid–base/serum ammonia is likely to be unstable in the perioperative period (this should *not* include the stable diabetic child)

Renal[1] or hepatic failure

---

[1]On active dialysis programme.

dures) must have a thorough understanding of the associated anatomy and pathophysiology. Such previous procedures constitute a relative contraindication to surgery in all but the largest DGHs that provide the services of fully trained paediatric anaesthetists (see later). With adequate preassessment and resources, however, it should be possible safely to offer such children appropriate day surgery with minimal disturbance to their life.

Airway abnormalities

Although most DGHs are well prepared to manage a difficult airway in an adult, the child with similar problems often has a syndrome and poses very different challenges to the anaesthetist. In particular, children with mucopolysaccharidoses are difficult to manage, even for staff in specialist centres,[30] and should be referred on for surgery from a DGH. Similarly, those with abnormal development of the first and second branchial arches or with craniosynostoses may have major airway problems perioperatively, requiring postoperative PICU/high-dependency unit (HDU) care. These facilities are usually only available in specialist centres. The question which always needs to be asked is: 'Can the whole team cope with all likely eventualities in the perioperative period?' If the answer is 'no', then these children must be referred to specialist centres, even for minor surgery.

Continuing clinical experience of surgeons and anaesthetists

Is high volume synonymous with a higher standard of care? Evidence for such relationships is not available for all aspects of paediatrics. However some does exist to support the regionalisation of neonatal care for babies less than 28 weeks' gestation[31] and for paediatric cardiac surgery.[32] Children with cancer (part of the management of which may include surgery) have also been shown to benefit from care in a regional centre with a high volume of cases.[33] Debate has occurred about evidence of the need to regionalise paediatric intensive care[34, 35] and whether children treated in a paediatric trauma centre have a better outcome compared with those treated elsewhere.[36] There is little published data on the outcomes of anaesthesia for children in specialist compared with non-specialist hospitals, however.

Lunn, in an editorial in 1992 on the implications of the 1989 NCEPOD report,[37] made recommendations for the number of children of different ages that an individual anaesthetist should manage each year to maintain skills (see Box 1.7). The 'Lunn criteria' have been widely accepted and applied as a standard by individual anaesthetists and departments wishing to maintain a paediatric interest. Although they do indeed provide basic guidance, they have not been assessed against any measurable outcomes. In particular, delivering anaesthetic care to 12 babies under 6 months of age per year may provide insufficient ongoing experience, given the diversity of pathology within this age group. Local policies might well dictate change to the basic criteria depending on the types of patients managed.

Good practice ought to be judged on the results of the team. With this in mind, it is reasonable to be concerned about surgical (as well as anaesthetic) outcomes whenever we anaesthetise a child. For paediatric surgery (as well as anaesthesia), there is little evidence of a strong relationship between a particular volume of work and the quality of outcome. However, there is evidence that some specific conditions in infancy are better managed by certain teams. For example, in pyloric stenosis, the incidence of duodenal perforation, wound problems and persistent vomiting would seem to relate to the volume of work of the individual surgeon.[38, 39] In a report of a large series of pyloric stenosis, the authors also found the rate for reoperation was higher for those surgeons operating on fewer babies.[40]

An important and potentially confusing confounding factor is that a specialist paediatric surgeon will tend to operate on many more neonates and small children than the general surgeon. Is it volume of work or training that is the most important factor determining outcome? In fact, it may be difficult to dissociate the effect of volume from other criteria affecting quality of care. In any case, a decision to refer a baby or child will not generally be made solely on the amount of work a centre does. However, volume of work is relevant to the economics of providing a service in that, clearly, it will be unviable unless a critical number of patients is referred to the centre each year.

Need for specialist services

Economics of providing specialist services

The potential cost of treating some major surgical conditions is enormous.[41] Only centres attracting large volumes of work can justify the expense of providing the full range of intensive care facilities for babies and children, such as ECMO or haemofiltration. Meaningful research into new and expensive techniques to determine their efficacy is similarly only feasible in large, specialised centres.

If paediatric surgery is based in such a large regional centre, it typically forms part of a hospital with over 1000 beds. However, providers should be aware of the potential for inefficiency in such large institutions. It has been demonstrated that centres with more than 600 beds may display so-called diseconomies of scale – bigger does not always mean more efficient.[42]

Intensive care

The anticipated need for intensive care (levels 2 or 3) is an important consideration for referral to a specialist paediatric hospital before surgery (See Box 3.1, Ch.3).

In a large prospective study of paediatric intensive care over 1 year from the north-west region of England,[43] 28% of admissions were related to surgery (excluding trauma). Most followed either cardiac or neurosurgery, but many also came from other surgical sub-specialities. In another study over 19 months from a large multidisciplinary PICU in Australia, the authors found that 85% of surgical admissions followed cardiac or neurosurgery with very few from general surgery.[44] This study also concluded that, although 5% of postoperative PICU admissions were unexpected, the vast majority might have been anticipated, and probably prevented, by a more careful preoperative assessment.

It is obviously extremely important that clinicians working in hospitals without PICU facilities on site assess children very carefully preoperatively in case surgery and/or anaesthesia is likely to precipitate a need for postoperative ventilation or other intensive care treatments.[10] At increased risk are those with complex or unstable cardiorespiratory, neurological or metabolic disease, or preexisting airway problems. Surgery of the upper abdomen or chest is also associated with a higher risk of admission to PICU postoperatively, particularly if the child is in the infant age range. Length of operative procedure may also be a factor. In my opinion, elective surgery should take place in a hospital with a PICU on site if the risks of postoperative intubation or ventilation are thought to exceed 5%. These risks may be difficult to quantify without considerable experience of the planned surgery and the particular child's physiological reserve. Units should, nevertheless, monitor closely the rate of unexpected postsurgical admissions to intensive care, which may be an important indicator of quality. All hospitals performing inpatient surgery in children should be capable of providing level 1 (high-dependency) care. These hospitals should also be able to establish level 2 intensive care in an emergency before referral to a regional PICU (see Chapter 4).

Choice of the parents or child

Occasionally it is necessary to refer a child to a particular specialist centre because of child or parental preference. Whenever practical, and most importantly advisable, this should be accommodated. If the child remains under the care of specialists in a remote tertiary centre, it is important that staff working at the local hospital are kept up to date about progress and the child or parents should carry a current medical summary in case of urgent admission locally.

PATTERNS OF PROVISION AND QUALITY OF SERVICE
Standards
Recommendations

As discussed, numerous authors in the last 10 years have suggested standards for the surgical care of children (see Ch. 1). Perhaps the most general of these are contained in *The Welfare of Sick Children in Hospital*.[45] A more specific review in 1994 by Action for Sick Children focuses exclusively on children's surgical issues and contains many examples of good practice from hospitals throughout the UK.[46] The authors' aims are for their extensive and detailed recommendations on all aspects of perioperative care to be adopted by all centres admitting children for surgery. A summary is presented in Box 2.4.

The Transfer of Infants and Children for Surgery, published by the BPA in 1993 (see Box 2.1) also deals with specific standards of care which should be achieved by all centres providing surgery for babies and children.[4] They include the need for appropriately trained consultants in anaesthesia and children's surgery to be supported by paediatricians, trained nurses and paramedical staff, as well as radiology and pathology services.

The National Health Service (NHS) reforms in the UK during the early 1990s gave an opportunity for the Royal Colleges and their specialist groups to publish their specific recommendations for the ideal organisation of paediatric surgical services. The British Association of Paediatric Surgeons' *Paediatric Surgery: Standards of Care*,[47] (which replaces its *Guidance to Purchasers*, first published in 1994) has recently been produced. It describes five categories of specialist paediatric surgery. These are: (1) surgery for neonates; (2) the surgical management of children with conditions requiring special expertise (e.g. tumours, hepatobiliary disorders); (3) surgery for children with associated disorders; (4) paediatric urology; and (5) adolescent/adult surgery requiring the expertise of a paediatric surgeon. It defines the children's surgical unit in terms of the type of surgery provided, the facilities available and the population served. The report accepts that much non-specialist surgery is provided in the DGH and defines a minimum standard in terms of staffing and facilities. A summary of recommendations is given in Box 2.5. The latest draft also for the first time defines more clearly the responsibilities of a specialist paediatric surgeon. This includes providing outreach clinics, already well established in some parts of the UK.

The RCA's most recent guidelines for the provision of anaesthetic services[10] includes a summary of recommendations for paediatric anaesthesia (Box 1.11). It also gives a comprehensive list of relevant previous recommendations. References cover the necessary support services, organisation, staffing and educational facilities.

Box 2.4 *Setting Standards for Children Undergoing Surgery*: standards recommended by Action for Sick Children (1994)[46]

- Information on all aspects of the condition, surgery and aftercare is given to parents and to children, according to their age and understanding
- Procedures for obtaining consent recognise the rights of children and their ability to understand and evaluate information
- Surgery on children should be undertaken by surgeons and anaesthetist with appropriate training and experience
- Arrangements for the admission of children for surgery, both elective and emergency, are as child- and family-centred as possible
- Each child is prepared for the operation, according to his/her maturity
- Routines and procedures for surgery minimise the anxiety for child and parents
- Arrangements for the child's travel and arrival at the theatre minimise the anxiety for child and parents
- The environment and procedures in the anaesthetic room minimise the anxiety for child and parents
- The environment and procedures in the recovery room minimise the anxiety for child and parents
- Children and parents are prepared for how the child will feel after the operation
- Children do not experience unnecessary pain
- Parents and children are involved before discharge in discussions about arrangements for their care
- Guidelines are agreed by the hospital, general practitioner and community staff on the responsibility for care of the child after discharge from hospital

Box 2.5 The requirements for specialist paediatric surgery[47]

- Trained and accredited paediatric surgeons and anaesthetists trained in paediatric anaesthesia
- A full range of specialist services for children, including paediatrics, neonatology, paediatric intensive care (at least level 2 care), paediatric radiology (with 24-h cover), paediatric neurosurgery, paediatric orthopaedics, paediatric plastic surgery, paediatric nephrology, paediatric cardiology, paediatric oncology and paediatric pathology
- Nursing staff trained in paediatric nursing, paediatric critical care and neonatal nursing
- Support services catering for the specific needs of children, including dieticians, physiotherapists, social workers, play leaders and teachers
- Separate facilities designed for children, notably the accident and emergency department, outpatients department, wards, operating theatres (including a dedicated emergency theatre for children), day-case unit, radiology suite and laboratory services
- Investigative/physiological laboratory services specifically staffed and equipped for children, such as gastrointestinal and gait analysis laboratories
- Accommodation for parents, who should have unrestricted access to their children

Training

It is no longer acceptable for surgeons or anaesthetists without adequate training and experience to manage children. The Senate of Surgery has issued recent recommendations for training general surgeons with an interest in children, including a minimum of 6 months in a paediatric surgical centre.[7] However, what constitutes an appropriate case load for a general surgeon with a paediatric interest? In 1986, Peter Jones (a general surgeon from Aberdeen) examined the likely number of emergency or elective operations by general surgeons on children under 13 years in a district hospital serving 200 000 people.[9] He concluded that this volume of work was best concentrated in the hands of one or two general surgeons. Nevertheless, the authors of the 1989 NCEPOD[1] reported that 24% of surgeons operating on children aged 3–10 years did fewer than 20 operations in this age group per year, and 83% operated on fewer than 20 babies under 6 months annually. In 1996, the RCPCH[8] sought to outlaw 'occasional paediatric surgical practice' and suggested that at least the equivalent of one operating list per week was essential. More recently, a working party of the Senate of Surgery[9] defined continuing (surgical) experience as equivalent to at least one operating session per fortnight.

Currently, however, there is a serious shortage of appropriately trained and experienced general surgeons[9] and few surgical trainees admit a paediatric interest. The difficulties will worsen when older surgeons retire. New training schemes have resulted in increasing specialisation and a generation of general surgeons who may have little experience of surgery in children. Even with the possible expansion of the number of adult surgeons with a paediatric interest, it is unlikely that most DGHs will be able to recruit or retain more than one such individual, leading to problems with cover out of hours and suspension of even elective activity during leave. This may further aggravate any inequalities of care between different parts of the country, particularly if there are long distances between specialist and non-specialist centres.[49]

For an anaesthetist, an appointment as a consultant with a paediatric interest (e.g. in a DGH) demands a minimum of 6 months' training in paediatric anaesthesia. A full-time career as a specialist paediatric anaesthetist requires at least 12 months' paediatric experience, including 6 months in a tertiary paediatric centre[50] (see Ch. 1). Ongoing experience has been defined in relation to the Lunn criteria and/or one paediatric list per week.[37]

Trainees in anaesthesia in the UK now have to undertake assessments in the work place based on competency. The purpose of this is to scrutinise both the content of the training programme and the performance of the trainee more carefully. In paediatric anaesthesia, as well as other subspecialities, the number of anaesthetics a trainee gives must represent part of this assessment process.

Organisation

Small district general hospitals

As a result of the various recommendations and further subspecialisation, staff in many smaller district hospitals may increasingly feel that they are unable to provide anything other than an elective service for young children and may have stopped anaesthetising babies altogether. Although small local units may be able to run a service during the day, providing a separate rota for children out of hours is often uneconomic and would, in any case, provide insufficient ongoing experience. These changes in practice have been further encouraged by the development of clinical accountability and pressure from government and society for professional groups to comply with guidelines and standards. The implications of the changes are only now being recognised by specialist children's hospitals, some of which are suddenly faced with the need to provide a service for all babies and small children having even minor surgery.

If further regionalisation of paediatric surgical services is adopted, how can clinicians working in non-specialist hospitals, particularly the smaller district hospitals, retain their skills for managing sick children? Recent commentators have suggested possible solutions to this problem. The 'hub-and-spoke' model (as described in Ch. 1) may be useful in some parts of the UK.[51] Senior staff spend time working in both the specialist children's and district hospitals. The anaesthetist, in particular, retains skills by performing regular lists in the specialist centre. This model does not generally provide cover for emergency surgery in the district hospital, so a robust system for transporting sick children to the specialist centre after appropriate resuscitation should be established in parallel. The 'hub-and-spoke' model probably works best if the distances between the two hospitals are relatively short (perhaps under 25 miles or 40 km). It also assumes that the rest of the local team other than the anaesthetist (e.g. paediatricians, surgeons, etc.) can retain a high level of clinical skill for diagnosing and managing surgical problems in childhood. Children with trauma, burns, pyloric stenosis, intussusception, obstructed hernia, appendicitis and ingested or inhaled foreign body form a large part of the emergency paediatric surgical work in most UK centres. When these conditions present to units without paediatric surgeons, clinicians must be able to recognise their serious nature and initiate appropriate treatment before transfer.

Geographically isolated hospitals

In 1996, a working party from the BPA published a report on the future configuration of paediatric services.[52] It defined an 'isolated unit' as one more than 1 h by road from its closest paediatric unit, and a 'small unit' as one with fewer than 1800 acute paediatric medical referrals per year.

Although the recommendations of the working party were written primarily as a guide to medical staffing and training in children's units, they have implications for surgery and anaesthesia. Paediatric surgery should not take place in small DGHs situated less than 30 min from a larger unit. The report proposes that in this situation the two units should amalgamate. However, they do accept that accessibility and local provision of acute paediatric care is a high priority and that there is a place for modified paediatric surgery occurring in isolated units. This is on the understanding that even these small units provide a suitable environment for children and the recommended levels of appropriate staffing.

Transfer from geographically isolated parts of the UK is not necessarily simple. Access to specialist care in these areas can vary during the year according to weather conditions. In addition, it is obvious that isolated hospitals will have the demands of paediatric medicine thrust upon them because they will be the first port of call for sick children in their catchment area. Medical and nursing staff will have to cope as well as possible before transferring children to appropriately staffed units. There is a need for these hospitals to provide a high-quality local service (including diagnosis, resuscitation, stabilisation and definitive surgery, if appropriate) for what is often a substantial population. Clearly, the quality of this service will depend primarily on the initial training and continuing experience and education of the clinicians serving the community. Resuscitation skills may be aided by easy access to multidisciplinary advanced paediatric life support courses. Small units should also be equipped to a high standard to allow initial optimal management before definitive surgery in the fit, older child. Children under 3–5 years (depending on the type of surgery) and most emergency cases will generally need transporting to a regional centre, if possible. This will require well-developed systems on the part of the receiving unit and the availability of the necessary skills for safe air transport.

Larger district or major acute general hospitals

Some large acute general hospitals serve local populations of 300 000–500 000. Most should be able to organise a satisfactory surgical service for children (e.g. paediatric orthopaedics, non-specialist general surgery, ear, nose and throat) and may also (depending on how close they are to a major paediatric surgical centre) be able to accept fit babies having more minor surgery (e.g. inguinal herniotomy, pyloromyotomy). They sometimes accept secondary referrals from smaller DGHs nearby. The quality of service provided must be consistent with nationally agreed standards (see Ch. 1) and should include experienced middle-grade paediatric medical cover. The ages of children, particularly babies, accepted for surgery and the type of operations undertaken will be influenced by the volume of work and the facilities available.

A working alternative model of provision in larger district or major acute general hospitals involves employing paediatric surgeons to provide a full surgical service (including trauma care) for children and young adults younger than 16 years, but not necessarily all neonates. It has been estimated that if specialist paediatric surgeons were to undertake all general surgery in children, there would be a need for at least 70 extra consultants in England and Wales alone.[9] This has major implications for training. Less isolated large acute units might, as an alternative, participate in the 'hub-and-spoke' model, already described. It is probable that no single option is appropriate for all geographical locations within the UK.

Specialist paediatric hospitals

Specialist paediatric centres provide care for children of all ages with significant medical problems having surgery, children who are very sick and others having complex surgery. They also deliver surgical services for many babies, particularly neonates or those born prematurely. A centre is likely to be provided only if there is a sufficient volume of work within the subspecialty to make it economically viable. The volume of work also influences the economics of running a service, as already described, and this may have a secondary effect on quality. The overall quality of care provided is important in the choice of referral centre and this must take into account the range of services available on site.

Ideally, a specialist paediatric centre should have good road and public transport links and be easily accessible within $1-1^1/_2$ h from all parts of the region it serves. The centre is best situated close to the middle of the region. For the youngest and sickest children requiring paediatric intensive care and/or surgery, the regional unit has a responsibility to provide a high-quality retrieval service 24 h a day if patients present at a peripheral unit.[53] A retrieval service is also an essential recommendation of the 1999 NCEPOD[26] report. Because of its distant location for many, specialist paediatric hospitals must also provide facilities for parents on site, including a long-stay car park and residential accommodation. Ideally, a surgical centre should be located adjacent to other tertiary services for children (e.g. cardiac, plastic and neurosurgery). Moreover, relationships should be well established with other subspecialists to provide a team approach to the care of babies with complex syndromes. An experienced general paediatrician or surgeon should take the lead in such cases, providing an overview of care and a named link with the peripheral unit where some of the child's surgery may eventually occur.

What other standards have been proposed for specialist paediatric surgical centres? In *Paediatric Surgery: Standards of Care*[47] (see Box 2.5), the British Association of Paediatric Surgeons has stated that a hospital admitting children for major surgery should have paediatric intensive care facilities. This has reiterated advice given by the Senate of Surgery in its document *The Provision of General Surgical Services for Children*.[9] The evidence behind this proposal has already been discussed.

Assessment of quality

The British Association of Paediatric Surgeons has proposed specific indicators of quality by which to judge a surgical service for children.[47] These indicators are divided into those related to the selection of children for operation (e.g. age at operation, number of operations or method of patient selection) and others primarily related to quality of treatment (e.g. postoperative complications, including transfer to a PICU or specialist surgical centre, length of stay in hospital and the availability and use of facilities for paediatric day care). The authors suggested that some operations (e.g. orchidopexy or circumcision) may be performed with less tight indications in district hospitals compared with paediatric surgical centres. Some other operations in children may also not be based on sound evidence. In particular, the benefits of myringotomy and grommet insertion are controversial.[54, 55] The incidence of these various procedures could usefully be monitored to provide a yardstick of quality.

CONCLUSIONS

Surgical services for children should be organised regionally, taking into account geography and existing resources. Facilities and standards of practice should be as consistent as possible with nationally agreed recommendations. Most district hospitals should be able to provide a range of non-specialist surgery for children older than 3 years.

For many regions, a three-centre model of care may best meet the future needs of children requiring surgery:

The small district general hospital

These hospitals should be able to provide resuscitation and stabilisation of all infants and children. They should also perform elective and emergency minor surgery for children older than 3 years. Such hospitals should have paediatric beds on site and appropriate middle-grade medical cover at all times. Babies and small children needing surgery are likely to be transferred to intermediate or tertiary centres.

The intermediate centre (larger district or major acute general hospital)

These hospitals should generally employ specialist paediatric surgeons and other specialist surgeons with an interest in children (e.g. ear, nose and throat, orthopaedics) and provide care for older babies and all children having surgery. This will include the management of trauma. The volume of work should be sufficient to justify separate on-call arrangements for paediatrics in both surgery and anaesthesia. Exceptions might include children having major general surgery (including cancer surgery) or those having cardiac or neurosurgery or likely to require postoperative care on a PICU. Such hospitals should provide paediatric radiology and pathology, neonatal intensive care unit (NICU) and paediatric HDU (level 1) on-site. Most neonates needing surgery should be resuscitated and stabilised before transport to a specialist paediatric (tertiary referral) centre. However, such centres should be able to care for babies with pyloric stenosis or inguinal hernias.

The specialist paediatric (or tertiary referral) centre

These centres should provide the full range of services, including neonatal, cardiac and neurosurgery, oncological medicine and surgery, PICU and NICU. These services should be supported by a fully funded retrieval team for transferring critically ill babies and children from other hospitals in the region.

The practical implications of moving all surgery for children into fewer (tertiary) centres are enormous. Latterly changes have often been made purely on the basis of age and because it is the simplest way of keeping 'within the rules'. Imaginative and well-funded proposals need to be worked out individually for regions within the UK depending on geography, existing services and training and staffing restrictions. If applied, this may eventually result in a uniformly high standard of surgical care for children in the UK.

REFERENCES

1. Campling EA, Devlin HB, Lunn JN. The Report of the National Confidential Enquiry into Perioperative Deaths (1989). London: NCEPOD: 1990.
2. Lancet. Editorial. NCEPOD and perioperative deaths of children. Lancet 1990; 23:1498–1500.
3. Atwell JD, Spargo PM. The provision of safe surgery for children. Arch Dis Child 1992; 67:345–349.
4. British Paediatric Association. The transfer of infants and children for surgery. London: British Paediatric Association/Royal College of Paediatrics and Child Health; 1994.

5. The Audit Commission Report: Children first: a study of hospital services. London: HMSO; 1993.
6. Department of Health. Health episode statistics 1997–98. London: Department of Health;1999.
7. Department of Health. Health episode statistics, vol. 2, 1994/95. London: Department of Health;1996.
8. Children's Surgical Services: Report of an ad hoc multidisciplinary children's surgical liaison group. London: Royal College of Paediatrics and Child Health; 1996.
9. Senate of Surgery of Great Britain and Ireland. The provision of general surgical services for children. London: Senate of Surgery of Great Britain and Ireland; 1998.
10. Royal College of Anaesthetists. Guidance on the provision of paediatric anaesthetic services. London: Royal College of Anaesthetists Bulletin; 2001; 8: 355–359.
11. Royal College of Surgeons of England. Surgical services for the newborn. London: British Association of Paediatric Surgeons/ The Royal College of Surgeons of England; 1999.
12. Nicholls G, Upadhyaya V, Gornall P, et al. Is specialist centre delivery of gastroschisis beneficial? Arch Dis Child 1993; 69:71–73.
13. Stoodley N, Sharma A, Noblett H, et al. Influence of place of delivery on outcome in babies with gastroschisis. Arch Dis Child 1993; 68:321–323.
14. Shaw KS, Filiatrault D, Yazbeck S, et al. Improved survival for congenital diaphragmatic hernia, based on prenatal ultrasound diagnosis and referral to a combined obstetric–pediatric surgical center. J Paediatr Surg 1994; 29:1268–1269.
15. UK collaborative randomised trial of neonatal extracorporeal membrane oxygenation. Lancet 1996; 348:75–82.
16. Cohen M. Pediatric anesthesia morbidity and mortality in the perioperative period. Anesth Analg 1990; 70:160–167.
17. Hughes DG, Mather SJ, Wolf AR. Handbook of neonatal anaesthesia. London: WB Saunders; 1996.
18. Hatch D, Sumner E, Hellman J. The surgical neonate: anaesthesia and intensive care. London: Edward Arnold; 1995.
19. Arul GS, Spicer RD. Where should paediatric surgery be performed? Arch Dis Child 1998; 79: 65–72.
20. Morray JP, Geiduschek JM, Caplan RA, et al. A comparison of pediatric and adult anaesthesia closed malpractice claims. Anaesthesiology 1993; 78:461–467.
21. Van der Walt JH, Sweeney DB, Runciman WB, et al. Paediatric incidents in anaesthesia: an analysis of 2000 incident reports. Anaesth Intens Care 1993; 21:655–658.
22. Keenan RL, Shapiro JH, Dawson MS. Frequency of cardiac arrests in infants: effect of pediatric anaesthesiologists. J Clin Anesth 1991; 3: 433–437.
23. Holzman RS. Morbidity and mortality in pediatric anesthesia. Pediatric Clin North Am 1994; 41:239–256.
24. Stoddart PA, Brennan L, Hatch DJ, et al. Postal survey of paediatric practice and training among consultant anaesthetists in the UK. Br J Anaesth 1994; 73:559–563.
25. Digivote (Association of Anaesthetists, proceedings of the Linkman conference), Bournemouth, September 1996.
26. Extremes of Age. The report of the National Confidential Enquiry into Perioperative Deaths (1997–98). London: NCEPOD; 1999.
27. Berry FA. The winds of change. Paediatr Anaesth 1995; 5:279–280.
28. Cote C. Who should be doing paediatric anaesthesia? Proc PGA 1997; A79:51.
29. Tikkanen J, Hovi-Viander M. Death associated with anaesthesia and surgery in Finland in 1986 compared to 1975. Acta Anesth Scand 1995; 39:262–267.
30. Walker RWM, Darowski M, Morris P, et al. Anaesthesia and mucopolysaccharidoses. Anaesthesia 1994; 49:1078–1084.
31. Field D, Hodges S, Mason E, et al. Survival and place of treatment after premature delivery. Arch Dis Child 1990; 66:408–411.
32. Jenkins KJ, Newburger JW, Lock JE, et al. In hospital mortality for surgical repair of congenital defects: preliminary observations of variation by hospital caseload. Pediatrics 1995; 95:323–330.
33. Stiller CA. Centralisation of treatment and survival rates for cancer. Arch Dis Child 1988;63:23–30.
34. Pearson G, Shann F, Barry P. Should paediatric intensive care be centralised? Trent vs. Victoria. Lancet 1997; 349:1213–1217.
35. Nicholl J, Willatts S. Paediatric intensive care – the way ahead? Anaesthesia 1998; 53:1141–1143.
36. Hall JR, Reyes HM, Meller JL, et al. The outcome for children with blunt trauma is best at a paediatric trauma centre. J Pediatr Surg 1996; 31:72–77.
37. Lunn JN. Implications of the National Confidential Enquiry into Perioperative Deaths for paediatric anaesthesia. Paediatr Anaesth 1992; 2:69–72.
38. Jahangeri M, Osborne MJ, Jayatunga AP, et al. Infantile pyloric stenosis: where should it be treated? Ann R Coll Surg 1993; 75:34–37.
39. Brain AJL, Roberts AS. Who should treat pyloric stenosis: the general or specialist paediatric surgeon? J Pediatr Surg 1996; 11:1535–1537.

40. Hulka F, Harrison MW, Campbell TJ. Complications of pyloromyotomy for infantile hypertrophic pyloric stenosis. Am J Surg 1997; 173:450–452.
41. Metkus AP, Esserman L, Soal A, et al. Cost per anomoly: what does a diaphragmatic hernia cost? J Pediatr Surg 1995; 30:226–230.
42. Hospital volume and health care outcomes, costs and patient access. Effective Health Care 1996; 2: number 8. Nuffield Institute for Health, University of Leeds and NHS centre for Reviews and Dissemination, University of York. London: Churchill Livingstone; 1996.
43. Haines L, Pollock J, Scrivener R. Report on a prospective study of intensive care utilisation in the north west region. London: Royal College of Paediatrics and Child Health Research Unit; 1996.
44. Downey GB, O'Connell AJ. Audit of unbooked paediatric post anaesthesia admissions to intensive care. Anaesth Intens Care 1996; 24:464–471.
45. Department of Health and Social Security. Welfare of children and young people in hospital. London: HMSO; 1991.
46. Action for Sick Children. Setting standards for children undergoing surgery. London: Action for Sick Children; 1994.
47. British Association of Paediatric Surgeons. Paediatric surgery: a standard of care. Final draft. London: Royal College of Surgeons of England; 2001. Professor D Lloyd, personal communication
48. Jones P. The general surgeon who cares for children. Br Med J 1986; ii: 1156–1158.
49. Wilkinson K, Crowle P. Where should paediatric surgery be performed (letter)? Arch Dis Child 1999; 80: 300.
50. Guidance for trainers. London: Royal College of Anaesthetists, issue 5; 2001.
51 Rollin AM. Paediatric anaesthesia – who should do it? The view from the district general hospital. Anaesthesia 1997; 52:513–516.
52. Report of a working party. Future configuration of paediatric services. London: British Paediatric Association; 1996.
53. NHS Executive. Paediatric intensive care. A framework for the future. UK: National co-ordinating group on Paediatric Intensive Care/NHS Executive; 1997.
54. The treatment of persistent glue ear in children. Effective Health Care 1992; 1 (4).
55. Lous J, Burton MJ, Felding JU et al. Grommets (ventilation tubes) for hearing loss associated with otitis media with effusion in children. In: The Cochrane Library, issue 2, 2002, Oxford.

CHAPTER 3

The critically ill child

Pauline M Cullen, Bruce L Taylor, Neil S Morton

INTRODUCTION

It is estimated that approximately 12 000 children per year will require admission to intensive care in the UK. Recommendations for the reorganisation of paediatric intensive care in England and Wales and for Scotland were published in 1996 and 1999.[1, 2] The core principle of these recommendations is that critically ill children should have access to the highest standards of intensive care irrespective of where they present.

The current evidence suggests that the sickest subgroup of critically ill children are less likely to die if treated in a paediatric intensive care unit (PICU) in a tertiary centre.[3] This has led to a centralisation of paediatric intensive care services and more children requiring to be moved to specialist units. About half of all children requiring intensive care will present initially to their district general hospital (DGH) so staff should be able to recognise, resuscitate and stabilise the critically ill child. The limits of provision in a given district setting must be recognised and agreed locally and regionally in accordance wherever possible with national guidelines and standards.

In the new structure of paediatric intensive care each geographical area should have a lead centre PICU to which DGHs will refer critically ill children according to clinical condition and locally agreed protocols. Some areas may also have designated major acute general hospitals (MAGHs), which will continue to provide some components of a locally agreed Paediatric Intensive Care service. Although these changes will lead to an increased number of retrievals, this does not diminish the key role that DGHs and MAGHs have in the initial (and often most hazardous) phase of the care of critically ill children. It is therefore crucial that the necessary staffing, skills and equipment are maintained or developed in these hospitals.

There is growing concern, however, that greater centralisation will lead to disinvestment in smaller hospitals, and that the skills and confidence of key staff will diminish over time. This deskilling may have been overemphasised, since children who will continue to be admitted to DGHs will require resuscitation and many aspects of paediatric intensive care. However, if general ICUs are discouraged from admitting and treating sick children, then loss of confidence and demotivation may become real issues. In time it may prove difficult to recruit staff with PIC skills to work in such hospitals, and in the longer term this may affect the quality of care that can be provided during the important phases of resuscitation and stabilisation.

Early recognition of the critically ill child, prompt resuscitation and thorough stabilisation of those who require transfer will improve the outcome provided they are accompanied by appropriately experienced personnel using suitable equipment.

DEFINITIONS OF LEVELS OF CARE

The classification of paediatric intensive care into levels (Box 3.1) is useful but the condition of a sick child may move very rapidly from one level to another. It is therefore important that good communication exists between DGH/MAGH and lead-centre clinicians, and that referral/transfer policies are established which build on existing facilities and expertise, while ensuring that all critically ill children receive the highest standards of care. The description of the level of care required by the paediatric patient takes account of nursing dependency, clinical context and number and nature of interventions.

EARLY RECOGNITION OF THE CRITICALLY ILL CHILD[4]

Impending cardiopulmonary arrest may be averted by early recognition and prompt intervention. Cardiac arrest in infants and children is rarely a sudden event. It is usually preceded by progressive deterioration in respiratory and circulatory function. It is vital to recognise the early signs of respiratory, circulatory and neurological failure. Once cardiac arrest occurs, the outcome in children is poor, with survival rates of 9–15%.[5-7] Often the child will be resuscitated, only to die of multiorgan failure in the intensive care unit. In addition, severe neurological sequelae occur in 30% of survivors. Efforts to improve outcome are best directed to the early recognition and prevention of cardiac arrests (Fig. 3.1).

Impending respiratory failure

Respiratory failure is the commonest underlying cause of cardiac arrest in children. It may result from upper or lower airway disease such as croup, tracheitis, epiglottitis,

Box 3.1 Classification of paediatric intensive care levels

Level 1: High-dependency care with nurse:patient ratio of 0.5:1
- A child who needs close monitoring and observation but not acute mechanical ventilatory support
- A child requiring long-term ventilatory support via a tracheostomy

Level 2: Intensive care with nurse:patient ratio of 1:1
- A child who needs continuous nursing supervision
- A child who is intubated and receiving ventilatory support, including continuous positive airways pressure
- A child who has recently been extubated
- An unstable level 1 case
- A level 1 case who is being nursed in a cubicle

Level 3: Intensive care with nurse:patient ratio of 1.5:1
- A level 2 case requiring multiple or complex interventions
- A level 2 case with multiple organ failure
- A level 2 case who is being nursed in a cubicle

Level 4: Intensive care with nurse:patient ratio of 2:1
- An unstable level 3 case
- A level 3 case who is being nursed in a cubicle
- A child on extracorporeal membrane oxygenation or ventricular assist device support
- A level 2 child receiving renal replacement therapy

Most level 2 care and all level 3 and 4 care should be provided in regional paediatric intensive care units but some level 1 and 2 care will be provided in district hospitals

bronchiolitis, asthma, pneumonia and foreign-body aspiration, or by prolonged convulsions, raised intracranial pressure, neuromuscular disease and drug overdose. Assessment of the work of breathing, respiratory rate and pattern, the presence of stridor or wheeze, the breath sounds and the colour of the skin and mucosae will identify the most important signs of impending respiratory failure (Box 3.2). Tachypnoea, recession, use of accessory muscles, grunting and tachycardia are all signs of increased work of breathing. Inspiratory stridor is a sign of upper-airway obstruction whilst wheezing denotes lower-airway disease. The onset of fatigue, or coincident neurological impairment, may diminish these important signs and produce a false impression of well-being. Hypoxic babies are generally unresponsive and floppy whilst hypoxic children may be agitated and/or drowsy. Pulse oximetry, capnography and capillary or arterial blood gases are useful.

Impending circulatory failure

The second principal cause of cardiac arrest in children is circulatory failure due to fluid loss or maldistribution. Circulatory failure (shock) is characterised by inadequate perfusion of organs and tissues. Clinical signs may vary depending on the underlying cause. Shock in children may result from:

- hypovolaemia caused by bleeding, trauma, burns and increased gastrointestinal losses;
- sepsis;
- cardiac disease, either congenital or acquired;
- a variety of medical conditions, including neurological disease and diabetic ketoacidosis.

Shock is traditionally classified as hypovolaemic, distributive, cardiogenic, obstructive or dissociative (Box 3.3).

Hypovolaemic shock is the commonest cause of shock in children, with sepsis second. Untreated shock is progressive and is divided into early (compensated shock), late

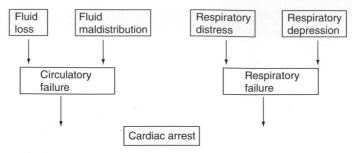

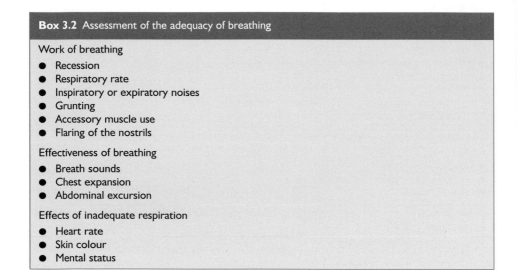

Fig. 3.1 Pathways leading to cardiac arrest in children.

Box 3.2 Assessment of the adequacy of breathing

Work of breathing

● Recession
● Respiratory rate
● Inspiratory or expiratory noises
● Grunting
● Accessory muscle use
● Flaring of the nostrils

Effectiveness of breathing

● Breath sounds
● Chest expansion
● Abdominal excursion

Effects of inadequate respiration

● Heart rate
● Skin colour
● Mental status

(uncompensated shock) and irreversible (fatal shock) according to severity. The journey from late shock to cardiac arrest can be brief. Even those children who do not progress to cardiac arrest may have dismal outcomes if advanced stages of shock persist without treatment. Most children have excellent compensatory mechanisms for hypovolaemia, making early recognition more difficult than in adults. Up to 50% of blood volume may be lost before a significant fall in blood pressure occurs.[8] The progression of shock to cardiopulmonary arrest can usually be prevented if the early signs of impending circulatory failure are recognised and appropriate therapy started (Box 3.4).

A raised heart rate is a common response to many types of stress, including fever, anxiety, pain or hypovolaemia. In shock, tachycardia is caused by catecholamine release, and is an attempt to maintain cardiac output by increasing heart rate in the face of a falling stroke volume. A heart rate of 180 beats min^{-1} is abnormal in all but neonates, and rates over 140 beats min^{-1} are abnormal in those aged 2–4 years. After 12 years, adult norms may be applied. Bradycardia in a shocked child is caused by *hypoxia* and acidosis and is a preterminal sign. The child's cardiovascular system compensates well in shock and blood pressure is initially maintained near normal. Hypotension is a late and often sudden sign of decompensation and if not reversed will rapidly be followed by cardiac arrest. Other early indications of shock include signs of vasoconstriction (pallor, cool extremities and

---

Box 3.3 Types and causes of shock

Hypovolaemic
- Haemorrhage
- Diarrhoea
- Vomiting
- Burns
- Peritonitis

Distributive
- Septicaemia
- Anaphylaxis
- Spinal cord injury

Cardiogenic
- Arrhythmias
- Cardiomyopathy
- Heart failure
- Valvular disease
- Myocardial contusion
- Myocardial infarction

Obstructive
- Tension pneumothorax
- Haemopneumothorax
- Flail chest
- Cardiac tamponade
- Pulmonary embolism
- Hypertension

Dissociative
- Profound anaemia
- Carbon monoxide poisoning
- Methaemoglobinaemia

Box 3.4 Rapid assessment of the adequacy of the circulation

Cardiovascular status
- Heart rate
- Pulse volume
- Capillary refill
- Blood pressure

Effects on other organs
- Respiratory rate and character
- Skin appearance and temperature
- Mental status
- Urinary output

---

weak thready distal pulses). In early septic shock there may be an initial high output state resulting in a warm periphery and bounding peripheral pulses. Slow capillary refill (> 2 s) is evidence of reduced skin perfusion. The extremity should be elevated slightly above the level of the heart when testing for capillary refill. Mottling, pallor, peripheral cyanosis and a core/peripheral temperature gradient of more than 2°C are signs of poor skin perfusion. All these signs may be difficult to interpret in children who have just been exposed to a cold environment. Urine flow is reduced or absent in shock. The volume of urine in the bladder is of little value in the immediate assessment of shock, but ongoing measurement of urine production provides an important insight into vital organ perfusion during resuscitation. A minimum flow of 1 ml kg^{-1} h^{-1} in children and 2 ml kg^{-1} h^{-1} in infants indicates adequate renal perfusion. Respiratory signs of early shock can be subtle. The acidosis produced by the poor tissue perfusion results in rapid deep breathing. Irregular respirations signal advanced shock.

Impending neurological failure

Mental status forms the other sign of early shock that is often overlooked. Early signs of brain hypoperfusion are agitation and confusion or even combativeness, often alternating with drowsiness. Infants may be irritable but drowsy with a weak cry and hypotonia. An early sign of reduced cerebral perfusion in the infant is failure to focus on the parent's face. As shock progresses the child becomes progressively more drowsy until consciousness is lost. Neurological status is determined by conscious level, posture and pupillary signs.

Conscious level assessment is kept simple and is based on the AVPU scale (Box 3.5).

A paediatric adaptation (Table 3.1^{8a}) of the Glasgow Coma Scale (GCS) (Table 3.2) may be more appropriate in cases of trauma.

PRIMARY ASSESSMENT AND RESUSCITATION

Resuscitation of the critically ill child requires a rapid and systematic response. A team approach works best. A rapid assessment of the airway, breathing, circulation and neurological status should be performed to identify life-threatening problems (Box 3.6).

The priorities of resuscitation are to secure the airway and provide adequate oxygenation and ventilation followed by vascular access and drug and fluid administration.

Airway

If trauma is suspected, the cervical spine must be completely immobilised. Children can have significant spinal cord injury without radiographic abnormality with devastating consequences if ignored. The patency of the airway should be assessed by the 'looking, listening and feeling' method. Relaxation of the muscles and passive displacement of the tongue posteriorly may obstruct the airway in the unconscious child. This is relieved by a head-tilt chin-lift manoeuvre or by the jaw thrust. If a cervical spine injury is suspected, head tilt is contraindicated and jaw thrust should be used. Other causes of airway obstruction include vomit, a foreign body or upper respiratory infections (for example, epiglottitis, bacterial tracheitis or croup). If airway obstruction is not relieved by positioning, the use of airway adjuncts and suctioning intubation will be required.

Foreign-body aspiration

The vast majority of deaths from foreign-body aspiration occur in preschool children. The diagnosis should be suspected if the onset of respiratory distress was sudden and associated

Box 3.5 Assessment of conscious level

- A Alert
- V Responds to voice
- P Responds to pain
- U Unresponsive

Table 3.1 Paediatric Coma Scale (age < 4 years)[8a]

Response	Score
EYES	
Open spontaneously	4
React to speech	3
React to pain	2
No response	1
BEST MOTOR RESPONSE	
Spontaneous or obeys verbal command	6
Localises pain	5
Withdraws with pain	4
Abnormal flexion to pain	3 (decorticate posture)
Abnormal extension to pain	2 (decerebrate posture)
No response	1
BEST VERBAL RESPONSE	
Smiles, oriented to sounds	6
Follows objects, interacts	5
Consolable, inappropriate	4
Inconsistently consolable, moaning	3
Inconsolable, irritable	2
No response	1

Table 3.2 Glasgow Coma Scale (age 4+ years)

Response	Score
EYES	
Open spontaneously	4
Verbal command	3
Pain	2
No response	1
BEST MOTOR RESPONSE	
Obeys verbal command	6
Localises pain	5
Flexion with pain	4
Flexion abnormal	3
Extension	2
No response	1
BEST VERBAL RESPONSE	
Oriented and converses	5
Disoriented and converses	4
Inappropriate words	3
Incomprehensible sounds	2
No response	1

with coughing, gagging and stridor.[9] Alternatively, the diagnosis may be suggested by an inability to deliver rescue breaths in an apnoeic child despite airway-opening manoeuvres. In the infant the larynx is conical; the narrowest part is at the level of the cricoid cartilage,

---

Box 3.6 Rapid clinical assessment

Airway and breathing
- Work of breathing
- Respiratory rate and pattern
- Stridor/wheeze
- Auscultation
- Skin colour

Circulation
- Heart rate
- Pulse volume
- Capillary refill
- Skin temperature
- Disability

Mental status
- Conscious level
- Posture
- Pupils

---

hence foreign bodies tend to impact at this level. In the older child the larynx is cylindrical; the narrowest part is the laryngeal inlet above the vocal cords, hence foreign bodies tend to lodge at this level or pass into the lower airways. If foreign-body aspiration is witnessed the child should be encouraged to cough as long as the cough remains forceful. Relief of obstruction should only be attempted when there are signs of complete upper-airway obstruction. Blind finger sweeps are not recommended as they may simply impact the foreign body deeper into the airway.

In infants there are two techniques recommended for dislodging foreign bodies. The infant is supported in the prone position straddling the rescuer's forearm, with the head lower than the trunk. Five sharp blows can then be given between the shoulder blades. If these fail to dislodge the foreign body, the child is turned supine, five chest thrusts are given, using the same landmarks as for chest compressions. In older children the back blows are followed by alternate cycles of chest thrusts and abdominal thrusts. If the child is conscious the Heimlich manoeuvre can also be used. Abdominal thrusts are not recommended in infants less than 1 year of age as damage to the abdominal contents may occur. After each cycle the mouth should be inspected and ventilation attempted. If the obstruction persists then an artificial airway will need to be established.

Breathing

A patent airway does not ensure adequate ventilation. High-flow oxygen should be given to all children with respiratory difficulty or hypoxia. In the non-intubated patient the high-flow oxygen should be delivered via a non-rebreathing mask with a reservoir bag. A pulse oximeter should be attached to the child and oxygen saturation monitored. If the child is not breathing adequately then ventilation should be commenced. Initially bag-mask ventilation should be performed. The assisted breaths should be slow and controlled, to avoid high peak airway pressures which will encourage gastric insufflation. A distended stomach both inhibits ventilation and increases the risk of regurgitation. Optimum tidal volumes are about 10–15 ml kg^{-1}, but adequacy of ventilation is more simply determined by observing chest movement. The ideal ventilation rate will depend on the age of the child, but 20 breaths min^{-1} will suffice for all age groups during the initial resuscitation. Generally speaking, a child who requires bag-mask ventilation will subsequently require intubation and positive-pressure ventilation. Once intubation has been achieved, the tube should be fixed carefully in place to prevent accidental removal or displacement. An orogastric or nasogastric tube should be inserted to prevent gastric dilatation. The laryngeal mask airway has been used successfully in adult resuscitation but its effectiveness in paediatric resuscitation has yet to be established.

Circulation

The circulatory status is assessed by palpation of a major pulse for 10 s. In infants the brachial pulse is preferred whilst in children the carotid or femoral pulse can be easily located. If the pulse is absent or slow, chest compressions should be started. In infants compression should be applied one finger's breath below an imaginary line between the nipples at a rate of 100 compressions per minute and a depth of one-third the depth of the chest.[10, 11] Two fingers may be used as direct pressure, or the hands can be placed around the chest, and the thumbs used to compress the sternum.[12, 13] The latter method is associated with a better cardiac output and blood pressure and is therefore the preferred technique.[14] When using this technique, care must be taken to allow the chest to reexpand fully during the decompression phase of the cardiopulmonary resuscitation (CPR) cycle. In older children compression is applied over the lower third of the sternum using the heel of the hand at a rate of 100 compressions per minute. Give one ventilation for every five compressions. Vital organ blood flow is severely reduced during CPR.[15, 16] A number of mechanical methods aimed at improving blood flow to vital organs during CPR have been investigated in adults. These include: (1) simultaneous compression–ventilation (SCV-CPR); (2) interposed abdominal compression (IAC-CPR); (3) active compression–decompression (ACD-CPR); and (4) vest CPR. As yet there are no data available on their use in peadiatric resuscitation and the results of ongoing trials are awaited. Extracorporeal membrane oxygenation (ECMO) has been used successfully to resuscitate children after open-heart surgery.[17] This technique requires sophisticated resources and technical skills, limiting its broader application.

Vascular access

Rapid access to the circulation is obviously vital for fluid and drug administration during paediatric resuscitation. In small children this may be extremely difficult because of the intense peripheral vasoconstriction.[18] Central venous drug administration is preferred since higher peak levels of drug are delivered more rapidly to the central circulation.[19, 20] In practice, the largest visible vein is used. Attempts at peripheral venous access should be limited to 90 s. Useful routes during resuscitation include the femoral vein and the external jugular vein, which is often distended during a cardiac arrest. The internal jugular, subclavian and intracardiac routes mean interruption of cardiac massage and are prone to serious complications in young children.

When venous access is not possible, the intraosseous route is safe, rapid and effective.[20–22] Drugs and fluids can be given by this route and gain rapid access to the central circulation. Fluid given by this route is best given as repeated boluses using a syringe attached to a length of extension tubing. Likewise, drugs require to be followed by a bolus of fluid to facilitate rapid delivery to the central circulation.

The intraosseous route is not just for patients in cardiac arrest. It should be considered whenever a life-threatening illness requires immediate drug or fluid therapy. The most popular site for intraosseous needle insertion is the proximal tibia; other possible sites include the distal tibia and distal femur. When establishing intraossseous access it is important to recognise the criteria for successful entry into the bone marrow. There should be loss of resistance as the marrow cavity is entered, the needle should remain upright without support, bone marrow should be aspirated and it should be easy to inject drugs and fluids without any subcutaneous infiltration. Complications include osteomyelitis, long bone fractures, extravasation of drugs and compartment syndrome.[23–27] These have been reported in fewer than 1% of cases; most can be avoided by careful insertion techniques.[28] Concern was raised that intraosseous administration would lead to fat embolism and alterations in gas exchange,[29] but more recent data show that pulmonary fat emboli occur as a result of CPR.[30]

Lipophilic agents, such as adrenaline (epinephrine), atropine, lidocaine (lignocaine) and naloxone may be given by the endotracheal route. Direct endotracheal instillation of adrenaline (epinephrine) followed by 5 ml of saline effectively distributes the drug into the lower airways.[31] The pharmacokinetics of drugs administered via the endotracheal routes are very variable. Animal studies suggest that peak blood levels are only 1/10 of those achieved following intravenous administration.[32–34] Hence a 10-fold increase in adrenaline (epinephrine) dosage is recommended for this route. This may produce profound hypertension in the postresuscitation phase due to the slow absorption of adrenaline (epinephrine) from the lung. This hypertension may be harmful to cerebral recovery,[35] and excessive afterload may further compromise cardiac function following arrest-induced myocardial ischaemia. We should therefore not rely solely on this route but continue to seek more reliable access during resuscitation.

DRUGS USED IN RESUSCITATION
Adrenaline (epinephrine)

Administration of adrenaline (epinephrine) plays a pivotal role in the advanced life support algorithms of paediatric resuscitation. Adrenaline (epinephrine) is indicated in all cardiac arrest settings (i.e. asystole, pulseless electrical activity and ventricular fibrillation). The importance of adrenaline (epinephrine) in raising peripheral vascular tone and thereby diverting blood flow to vital organs during CPR is universally accepted. However, adrenaline (epinephrine) can greatly increase myocardial oxygen demand, increase afterload and precipate ventricular dysrhythmias. For these reasons the use of high-dose adrenaline (epinephrine) remains controversial. In animal studies, high-dose adrenaline (epinephrine) has been shown to increase cerebral and myocardial blood flow and increase the rate of return of spontaneous circulation.[36, 37] Three large multicentre studies in adults, however, found no beneficial effect of high-dose adrenaline (epinephrine) over standard doses.[38–40] Similarly, no benefit of high-dose adrenaline (epinephrine) was found in out-of-hospital or in-hospital resuscitation in children.[41, 42] To achieve a balance between the potential benefit of more rapidly restarting the heart against the potential toxicity of high-dose adrenaline (epinephrine), the current recommendations have been devised. The initial dose is 0.01 mg kg^{-1} of adrenaline (epinephrine). If this dose is not effective in 3–5 min, a dose of 0.1 mg kg^{-1} should be used. As the action of adrenaline (epinephrine) is short-lived, this dose should be repeated every 3–5 min until the return of spontaneous cardiac activity.

Bicarbonate: acidosis in cardiac arrest

A combination of low blood flow and poor ventilation leads to a mixed respiratory and metabolic acidosis during cardiac arrest. Severe acidosis blunts the responsiveness of the cardiovascular system to catecholamines, depresses myocardial contractility, increases pulmonary vascular resistance and dilates systemic vascular beds.[43–46] Intubation and ventilation correct hypoxaemia, but tissue blood flow remains severely compromised during cardiac massage. During CPR, poor tissue blood flow results in substantial gradients of pH and carbon dioxide concentrations between arterial and venous blood.[47] This is the result of impaired CO_2 elimination from the tissues in the low-flow circulation.

The key to improving the acidosis is to restore tissue perfusion by restoring cardiac activity and supporting circulatory function. The role of buffers such as sodium bicarbonate remain unclear. Bicarbonate administration is unlikely to improve the situation as hydrogen ions are buffered in a reaction that results in the production of carbon dioxide to the tissues:

$$NaHCO_3 + H \rightarrow Na + H_2CO_3 \rightarrow H_2O + CO_2$$

Administration of bicarbonate during cardiac arrest may worsen intracellular acidosis, adversely affecting cellular function.[48, 49] For these reasons and the lack of data showing it has a beneficial effect, the early use of bicarbonate is not currently recommended in cardiac arrest.[50] In the post-resuscitation phase, the administration of bicarbonate appears to correct metabolic acidosis without adverse effects.[51]

Calcium

In the normal heart calcium increases myocardial contractile function. In the ischaemic heart energy sources are depleted and calcium accumulates in the cytoplasm, causing toxic effects. Studies have shown that calcium entry into the cell cytoplasm is the final common pathway in cell death, and calcium administration during cardiac arrest may actually cause injury.[52] Calcium administration causes coronary spasm and may produce cardiac arrest in systole unresponsive to further drug therapy. Administration of calcium may also cause spasm of the coronary vessels and so increase post-arrest neurological deficit. Recent data suggest that calcium may antagonise the action of adrenaline (epinephrine) and other adrenergic agents and raise blood pressure by producing systemic vasoconstriction rather than by a positive inotropic effect.[53] There is currently no evidence to support the use of calcium in asystole and its use in electromechanical dissociation is challenged.[54, 55]

Ionised hypocalcaemia is relatively common in paediatric intensive care patients. One large study demonstrated significant hypocalcaemia in 18% of paediatric intensive care patients.[56, 57] Hypocalcaemia also occurs when cardiac arrest is secondary to septic shock or following massive blood transfusion. For these reasons, calcium is only indicated to correct documented ionised hypocalcaemia, to antagonise the adverse cardiovascular effects of hyperkalaemia and hypermagnesaemia and to reverse the toxic effects of calcium-channel blockers.

TREATMENT SUMMARY[58, 59] (Figs 3.2 and 3.3)

Profound bradycardia or asystole is the most common rhythm associated with cardiac arrest in children. Profound bradycardia may precede asystole and should be treated similarly. Treatment is an initial dose of adrenaline (epinephrine) 0.01 mg kg^{-1}. If there is no response, a dose 10 times the original dose should be given (0.1 mg kg^{-1}). This dose should be repeated every 3–5 min during the arrest. Treatable causes of cardiac arrest should be sought, e.g.. hypoxia, hypovolaemia, tension pneumothorax, cardiac tamponade, drug overdose, hypothermia and electrolyte imbalance. Resuscitation attempts should not be abandoned until a reasonable attempt has been made to correct potentially reversible causes of cardiac arrest.

Ventricular fibrillation and tachycardia, although common in adults, are relatively uncommon in children. The reported incidence of ventricular fibrillation in children is 0–10%.[60, 61] The recommended sequence is to give two rapid defibrillatory shocks of 2 J kg^{-1}, followed by a single shock of 4 J kg^{-1}. All further shocks should be 4 J kg^{-1} and repeated three times in rapid succession. After the first cycle of three shocks, adrenaline (epinephrine) 0.01 mg kg^{-1} should be given and a dose of 0.1 mg kg^{-1} after the second cycle of three shocks and between all subsequent cycles. This sequence of adrenaline (epinephrine) followed by three shocks and 1 min of CPR is continued until either the return of sinus rhythm or resuscitation is abandoned. When ventricular fibrillation occurs in children there is often an underlying cause and treatment of hypothermia, drug overdose and electrolyte imbalance should be attempted.[58, 59, 62]

Arrhythmia management

Supraventricular tachycardia is the most common arrhythmia seen in children. If the child is in shock, the treatment of choice is synchronised cardioversion 0.5–2 J kg^{-1}. Intravenous adenosine is rather like giving a 'medical shock' and is used in some centres in preference

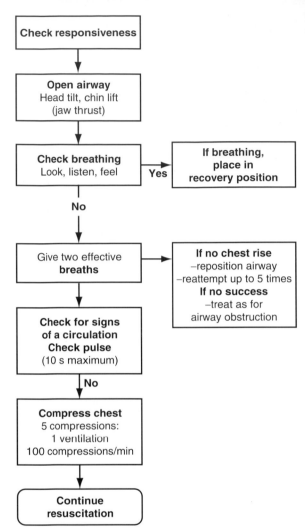

Fig. 3.2 Algorithm for basic paediatric life support.[58]

Check responsiveness

Open airway
Head tilt, chin lift
(jaw thrust)

Check breathing
Look, listen, feel — **Yes** → If breathing, place in recovery position

No

Give two effective breaths → If no chest rise
−reposition airway
−reattempt up to 5 times
If no success
−treat as for
airway obstruction

Check for signs
of a circulation
Check pulse
(10 s maximum)

No

Compress chest
5 compressions:
1 ventilation
100 compressions/min

Continue
resuscitation

to cardioversion as first-line treatment. The dose of adenosine is 50 μg kg^{-1}, increasing over three doses to 500 μg kg^{-1}. The half-life of the drug is about 6 s, so it needs to be injected as close to the heart as possible or followed by a bolus of fluid. Brief asystole is often seen, but sinus rhythm usually returns in seconds.

FLUID RESUSCITATION
Hypovolaemic shock

Expansion of the circulating blood volume is a critical component of paediatric resuscitation in children who have sustained trauma and acute blood loss.[63] It may also be life-saving in shock due to sepsis or other conditions causing fluid depletion (diabetic ketoacidosis, gastroenteritis, burns). Early restitution of circulating blood volume is important to prevent progression to overt circulatory failure and cardiac arrest.

Crystalloid or colloid fluids are available for volume resuscitation. When using crystalloids, only those fluids at least isotonic to serum have a role in shock. The use of paediatric maintenance fluids (e.g. 5% dextrose 0.225% saline) should never be used for bolus resuscitation. The

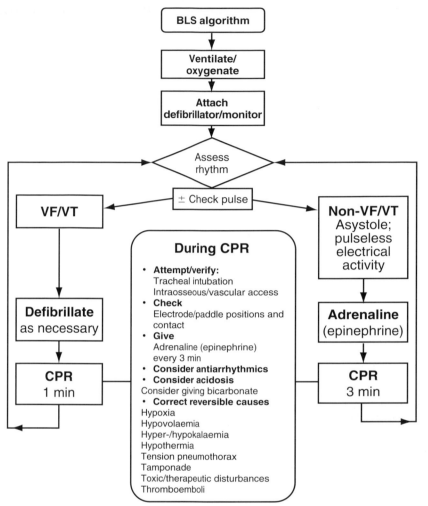

Fig. 3.3 Algorithm for advanced paediatric life support. BLS, basic life support; VF, ventricular fibrillation; VT, ventricular tachycardia; CPR, cardiopulmonary resuscitation.[59]

use of diluted fluids is not only ineffective but may reduce serum sodium concentration abruptly. Commonly used fluids include lactated Ringer's solution, 0.9% normal saline or 5% albumin. Lactated Ringer's is the crystalloid fluid of choice in shock.[64] An initial fluid bolus of 20 ml kg^{-1} is given as rapidly as possible. The circulatory status is then reassessed and, if there is no improvement in vital signs, a second bolus of 20 ml kg^{-1} is given. The most common mistake in the treatment of hypovolaemia in shocked children is failure to give enough fluid. There has been much debate about the fluid of choice for initial resuscitation. Proponents of colloid suggest that it is more likely to stay within the intravascular space. Opponents argue that colloid infusions will result in increased pulmonary and cerebral oedema, as the colloid leaks into injured tissues.[65] In a recent paper, the Cochrane Injuries Group Albumin reviewers concluded from their meta-analysis of 30 studies using albumin that its administration to critically ill patients might be responsible for an increased mortality.[66] The results of this study were severely criticised because of the study design and it is not generally felt that the weight of evidence is adequate to justify acute changes in practice as yet. Compared with other colloidal solutions and with crystalloid solutions, human albumin solutions are expensive. Volume for volume, human albumin solution is twice as expensive as hydroxyethyl starch and over 30 times more expensive than crystalloid solutions such as sodium chloride or Ringer's lactate.

When crystalloids are used the volume required is two to four times that of colloid, as only 25% of the volume infused will remain in the intravascular compartment. The remainder will fill the extracellular and interstitial compartments.[67, 68] Theoretically, this would lead to increased tissue oedema. There is disagreement as to whether the oedema is detrimental to tissue oxygenation or not. The main advantages of using crystalloids for resuscitation are the availability and cost-effectiveness of these solutions. Clearly the decision to use a particular type of fluid to replace volume loss needs to take into account the cause of the hypovolaemia. Often, the use of both crystalloid and colloid is appropriate. In the trauma patient blood will be required after the second bolus of resuscitation fluid if signs of hypovolaemia persist.

The one contraindication to aggressive fluid therapy in shock is congestive heart failure. This diagnosis should be evident from a quick examination of the heart and lungs and either palpation of the liver margin or evaluation of the neck vein distension. The liver in the young child is easily distensible and thus an excellent gauge of venous congestion. An echocardiogram will confirm the diagnosis.

Discontinuing resuscitation

Currently there are no guidelines for discontinuing resuscitation. Due to the extremely poor prognosis of out-of-hospital cardiac arrests in children, prolonged efforts at resuscitation would seem inappropriate. It has been suggested that, except when treating children with extreme hypothermia (< 30°C), resuscitative efforts in the emergency department after out-of-hospital cardiac arrest should be limited to 20 min and two doses of adrenaline (epinephrine).[5]

POSTRESUSCITATION STABILISATION

Following resuscitation, normal cardiac output and tissue oxygen delivery must be restored as rapidly as possible. The child who has been successfully resuscitated from cardiac arrest is often poorly perfused, hypotensive and acidaemic. A common reason for persistent poor perfusion is cardiogenic shock resulting from arrest-associated myocardial ischaemia.[69, 70] Once stable return of spontaneous cardiac activity is achieved, children often require ongoing pharmacological support to maintain tissue perfusion.

The choice of inotropic drug will depend on the circulatory status and the underlying cause of the arrest. Adrenaline (epinephrine) is the drug of choice for myocardial dysfunction and shock in the postresuscitation period, especially if the child is hypotensive.[71] Dobutamine may be an effective agent in the normotensive, post-arrest patient who remains poorly perfused secondary to a low cardiac output state.[72, 73] In the hypotensive patient, dobutamine may further lower blood pressure by decreasing systemic vascular resistance.[73] In children with cardiogenic shock, dobutamine has been shown to increase cardiac output and reduce pulmonary wedge pressure, central venous pressure and pulmonary and systemic vascular resistances.[74, 75] Dopamine may be used in children with less severe shock and hypotension. The decision to use dopamine over dobutamine is often arbitrary and based on personal preference.

In all poorly perfused or hypotensive patients further fluid resuscitation may be beneficial. The fluid should be administered slowly with careful observation for fluid overload. Overenthusiastic fluid resuscitation may adversely affect cardiac function. Mechanical ventilation of the lungs is usually continued in the immediate postresuscitation period as a means of best ensuring optimal blood gases. Controlled ventilation will help ameliorate cerebral oedema and correct the mixed respiratory and metabolic acidosis resulting from the arrest.

Appropriate investigations include arterial blood gases, electrolytes, blood glucose, full blood count and clotting screen and blood cultures. In cases of haemorrhage, blood should be cross-matched. A chest X-ray should be performed to determine the correct positioning of the endotracheal tube and exclude complications. In trauma victims, X-rays of skull, cervical spine and pelvis should be requested and neurological monitoring commenced using the modified GCS. Post-resuscitation care consists of frequent assessments of cardiopulmonary function to monitor treatment progress. Treatment should be directed to correct ongoing hypovolaemia or hypotension, metabolic acidosis, electrolyte abnormalities and seizure activity.

Primary assessment and resuscitation are concerned with the maintenance of vital functions, while secondary assessment and emergency treatment allow more specific urgent therapies to be started. Once the initial resuscitative measures are completed, a full assessment of the patient should be performed. This should include a full medical history, a clinical examination and specific investigations to establish which emergency treatments might benefit the child. Time is limited and a focused approach is essential. The history and examination may provide useful information about the possible aetiology of the disease process, and aid definitive treatment. With the exception of a brief respiratory arrest following overenthusiastic analgesia, all children who have suffered a cardiorespiratory arrest should be transferred to a PICU. For some children this will involve transfer to a tertiary referral unit.

EARLY FEATURES OF SPECIFIC CONDITIONS AND THEIR MANAGEMENT

Septic shock

Early septic shock is characterised by raised cardiac output, decreased systemic vascular resistance, warm extremities and a wide pulse pressure. This hyperdynamic state is recognised by hyperpyrexia, hyperventilation, tachycardia and mental confusion. These signs can easily be overlooked. Alteration of conscious level is a very useful early sign of septic shock. Mild arterial desaturation may be present and arterial blood gases will show a metabolic acidosis with an attempt at respiratory compensation. As shock progresses, hypotension develops and signs of peripheral circulatory failure become evident. The clinical manifestations of late septic shock are indistinguishable from those of other forms of shock.[76, 77] The hypovolaemia is exacerbated by increased capillary permeability and arteriolar and venous dilation with peripheral pooling of blood. The key to successful intervention in sepsis is recognition before hypotension occurs. Survival in septic shock depends on maintenance of the hyperdynamic state.[78] Infants, who have poor cardiac reserves, often present with hypotension and a hypodynamic state. These infants can be a diagnostic challenge but sepsis must be assumed and treated aggressively. The main pathogens in septic shock are Gramnegative bacteria, but β-haemolytic streptococci, staphylococci and other Gram-positive bacteria are also important. *Neisseria meningitidis* and *Haemophilus influenzae* are the two most common bacterial cause of septic shock in previously well children.[79, 80] In meningococcal sepsis the Glasgow Meningococcal Prognostic Score (Table 3.3) may be useful to guide decision-making: a score of 8 or a rapidly deteriorating score despite resuscitation is an index of severity of illness and the need for rapid institution of full intensive care support.[81]

Table 3.3 Glasgow Meningococcal Prognostic Score[81]	
Criteria	**Score**
Systolic blood pressure < 75 mmHg if < 4 years; < 85 mmHg if > 4 years	3
Skin–rectal temperature gradient > 3°C	3
Glasgow Coma Score < 8 at any time or deterioration of 3 or more in 1 h	3
Extent of purpura: widespread/extending	1
Parental questioning: 'Has your child's condition become worse in the last hour?'	2
Base deficit (capillary) > 8	1
Absence of meningism	2
Total	**15**

The initial management should centre on the failure of cellular oxygenation. Oxygen delivery can be increased by increasing oxygenation, cardiac output or haemoglobin concentration. As high a concentration of oxygen as possible should be administered to any patient at risk of shock. Up to 80% of children with septic shock will require assisted ventilation to maintain adequate gas exchange. Intubation should be performed on the basis of clinical evidence of respiratory distress but also to facilitate treatment.

Virtually all children with sepsis and septic shock require immediate volume resuscitation.[82] This can be given in 20 ml kg^{-1} volume boluses to a total of 40–60 ml kg^{-1} in the first 10 min of presentation. Some children may require as much as 200 ml kg^{-1} in the first hour of treatment.[63] Despite aggressive volume resuscitation, most children with septic shock have cardiovascular dysfunction that requires the addition of inotropes. Children can have predominant cardiac failure, predominant vascular failure or a combination of both.[83–85] Although various inotropes and vasopressors can be titrated to desired effect, a more simplified approach during resuscitation is the use of adrenaline (epinephrine). A useful starting dose would be 0.05 μg kg^{-1} min^{-1} increasing up to 0.5 μg kg^{-1} min^{-1} in resistant cases. Other commonly used cardiovascular drugs include dopamine, dobutamine and noradrenaline (norepinephrine). The pharmacology of these agents is beyond the scope of this chapter.

Appropriate antibiotic therapy should be given according to the age of child. It is customary to give a third-generation cephalosporin such as cefotaxime until sensitivities are known. In neonates a combination of ampicillin and gentamicin or ampicillin and cefotaxime are used. Adequate ongoing treatment of septic shock depends on aggressive ventilatory management and complex invasive monitoring, including indwelling arterial, central venous and pulmonary artery catheters. This allows precise titration of fluids and inotropic and vasodilator drugs. Further management is primarily directed at preventing and ameliorating the development of multiple organ failure.

Diabetic ketoacidosis

Diabetic ketoacidosis is frequently the initial manifestation of diabetes mellitus in children. The condition is due to relative or absolute lack of insulin resulting in an inability to metabolise glucose. This leads to hyperglycaemia and glucosuria. When the amount of glucose in the urine exceeds the reabsorptive capacity of the proximal tubules, an osmotic diuresis ensues with loss of water and electrolytes, resulting in dehydration. Fat is utilised as a source of energy, resulting in the production of large quantities of ketones, leading to a metabolic acidosis. The latter is initially compensated for by hyperventilation.

Fever, vomiting and hyperventilation contribute to the dehydration. The serum sodium may be high in severe dehydration but may also be normal or low. Despite this, the child will have lost a great deal of sodium. Hypokalaemia may not be apparent in the acute presentation; however, total body potassium is low and will need to be corrected as treatment progresses. Children presenting with diabetic ketoacidosis are usually severely dehydrated. The hyperosmolar state may result in underestimation of the severity of the dehydration.

The initial therapeutic approach should be to assess the airway, breathing and circulation. A shocked patient should be given 100% oxygen and will require immediate and aggressive fluid resuscitation. A fluid bolus of 20 ml kg^{-1} of isotonic crystalloid (normal saline) or colloid should be given to reverse the signs of shock and repeated as necessary until haemodynamic stabilisation has been achieved. This is followed by a gradual correction of the remaining fluid and electrolyte deficit over 48 h. Maintenance fluids plus half the deficit should be given over the first 24 h and the remainder over a further 24 h. The initial fluid should not contain glucose, therefore normal saline is usually recommended until the blood sugar starts to fall, when the fluid should be changed to 0.45% saline in 5% dextrose. Potassium replacement should be started (20–40 mmol l^{-1}) once a urine output has been confirmed. The osmotic diuresis will persist until the blood sugar falls, therefore calculated fluid requirements will underestimate ongoing fluid losses unless the urine volume is taken into account.

Once shock has been treated and the serum potassium normalised, an insulin infusion should be started. The initial dose is 0.1 units kg^{-1} h^{-1}. This initial dose may need to be increased or decreased according to frequent blood sugar estimations. This initial dose is often reduced to 0.05 units kg^{-1} h^{-1} of insulin as soon as the blood sugar starts to fall. The insulin should be administered through a separate infusion. The acidosis of diabetic ketoacidosis is initially compensated for by hyperventilation. Fluid resuscitation with improved tissue perfusion and insulin therapy usually corrects the acidosis. Bicarbonate therapy is only indicated if the pH is < 7.0 following the initial resuscitation and not improving after the first few hours of fluid and insulin therapy.[86]

Rapid infusion of isotonic fluids has been implicated in the development of cerebral oedema in diabetic ketoacidosis.[87, 88] However, no correlation between fluid administration and the development of cerebral oedema was found in two studies[89, 90] and cerebral oedema has occurred in children who have not been given any fluid resuscitation.[91] Until we know the cause of cerebral oedema in diabetic ketoacidosis it is recommended that that we avoid rapid changes in serum sodium or osmolarity and rehydrate over 48 h. Early recognition of reduced conscious level should lead to measures to reduce intracranial hypertension, and transfer to a unit capable of performing intracranial pressure measurement.

Children who present with severe diabetic ketoacidosis will require frequent monitoring of cardiovascular variables, fluid balance, blood sugar, acid–base status, urea and electrolytes as well as hourly neurological observations during the first 48 h. This is most easily performed in a high-dependency or intensive care unit. Complications include cerebral oedema, renal failure, thrombosis and acute respiratory distress syndrome.

Trauma

Trauma continues to be the leading cause of death in children older than 1 year. The most common causes of childhood trauma are motor vehicle accidents, falls, bicycle accidents, drowning and burns. Poor resuscitation has been identified as a major cause of preventable death in paediatric trauma victims.[97] Mortality associated with paediatric trauma occurs at three distinct peaks: (1) upon impact; (2) within 2 h of the injury; and (3) from complications during the recovery period. Approximately 50% of all deaths occur at the time or within moments of impact.[98] These deaths are due to laceration of major intrathoracic or intra-abdominal vessels, high division of the cervical spine, rupture of cardiac chambers and severe head injury. The second mortality peak, which accounts for 30% of all trauma deaths, occurs within the first 1–2 h after impact. These deaths are often related to inadequate resuscitation and stabilisation and may be preventable. Causes include uncontrolled haemorrhage, airway obstruction, respiratory failure and intracranial bleeding. Triage and appropriate intervention have the greatest impact on survival during this period. The third mortality peak, which accounts for 20% of deaths, occurs during the recovery period, and is due to sepsis, progressive respiratory insufficiency or multiorgan failure.

The initial stabilisation of the paediatric trauma victim requires an organised, systematic approach in order to diagnose and treat the multiple life-threatening injuries that may be present. This should comprise:

- the primary survey and resuscitation;
- secondary survey;
- emergency treatment;
- definitive care.

The primary survey

The primary survey is designed to identify and simultaneously treat life-threatening conditions. This assessment follows the familiar ABCDE pattern:

- A = airway and cervical spine;
- B = breathing;
- C = circulation and haemorrhage control;
- D = disability (neurological evaluation);
- E = exposure

Immediate goals of the primary survey include systematic identification of all life-threatening injuries and prioritisation of their management. This survey, which should only be interrupted in the case of complete airway obstruction, includes assessment and management of the airway (with attention to possible cervical spine injury), ensuring adequate oxygenation and ventilation, maintenance of circulatory status (including control of bleeding and fluid resuscitation) and evaluation of neurological status.

Inadequate airway management is the single most important cause of morbidity and mortality in an otherwise salvageable patient.[99] All trauma victims should have supplemental oxygen administered. The cervical spine should be presumed to be injured, especially if there is obvious injury above the clavicle. Children can have significant spinal cord injury without radiographic abnormality. Consequently, all children with altered level of consciousness, head trauma, abnormal neurological signs or high-speed/impact mechanism of injury should be suspected of having spinal cord injury. The neck should be immobilised with a hard collar in the conscious or uncooperative child or with inline manual stabilisation (a semirigid collar, and sandbags) in the unconscious child. Particular care of the neck should be taken during intubation or when turning the child. Indications for intubation include airway obstruction, respiratory arrest or respiratory inadequacy, GCS < 9, and the need for prolonged ventilatory support. Immediate intubation and ventilation may be required in children with severe head, facial, chest or abdominal injuries.

All paediatric patients who have sustained significant trauma require immediate placement of two large-bore intravenous cannulae. Useful sites include antecubital fossa and femoral veins. When it is not possible to achieve rapid intravenous access, the intraosseous route may be used. Fluid boluses of 20 ml kg^{-1} should be given based on a rapid circulatory assessment. Blood transfusion will be required if signs of hypovolaemia persist after the second bolus of resuscitation fluid. A surgical opinion should also be sought urgently. Packed red blood cells should be administered in 10-ml boluses according to circulatory status. Type-specific blood is used if available, but typing should not delay resuscitation. Uncross-matched O-negative 'universal donor' blood should be immediately available in dire emergencies. Once fluid resuscitation is underway, attention is turned to control any obvious sites of haemorrhage.

Shock in the injured child is almost always secondary to acute blood loss. Occasionally, however, other causes of haemodynamic compromise may be present, such as tension pneumothorax, massive haemothorax, cardiac tamponade, myocardial contusion or spinal shock.

LIFE-THREATENING INJURIES

Some life-threatening conditions must be dealt with immediately during the primary survey and resuscitation. In the child with chest injuries, life-threatening conditions include tension pneumothorax, open pneumothorax, massive haemothorax, flail chest and cardiac tamponade. The paediatric chest wall is extremely compliant, so severe blunt chest trauma may be sustained without associated rib fractures.[100] The presence of rib fractures indicates that severe chest trauma has occurred, and injury to underlying organs, such as liver, spleen, lungs and heart, is more likely. Urgent treatment of tension pneumothorax requires needle decompression followed by placement of a chest drain. Both massive haemothorax and open pneumothorax will likewise require insertion of a chest drain. In addition, in open pneumothorax, the wound should be covered by an occlusive dressing but closed only on 3 sides.

Flail chest will usually require a period of mechanical ventilation. Cardiac tamponade usually results from penetrating chest trauma and is extremely rare in children but if present requires emergency surgical drainage and repair. Most immediately life-threatening chest injuries can be successfully managed in the accident and emergency department; however, some conditions, such as continued haemorrhage after chest drain insertion, massive air leak, disruption of the great vessels and cardiac tamponade, will require cardiothoracic referral.

Children whose circulation is not stable after replacement of 40 ml kg^{-1} of fluid are probably bleeding into the thoracic or abdominal cavities. Signs of intraabdominal bleeding caused by organ rupture include abdominal distension that does not improve following nasogastric decompression, abdominal tenderness, blood or bile-stained nasogastric aspirate and shock. Abdominal ultrasound or computed tomography (CT) scan of the abdomen may help establish the diagnosis. Intraabdominal bleeding, particularly if associated with shock, is a life-threatening surgical emergency and will require urgent laparotomy. Likewise, all children with penetrating abdominal injuries and those with definite signs of bowel perforation will require urgent laparotomy. Children with hepatic or splenic injury who are haemodynamically stable may be managed non-operatively with admission to a PICU for careful monitoring. Up to 90% of children with blunt hepatic or splenic injury may be managed conservatively.[101]

Isolated long bone or pelvic fractures may also cause significant blood loss in children, but these fractures rarely result in hypovolaemic shock unresponsive to initial volume resuscitation.[102] Closed fracture of the femur may cause loss of approximately 20% of blood volume, and an open fracture significantly more. Multiple fractures may infrequently cause severe shock. Isolated head injury rarely causes sufficient blood loss to produce shock, although scalp lacerations may cause significant blood loss.

Blood samples for cross-matching, haematology, biochemistry, blood gases, blood sugar and liver enzymes should be taken as soon as intravenous access has been established. A lateral view of the cervical spine and radiographs of chest, pelvis and skull should be performed. A CT scan of the head is usually indicated in any child with alteration of conscious level following injury. In some centres, routine chest and abdominal CTs are also performed. Urinary catheterisation should be performed once urethral damage has been excluded. A nasogastric or orogastric tube should be inserted to decompress the stomach as acute gastric dilatation is common in injured children. Analgesia should be administered and titrated against the child's response. Local anaesthetic techniques such as femoral nerve block may be useful.

SECONDARY SURVEY AND DEFINITIVE CARE

A secondary survey is performed after the primary survey is completed and resuscitative efforts are underway. As part of the secondary survey, the child should be completely undressed and examined from head to toe for injuries that may have been overlooked during the primary survey. A more detailed assessment of neurological status using the GCS or Paediatric Coma Score should be performed. During this examination, the vital signs and neurological status should be continually monitored, and any deterioration should lead to immediate reassessment of airway, breathing and circulation, and appropriate resuscitative measures should be commenced.

Once the secondary survey has been completed, an emergency treatment plan should be drawn up to treat injuries detected during the examination. These may include such conditions as simple pneumothorax, lung contusion, diaphragmatic rupture, abdominal visceral injuries, renal or bladder trauma, long bone and pelvic fractures. Many teams may be involved in the definitive care of the seriously injured child. It may be necessary to transfer the child either within the hospital or to a tertiary referral centre for specialised treatment. Secondary transfer should not be undertaken until all life-threatening problems have been addressed and the child is stable.

Special problems of head injury in children[4, 103, 104]

Head injury is the most common single cause of death in children aged 1–15 years.[99, 105] Children are more likely to suffer increased intracanial pressure and diffuse cerebral injury than adults. Intracranial bleeding occurs in 20–25% of children compared to 40–50% in adults. Subdural haematomas are the most common and are generally associated with severe brain injury. Extradural and intracerebral haematomas occur less frequently. In infants with unfused sutures, large extradural and subdural haematomas may occur before neurological symptoms and signs develop. Factors indicating a potentially serious head injury are as follows:

- involvement in a road traffic accident or a fall from a height;
- a history of loss of consciousness;
- obtunded child;
- obvious neurological signs;
- evidence of penetrating injury;
- evidence of skull fracture.

Attention to airway and cervical spine, breathing and circulation and avoidance of factors that raise intracranial pressure are the first priorities to prevent secondary brain injury. Pupil size and reactivity should be examined, and a rapid assessment of conscious level (AVPU: see Box 3.5) should be made. Appropriate resuscitative measures should be commenced. A history of the event should be sought from the parents and ambulance personnel. The secondary survey should involve a more detailed examination for bruises, lacerations or depressed skull fractures. Leakage of blood or cerebrospinal fluid from the nose or ear suggests the presence of a basal skull fracture. The conscious level should be assessed using the relevant children's coma score. Pupillary size and reactivity are tested and the fundi examined using an ophthalmoscope. Tone, movement and reflexes are assessed and any evidence of lateralising signs documented. Indications for a skull radiograph are given in Box 3.7.

A CT scan of the head is indicated in all children with reduced conscious level or neurological signs or symptoms.

All patients with a GCS < 8 should be intubated and ventilated immediately. Others may require intubation and ventilation for CT scan, for associated injuries and for transport to a specialised centre.

A deteriorating conscious level is due to increased intracranial pressure, as a result of either expanding intracranial haematoma or cerebral oedema, and requires urgent neurological referral (Box 3.8) and treatment to improve cerebral perfusion temporarily (Box 3.9).

Box 3.7 Indications for skull radiograph

- Loss of consciousness or amnesia at any time
- Neurological symptoms and signs
- Cerebrospinal fluid or blood from nose or ear
- Suspected penetrating injury/foreign body
- Scalp bruising/swelling
- Significant mechanism of injury
- Children under 2 years of age with expansile skull sutures
- Difficulty in assessing the child
- Non-mobile infants
- Children in whom an adequate history is not available
- Alcoholic intoxication

Box 3.8 Indications for neurosurgical referral

- Deteriorating conscious level
- Focal neurological signs
- Depressed skull fracture
- Basal skull fracture
- Penetrating injury
- Coma score < 12

Box 3.9 Measures to increase cerebral perfusion temporarily

- Nurse 30° head-up to improve cerebral venous drainage
- Ventilation to a normal or slightly reduced arterial carbon dioxide level to reduce intracranial pressure
- Infusion of intravenous mannitol 0.5–1 g kg^{-1}
- Combat hypotension with colloid infusion

Seizure activity raises intracranial pressure and should be controlled by the use of anticonvulsants. Diazepam is the drug of choice, but phenytoin is indicated if prolonged convulsions occur. Adequate analgesia and sedation should be prescribed. Definitive care usually involves transfer to a specialised neurosurgical unit.

Burns

Severe burn injury represents one of the most acute challenges in paediatric resuscitation. Most fatal burns occur in house fires and smoke inhalation is the usual cause of death. Seventy per cent of those burnt are preschool children. Scald injuries are the most common type of burn and occur mostly in the age group 0–4 years. As with other types of injury the structured approach works best: airway and cervical spine, breathing, circulation, disability and exposure.

The airway may be compromised either because of inhalation injury, or through severe facial burns. The latter are usually obvious, whereas the former may only be detected on close airway inspection. Inhalation injury should be suspected in the following circumstances: (1) history of closed-space burn; (2) history of altered consciousness; (3) hoarseness, stridor, facial burns, singed nasal and facial hair and carbonaceous sputum; (4) the presence of crepitations or wheezing on auscultation of the chest. The initial assessment may reveal few signs of respiratory distress. Once fluid resuscitation begins, upper-airway obstruction may develop rapidly, making intubation difficult. Thus even suspicion of airway compromise should lead to immediate consideration of intubation. All but the most experienced should seek expert help unless apnoea requires immediate intervention. If there is any suspicion of cervical spine injury, the neck should be immobilised and appropriate precautions taken. Carbon monoxide poisoning is the most frequent immediate cause of death, therefore all burned patients must receive 100% oxygen. The addition of 100% oxygen decreases the half-life of carbon monoxide from 250 to 50 min. If there is evidence of respiratory distress then ventilation will be required. Inhalation injury increases burn mortality significantly.

In the first few hours following the burn injury, signs of hypovolaemic shock are rarely exclusively attributable to the burns and other causes such as haemorrhage should be excluded. Children with burns of 10% or greater will require intravenous fluids as part of their burn care, in addition to their maintenance fluids.[92] Intravenous access should be established as soon as possible. Percutaneous access through unburned tissue is preferred. In severe burns the intraosseous route may be used during the initial resuscitation. A bolus of crystalloid of 20 ml kg^{-1} should be given if there are clinical signs of hypovolaemia. Most burnt children will be in severe pain and should be given 0.1 mg kg^{-1} of intravenous morphine as soon as possible. This should be followed by an infusion of morphine of 10–20 µg kg^{-1} h^{-1}.

As soon as the initial resuscitation is in progress, a thorough head-to-toe secondary assessment should be performed. In addition to the burn injury, the child may have suffered the effects of an explosion, may be injured from falling objects, or may have fallen trying to escape from the fire. An altered level of consciousness may be due to hypoxia following smoke inhalation or an associated head injury. The relative surface area and depth of the burn injury need to be assessed. The surface area is usually estimated using a paediatric burns chart. It is important to note that infants and small children have proportionally large head and neck surface area and smaller limbs. If no paediatric burns charts are available, it may be useful to remember that the child's hand represents 1% of body surface area and is always related to the size of the child. The rule of nines cannot be applied to young children.

The depth of the burn is usually classified as superficial, partial-thickness or full-thickness. First-degree burns cause injury only to the epidermis and clinically the skin appears red without blister formation. This type of injury is associated with severe pain and minimal fluid loss. Partial-thickness burns cause some damage to the dermis and are associated with blistering, fluid loss and pain. Full-thickness burns damage both the epidermis and dermis and may cause damage to deeper structures. The skin looks white and charred, and is painless and leathery to touch. Full-thickness circumferential extremity burns require escharotomy prior to transfer to tertiary centres if the peripheral circulation is compromised. Burns should be covered with sterile towels initially. Later these can be replaced by Sofratulle or other such lubricated gauze, topped with sterile dry dressings. Children should never be transferred with cold soaks in place.

Initial fluid losses result in marked hypovolaemia and require aggressive fluid replacement. The acute hypovolaemia is most marked in the first 48 h. This is followed by a more chronic phase of hypermetabolism and large evaporative losses (1–2 ml kg^{-1} day^{-1} per % burn) lasting for several days. Extensive burns are associated with a systemic loss of capillary integrity. This is greatest in the first 1–2 days following injury, resolving over several days.[93]

Aggressive early fluid resuscitation has been the largest factor in increasing survival of burned children to nearly 95%. Numerous schedules for fluid replacement in paediatric burns have been advocated. Perhaps the simplest and most widely used is the Parkland formula:[94]

$$\text{Percentage burn} \times \text{weight (kg)} \times 4 = \text{fluid in ml over 24 h}$$

The fluid here refers to crystalloid: half should be given over the first 8 h and the remainder over the next 16 h. The Parkland formula is very effective in maintaining blood volume and tissue perfusion at the expense of significant tissue oedema. More recent studies suggest better outcome if half the estimated 24-h volume is given over 4 h rather than the recommended 8 h.[95] Regardless of the replacement schedule used, continuous adjustments of fluid rate and electrolyte content are necessary to individualise therapy. Maintenance of intravascular volume and tissue perfusion is best accomplished by using urine output as an indicator of renal perfusion. When to use colloid and the use of hypertonic saline are controversial.[96] It has been suggested that the early use of colloid may increase tissue oedema. The integrity of the microvascular circulation is significantly improved after the first 12–24 h and colloid 10–20 ml kg^{-1} day^{-1} may be given to maintain intravascular volume and urine output. Ongoing fluid therapy is guided by renal function tests, serum sodium levels and assessment of tissue perfusion. Definitive care of the child with significant burns requires transfer to a paediatric burns facility.

ORGANISATION OF PAEDIATRIC INTENSIVE CARE SERVICES
Reception of critically ill children[106]

All hospitals admitting children must be able to resuscitate and stabilise them. Only accident and emergency departments on the same hospital site as inpatient facilities should accept children but all hospitals should have in place a protocol for use in the event of a child presenting to them. All DGHs with paediatric inpatient wards or with emergency departments that treat children must be able to provide facilities for resuscitation, stabilisation and treatment of critically ill children before referral to a PICU team on site or in the lead centre. The location of these facilities will depend on local admission practices (e.g. emergency department, general intensive care unit, paediatric admission ward) but readily portable equipment should also be available to allow advanced life support to be initiated in isolated areas, e.g. radiology department. A paediatric emergency response team of suitably trained and experienced medical and nursing staff should be continuously available.

Box 3.10 Reception of critically ill children[112]

Environment and support for parents and children
- Compliance with paediatric accident and emergency standards
- Child- and family-focused environment
- Separation from adult patients
- Parental access to the child at all times
- Keep parents fully informed about child's condition, treatment plan and retrieval/transfer as appropriate
- Access to support services for family

Medical staffing
- Lead consultant for paediatric accident and emergency issues
- Named consultant responsible for protocols for management of critically ill children
- 24-h on-site medical staff cover with at least one of the on-call team certified with Advanced Paediatric Life Support/Paediatric Advanced Life Support (APLS/PALS)

Nurse staffing
- Lead nurse for paediatric issues with responsibility for ensuring training of nurses in APLS/PALS, good liaison with hospital and community paediatric services
- At least one APLS/PALS-certified nurse on duty at all times
- Acutely ill children should not be cared for in nurse-led minor-injury units, but there should be a staff member on each shift with basic paediatric airway skills, training in paediatric resuscitation and access to local protocols for managing the acutely ill child

Access and provision of advice between lead centre and referring hospital
- Advice from medical paediatric inpatient unit and lead centre for paediatric intensive care
- Agreed protocol for accessing advice 24 h per day 7 days per week

Equipment and facilities
- Separate designated and equipped area for resuscitation and stabilisation of critically ill children of all ages
- Critically ill children awaiting retrieval should be cared for in a high-dependency area

Quality and management of services
- Appropriate alert system
- Agreed protocols
- Critical incident reporting
- Audit and quality assurance analysis of those cases referred for intensive care

This team should be supported at all times by appropriate consultant medical staff who are readily available to attend. Whenever possible, resuscitation and treatment should occur in a purpose-designed area fully equipped with a comprehensive range of equipment for children of all ages (Box 3.10).

In all DGHs and MAGHs there should be a designated lead consultant in paediatric intensive care and a corresponding lead nurse. The planning of equipment and organisation of emergency responses should be the responsibility of the lead consultant, with support from other appropriate individuals, e.g. resuscitation committee, resuscitation training officer(s), senior nursing staff. There should be a rolling programme of training in paediatric resuscitation and the management of paediatric emergencies for medical and nursing staff. Training in advanced paediatric life support (APLS/PALS) should be encouraged for all staff who are likely to care for sick children, but it should be emphasised that successful completion of such courses is an adjunct (and not a substitute) for supervised clinical experience and training.

The lead consultant and lead nurse are responsible for ensuring that there is regular and reliable communication with the lead centre, and with single-speciality centres, e.g. burns units, if they are not incorporated in the lead centre. Clinical pathways should be established for all anticipated paediatric emergencies, and, if appropriate, for the method and timing of referral. It is important that all key staff are aware of these arrangements, in order that attention is not diverted from clinical care when a child becomes seriously ill.

PROVISION OF HIGH-DEPENDENCY CARE (LEVEL I CARE) IN THE DISTRICT HOSPITAL[106, 107]

Level I high-dependency care

In all DGHs and MAGHs there should be a purpose-designed and equipped area to which children who require high-dependency care should be admitted. Around 5–15% of all DGH admissions need high-dependency care, with a few of these requiring step-up care to level 2 or higher care. Around 0.5–1% of admissions need initiation of level 2 care pending retrieval and transfer to a PICU.

Local factors will influence whether such facilities should be located in the general ICU or within the paediatric inpatient structure. There should be piped medical gases and ample power outlets supported by a generator electrical supply. A monitoring system should be available which will allow continuous display of electrocardiograph, pulse oximetry and respiratory rate, and ideally it should be possible to measure invasive pressures as well as intermittent blood pressure.

In addition to all the necessary equipment required to deliver high-dependency care, there must also be immediate availability of suitable equipment to initiate level 2 or even level 3 care if a child's condition deteriorates. A range of such equipment must be provided for children of all ages, including infants. This should include the availability of a suitable ventilator, together with capnography and airway pressure alarms (Box 3.11).

Criteria for provision of high-dependency care[107]

The criteria for needing high-dependency care are based on the disease, the interventions needed and a number of conditional factors. Thus, respiratory, cardiovascular, neurological and renal functions are all factors in determining need (Box 3.12).

PROVISION OF PAEDIATRIC CRITICAL CARE (LEVEL 2 CARE) IN THE DISTRICT HOSPITAL

Other than for a period of stabilisation prior to transfer, the level of care within a general paediatric ward should not exceed high-dependency care. Local agreements should be made as to when and where children who require higher levels of care are transferred, but in general DGHs should not be expected to provide level 2 or 3 care for prolonged peri-

Box 3.11 Standards for paediatric high-dependency units (HDUs)[112]

Medical staffing
- Lead consultant: resuscitation, HDU care, initiation of paediatric intensive care
- 24-h consultant paediatric cover with advance resuscitation skills
- 24-h consultant anaesthetic cover with advanced paediatric resuscitation skills
- 24-h resident cover on site by doctors with Advanced Paediatric Life Support/Paediatric Advanced Life Support (APLS/PALS) training

Nurse staffing
- 24-h cover by a fully trained paediatric intensive care nurse
- Trained children's nurses
- One nurse per shift with APLS/ PALS skills
- Nurse staffing ratio 0.5:1 or 1:1 if the child is in a cubicle

Access on site to other paediatric subspecialties and services
- General paediatric inpatient unit
- Neonatal unit
- General intensive care unit
- 24-h access to biochemistry, haematology, microbiology and radiology services
- Paediatric physiotherapy, pharmacy, dietetics

Equipment and facilities
- Designated paediatric high-dependency facilities
- Suitable for child awaiting retrieval

Environment and support services for parents, carers and children
- Parental access
- Child-friendly environment
- Multidisciplinary care
- Information and support services

Advice from lead centre
- Access throughout 24 h

Education and training
- Access to APLS/PALS training
- Ongoing training
- Access to RN Part 15 and ENB 415 or equivalent
- Access to a hospital-based Basic Life Support training programme
- Quality and management of services
- Agreed protocols
- Clinical audit
- Critical incident reporting

Operational issues
- Anticipate seasonal increase in winter months

ods. If, however, the child's condition is such that the requirement for mechanical ventilation is likely to be short, it may be preferable to continue care in the DGH. Under such circumstances the child should usually be admitted to the ICU, where appropriate facilities for his or her age (and family) should be provided according to published recommendations.[107] Children who require a higher level of care in the MAGH should normally be admitted to the general ICU which should have purpose-designed facilities for children of all ages. Local agreements with the lead centre should influence the duration and levels of

Box 3.12 Clinical categories of children who are suitable for high-dependency (HD) care in a district general hospital (DGH)[107]

HD unit or HD beds in children's ward in DGH

- Prolonged/recurrent convulsions
- Bacterial meningitis
- Glasgow Coma Scale 8–12
- Circulatory instability due to hypovolaemia other than meningococcal disease
- Diabetic ketoacidosis with drowsiness
- Patient whose pain is difficult to control
- Meningococcal disease in a stable state
- Intravenous fluid resuscitation > 10 ml kg^{-1} and < 30 ml kg^{-1}
- Continuous intravenous drug infusion (except analgesia alone)
- Acute renal failure (urine output < 1 ml kg^{-1})
- Bronchiolitis with $FIO_2 > 50\%$ via head box or face mask or continuous positive airways pressure
- Recurrent apnoeas
- Upper-airway obstruction – close observation
- Asthma on intravenous drugs or hourly nebulisers
- Poisoning/substance misuse with potential for significant problems
- After/during sedation for a procedure
- Pre- or postoperative patients with complex fluid management, analgesia, bleeding, complex surgery
- Cardiac arrythmia which has responded to first-line therapy (other than cardioversion)
- Stable long-term ventilation

Specialist HD unit

- Multiple drug therapy (e.g. complex chemotherapy)
- Bone marrow transplant/severe neutropenia
- Acute renal replacement therapy
- Hourly cycle peritoneal dialysis

care undertaken in the MAGH ICU. In both DGHs and MAGHs the age of the child should also influence the decision as to whether to treat locally or to transfer. Many adolescents who fall into the category of paediatrics may require intensive care for conditions which are equally commonly dealt with by general ICUs, e.g. acute intoxication, drug overdose, trauma. If there is no clinical necessity to transfer such patients it may be sensible to continue their management in the general ICU and preserve lead centre PICU beds for the children who really need them.

CRITERIA FOR REFERRAL TO A PICU

The Paediatric Intensive Care Society produced referral criteria for paediatric intensive care in 2001 and these have been annotated and clarified by the Department of Health Paediatric HDU Working Group recently[107] (Boxes 3.13–3.15).

TRANSPORT OF THE CRITICALLY ILL CHILD[2, 106, 108]

Centralisation of paediatric intensive care facilities means that more children will need to be moved to specialist units. It has been clearly shown that this results in improved morbidity and mortality rates for the sickest children and that properly conducted transportation does not cause a deterioration in the patient's condition and outcome.[3, 109–111] By recognising critically ill children early, by thoroughly assessing and stabilising their condi-

Box 3.13 Criteria for referral for paediatric intensive care[107, 112]

- Meningococcal disease with shock
- Advanced respiratory support (other than short-term postoperative support)
- An intensive care-dependent procedure is highly likely (see Box 3.14)
- Symptoms or evidence of shock, severe respiratory distress or respiratory depression
- Potential to develop airway compromise
- Has required or continues to require resuscitation
- Significant major injury
- Prolonged or medium-/high-risk or specialist surgery even if elective
- Potential or actual severe metabolic, fluid or electrolyte derangement or imbalance
- Acute organ or organ system failure
- Established chronic disease plus acute clinical deterioration or secondary failure in another organ system
- Needs 1:1 nursing because of the complexity of an acute or acute-on-chronic illness

Box 3.14 Intensive care-dependent procedures which need a paediatric critical care environment[112]

- Nasopharyngeal and endotracheal intubation
- Endotracheal continuous positive-airways pressure
- Artificial/mechanical ventilation
- Continuous invasive cardiovascular monitoring
- Antiarrhythmic, inotropic or vasoactive drug infusions
- Acute renal support
- Cardioversion or DC countershock
- Acute or external cardiac pacing
- Mechanical circulatory support
- Intracranial pressure monitoring (in acute illness, this may be possible in wards or high-dependency units)
- Complex intravenous nutrition or drug scheduling (in specialist wards such as oncology units this level of care can be provided)
- Complex anticonvulsant therapy
- Frequent or pressurised infusions of blood products
- Active or forced diuresis
- Induced hypothermia
- Balloon tamponade of oesophageal varices
- Emergency thoraco- or pericardiocentesis

tion prior to transfer and by ensuring that appropriately experienced personnel accompany the child using appropriate equipment, secondary insults during transport can be avoided.[111]

The rank order of frequency of primary diagnoses in patients requiring transport to intensive care is different in adults and children (Table 3.4).

The main reason is the higher incidence of infective causes of respiratory failure in children. This includes croup, tracheitis, epiglottitis, bronchiolitis, asthma and pneumonia. Neurological dysfunction is a commoner reason for transport and may be due to primary

> **Box 3.15** Clinical categories of children who need paediatric intensive care[107]
>
> - Arrhythmia which fails to respond to first-line therapy
> - After cardiac surgery
> - Possibility of progressive deterioration to the point of needing ventilation (e.g. recurrent apnoeas, airway obstruction)
> - Vasoactive infusions to support cardiac output or control blood pressure
> - Nebulised adrenaline (epinephrine) for upper-airway obstruction after two doses or more
> - Recently extubated after prolonged intubation
> - Postoperative patient with multiple drains requiring hourly fluid replacement
> - Any airway intervention
> - Ventilated or assisted respiration other than during recovery from anaesthetic
> - Cardiopulmonary resuscitation
> - Central nervous system depression sufficient to compromise the airway protective reflexes/respiratory drive or potential to progress
> - Uncontrolled shock needing repeated volume and/or inotropes or greater than 30 ml kg^{-1} resuscitation fluid volume
> - Diabetic ketoacidosis with deteriorating level of consciousness after start of therapy
> - Tracheostomy for acute illness

central nervous system infection or secondary to sepsis, poisoning, hypoxia, ischaemia, trauma, epilepsy or metabolic disorders.

Priorities before transport

The priorities are the ABCDE of resuscitation with some important additions. The airway must be secure for transport and endotracheal intubation and stabilisation of the cervical spine should be performed if appropriate. Ventilation must be controlled for transport if the patient is intubated. Bleeding must be controlled and the circulation must be optimised using fluids, inotropes, vasodilators and prostaglandins as appropriate, delivered via appropriate intravascular lines and with intra-arterial blood pressure monitoring. In critically ill infants, hypoglycaemia is a possibility and should be sought and corrected. Intracranial hypertension should be treated in those at risk by controlling ventilation and by judicious use of diuretics, but urgent neurosurgical intervention may be required (see below). Prior to transfer, open wounds should be dressed and sutured if appropriate and fractures should be stabilised in suitable splints or plaster casts. For children with infectious diseases, cultures should be taken and antibiotic and antiviral chemotherapy should be started. This is especially important in meningococcal disease, meningitis and encephalitis. In small infants temperature

Table 3.4 Range of diseases requiring critical care transport

Rank	Adult	Paediatric
1st	Trauma	Respiratory failure
2nd	Respiratory failure	Neurological dysfunction
3rd	Gastrointestinal disease or surgery	Major sepsis
4th	Major sepsis	Drug overdose or poisoning
5th	Neurological dysfunction	Burns or smoke inhalation
6th	Cardiovascular disease	Cardiovascular disease
7th	Drug overdose or poisoning	Trauma

maintenance is a major problem during transport and active warming measures, adequate covering with insulating layers and a heated incubator for neonates are important measures. Communication must be very good between the referring and receiving hospitals and adequate records of the patient and the management to date must be exchanged. The charts, clinical notes, results of investigations and copies of X-rays and scans must be passed on to the receiving hospital. A detailed history from the parents/guardians must be obtained and parental transport and advice about the location of the receiving hospital intensive care unit should be given. Parents are usually not advised to travel along with their child but in certain circumstances this is the best option.

Monitoring during transport

The most important safety feature during transportation of critically ill children is the presence of trained, experienced personnel monitoring the child and the equipment. Pulse oximetry is perhaps the single most useful monitor during transport but reliable information depends on the oximeter possessing the ability to reject artefacts due to motion. A portable electronic monitor incorporating pulse oximetry, electrocardiogram, dual pressure monitoring, temperature measurement and capnography is very helpful. Non-invasive blood pressure recording is unreliable during transport as it is subject to movement artefact. Ventilation can be controlled by hand using an anaesthetic T-piece circuit as long as a doctor who is familiar with this technique is present. A mechanical ventilator can be used as appropriate for the child's age.

Organisation of paediatric critical care transport and referral protocols

PICUs should provide a retrieval team for secondary transport of critically ill children from referring hospitals. The team should comprise a trained paediatric anaesthetist or intensivist and an experienced PICU nurse if possible. Even with dedicated transport teams, the response time is not immediate and so it is the responsibility of the referring hospital to perform the resuscitation and stabilisation of the child. This often involves securing the airway and vascular access, and early involvement of senior anaesthetic or intensive care personnel at the referring hospital is to be encouraged. The consultation and referral of critically ill children for transport to the regional PICU must be at consultant-to-consultant level and there should be an efficient telephone contact system to the duty PICU consultant involving one or at most two calls. Advice can be given by phone to assist the referring staff pending arrival of the transfer team and portable phone contact is useful to keep the transfer team members updated on progress or deterioration and to give an estimated time of arrival. The child is the responsibility of the referring consultant until care is formally handed over to the transfer team at the bedside. Depending on the child's condition, the transfer team may have to spend some time on stabilisation prior to departure. The PICU should be contacted, the most appropriate transport mode discussed and an estimated time of return given. It may not be possible to stabilise some children sufficiently for transport and this must be explained to relatives. Sometimes a transport team may already be on a call or may not be available and the referring staff may need to undertake the transfer but this should not be delegated to junior staff and an anaesthetist or experienced critical care staff should be involved in the transport in these circumstances.

Special problems of children with head injuries

Head-injured children need special measures and every effort must be made to minimise delay in reaching neurosurgical care. This means many of these cases require primary transport by staff from the referring hospital for specialist neurosurgical care. In such cases it may not be appropriate to await the availability and arrival of a retrieval team and a team from the referring hospital may have to undertake the transport. An anaesthetist of suitable training and experience should be part of this team because these children often require intubation, controlled ventilation and careful monitoring. Those who need immediate intubation and controlled ventilation include those with a GCS of 8 or less, those who have lost protective laryngeal reflexes, those who are hypoxaemic or hypercarbic or in whom spontaneous overventilation, periodic breathing or apnoea is noted. Some children are intubated and ventilated for the transfer and this includes those with deteriorating consciousness, facial or mandibular fractures, bleeding into the mouth or seizures.

Head-injured children who require immediate referral and transport to a neurosurgeon include those with a skull fracture plus a GCS < 15, or focal neurological signs, or fits, or other neurological signs; those with persisting coma; or whose conscious level is deteriorating; or those with focal pupillary or limb signs. Those head-injured children who should be referred urgently include those in whom confusion persists for more than 6 h, those with compound depressed skull fractures, or penetrating injuries, those with cerebrospinal fluid leaks from the ear or the nose and those with persisting or worsening headache or vomiting. Particular care is required when transporting children with head injuries to minimise changes in intracranial pressure and cerebral blood flow due to acceleration, deceleration, hypoxaemia and air expansion at altitude.

Special problems of mode of transport

Road transport by ambulance carries with it the problems of acceleration and deceleration forces, movement artefact on monitors and motion sickness for staff and conscious patients. These are also problematic at sea and in air transport by fixed wing or helicopter. Temperature maintenance is a problem in small infants with all transport modes but particularly in military helicopters and at sea. Altitude is associated with a fall in ambient temperature but, more importantly, with falls in both the ambient oxygen tension and the ambient pressure. This latter effect means that gas in closed spaces expands with increasing altitude and thus a given volume of air or gas in the thoracic cavity, cranium, mediastinum, pericardium, peritoneum or obstructed viscus will try to increase in size but if contained, the pressure in the cavity will rise. Unpressurised aircraft will be especially risky but even pressurised aircraft fly with cabin pressures equivalent to an altitude of around 2500 m: by special request some air ambulances can be pressurised to the equivalent of sea level although this reduces the airframe life. Helicopters produce a lot of vibration artefact on monitors and are very noisy, giving communication problems. Space and visibility to work are often very limited in helicopters and fixed wing aircraft. Another important problem in all aircraft is electrical interference from medical equipment with the aircraft's electronic systems and vice versa.

REFERENCES

1. Department of Health. Paediatric intensive care – a framework for the future. London: Department of Health; 1996.
2. Scottish Office Department of Health. SPICA – Scottish paediatric intensive care audit. Edinburgh: Scottish Office Department of Health; 1999.
3. Pollack MM, Alexander SR, Clark N, et al. Improved outcomes from tertiary centre pediatric intensive care: a statewide comparison of tertiary and non tertiary care facilities. Crit Care Med 1991; 19:150–159.
4. Advanced Life Support Group. Advanced paediatric life support. 3rd edn. London: British Medical Journal Publishing Group; 2001.
5. Schindler MB, Bohn D, Cox PN, et al. Outcome of out-of-hospital cardiac or respiratory arrest in children. N Engl J Med 1996; 335:1473–1479.
6. Zaritsky A. Outcome of pediatric cardiopulmonary resuscitation. Crit Care Med 1993; 21(suppl):S325–S327.
7. Ronco R, King W, Konley DK, et al. Outcome and cost at a children's hospital following resuscitation for out-of-hospital cardiopulmonary arrest. Arch Pediatr Adolesc Med 1995; 149:210–214.
8a. Gentleman D, Dearden M, Midgley S, Maclean D (1993) Guidelines for resuscitation and transfer of patients with serious head injury. Br Med J; 307: 547–552.

8. Schwaitzberg SD, Berman KS, Harris BH. A pediatric trauma model of continuous hemorrhage. J Pediatr Surg 1988; 23:605.

9. Committee on Pediatric Emergency Medicine. First aid for the choking child. Pediatrics 1993; 92:477–479.

10. Philips GW, Ziderman DA. Relation of the infant heart to the sternum; its significance in cardiopulmonary resuscitation. Lancet 1986; I:1204–1205.

11. Orlowski JP. Optimum position for external cardiac massage in infants and children. Crit Care Med 1984;12:224.

12. Todres ID, Rogers MC. Methods of external cardiac massage in the newborn infant. J Pediatr 1975; 86:781–782.

13. David R. Closed chest cardiac massage in the newborn infant. Pediatrics 1988; 81:552–554.

14. Menegazzi JJ, Auble TE, Nichhhklas KA, et al. Two thumb versus two finger chest compression during CPR in a swine model of cardiac arrest. Ann Emerg Med 1993; 22:240–243.

15. Paradis NA, Martin GB, Rivers EP, et al. Coronary perfusion pressure and return of spontaneous circulation in human cardiopulmonary resuscitation. JAMA 1990; 263:1106–1113.

16. Goetting MG. Effect of basic life support and epinephrine on coronary perfusion pressure in pediatric cardiac arrest. Crit Care Med 1994; 22:A153.

17. del-Nido PJ, Dalton HJ, Thompson AE, et al. Extracorporeal membrane oxygenator rescue in children during cardiac arrest after cardiac surgery. Circulation 1992; 86:11300–11304.

18. Rossetti VA, Thompson BM, Aprahamian C, et al. Difficulty and delay in intravascular access in pediatric arrests. Ann Emerg Med 1984; 13:406.

19. Hedges JR, Barson WB, Doan LA, et al (1984). Central versus peripheral intravenous routes in cardiopulmonary resuscitation. Am J Emerg Med 1984; 2:385–390.

20. Emerman CL, Pinchak AC, Hancock D, et al. Effect of injection site on circulation times during cardiac arrest. Crit Care Med 1988; 16:1138–1141.

21. Andropoulos DB, Soifer SJ, Schreiber MD. Plasma epinephrine concentrations after intraosseous and central venous injection during cardiopulmonary resuscitation in the lamb. J Pediatr 1990; 116:312–315.

22. Orlowski JP, Porembka DT, Gallagher JM, et al. Comparison study of intraosseous, central intravenous, and peripheral intravenous infusions of emergency drugs. Am J Dis Child 1990; 144:112–117.

23. Christensen DW, Vernon DD, Banner WJ, et al. Skin necrosis complicating intraosseous infusions. Pediatr Emerg Care 1991; 7:289–290.

24. Galpin RD, Kronick JB, Willis RB, et al. Bilateral lower extremity compartment syndromes secondary to intraosseous fluid resuscitation. J Pediatr Orthop 1991; 11:773–776.

25. LaFleche FR, Slepin MJ, Vargas J, et al. Iatrogenic bilateral tibial fractures after intraosseous infusion attempts in a three month old infant. Ann Emerg Med 1989; 18:1099–1101.

26. Simmons CM, Johnson NE, Perkin RM, et al. Intraoosseous extravasation complication reports. Ann Emerg Med 1994; 23:363–366.

27. Rimar S, Westry J, Rodriguez R. Compartment syndrome in an infant following emergency intraosseous infusion. Clin Pediatr 1988; 27:259–260.

28. Heinild S, Sodergaurd T, Tudvad F. Bone marrow infusions in childhood: experience from a thousand infusions. J Pediatr 1947; 30: 400–411.

29. Orlowski JP, Julius CJ, Petras RE, et al. The safety of intraosseous infusions: risks of fat ond bone marrow emboli to the lungs. Ann Emerg Med 1989; 18:1062–1067.

30. Fiallos M, Kissoon N, Abdelmoneim T, et al. Fat embolism with the use of intrasseous infusion during cardiopulmonary resuscitation. Am J Med Sci 1989; 314:73–79.

31. Johnston C. Endotracheal drug delivery. Pediatr Emerg Care 1992; 8:94–97.

32. Quinton DN, O'Bynne G, Aitkenhead AR. Comparison of endotracheal and peripheral intravenous adrenaline in cardiac arrest: is the endotracheal route reliable? Lancet 1987; I:828–829.

33. Hornchen U, Schuttler J, Stoeckel H, et al. Endobronchial instillation of epinephrine during cardiopulmonary resuscitation. Crit Care Med 1987; 15:1037–1039.

34. Ralston SH, Tacher WA, Showen L, et al. Endotracheal versus intravenous epinephrine during electromechanical dissociation with CPR in dogs. Ann Emerg Med 1985; 14:1044–1048.

35. Bleyaert AL, Sands PA, Safar P, et al. Augmentation of postischemic brain damage by severe intermittent hypertension. Crit Care Med 1980; 8:41–45.

36. Kosnik JW, Jackson RE, Keats S, et al. Dose related response of centrally administered epinephrine on the change in aortic diastolic pressure during closed-chest massage in dogs. Ann Emerg Med 1985; 14:204–208.

37. Brown CG, Werman HA. Adrenergic agonists during cardiopulmonary resuscitation. Resuscitation 1990; 19:1–16.

38. Brown CG, Martin DR, Pepe PE, et al. A comparison of standard-dose and high-dose epinephrine in cardiac arrest outside the hospital. N Engl J Med 1992; 327: 1051–1055.

39. Callahan M, Madsen CD, Barton CW, et al. A randomised trial of high-dose epinephrine and norepinephrine versus standard dose epinephrine in pre-hospital cardiac arrest. JAMA 1992; 268:2667–2672.

40. Steill IG, Hebert PC, Weitzman BN, et al. High-dose epinephrine in adult cardiac arrest. N Engl J Med 1992; 327:1045–1050.

41. Carpenter TC, Stenmark KR. High-dose epinephrine is not superior to standard-dose epinephrine in pediatric in-hospital cardiopulmonary arrest. Pediatrics 1997; 99:403–408.

42. Diekman RA, Vardis R. High-dose epinephrine in pediatric out-of-hospital cardiopulmonary arrest. Pediatrics 1995; 95:901–913.

43. Steinhart CR, Permutt S. Gurtner GH, et al. β-adrenergic activity and cardiovascular response to severe respiratory acidosis. Am J Physiol 1983; 1: H46–H54.

44. Steenberger C, Deleeuw G, Rick T, et al. Effects of acidosis and ischaemia on contractility and intracellular pH of rat heart. Circ Res 1977; 41:849–858.

45. Wood WB, Manley ES, Woodbury RA. The effects of CO_2 induced respiratory acidosis on the depressor and pressor components of the dog's blood pressure response to epinephrine. J Pharmacol Exp Ther 1963; 139:238–247.

46. Zaritsky AL, Gomez R. Acidosis, epinephrine, and the model. Crit Care Med 1993; 21:1821–1823.

47. Weil M, Rackow E, Trevino R, et al. Difference in acid–base state between venous and arterial blood during cardiopulmonary resuscitation. N Engl J Med 1986; 315:153–156.

48. Graf H, Leach W, Arieff AL. Metabolic effects of sodium bicarbonate in hypoxic lactic acidosis in dogs. Am J Physiol 1985; 249:F630–F635.

49. Ritter JM, Doktor HS, Benjamin N. Paradoxical effect of bicarbonate on cytoplasmic pH. Lancet 1990; 335:1243–1246.

50. Dybvik T, Strand T, Steen PA. Buffer therapy during out-of-hospital cardiopulmonary resuscitation. Resuscitation 1995; 29:89–95.

51. Sessler D, Mills P, Gregory G, et al. Effects of bicarbonate on arterial and brain intracellular pH in neonatal rabbits recovering from hypoxic lactic acidosis. J Pediatr 1987; 111:817–823.

52. Katz AM, Reuter H. Cellular calcium and cardiac cell death. Am J Cardiol 1979; 44:188–190.

53. Zaloga GP, Strickland RA, Butterworth JF, et al. Calcium attenuates epinephrine's β-adrenergic effects in post-operative heart surgery patients. Circulation 1990; 81:196–200.

54. Stueven H, Thompson B, Aprahamian C, et al. The effectiveness of calcium chloride in refractory electromechanical dissociation. Ann Emerg Med 1985; 14:626–629.

55. Stueven H, Thompson B, Aprahamian C, et al. Lack of effectiveness of calcium chloride in refractory asystole. Ann Emerg Med 1985; 14:630–632.

56. Cardenas-Rivero N, Chernow B, Stoiko MA, et al. Hypocalcaemia in critically ill children. J Pediatr 1989, 114.946–951.

57. Zaritsky A, Nadkarni V, Getson P, et al. CPR in children. Ann Emerg Med 1989; 16:1110.

58. Phillips B, Zideman D, Garcia-Castrillo L, et al. European Resuscitation Council guidelines 2000 for basic paediatric life support. Resuscitation 2001; 48:223–229

59. Phillips B, Zideman D, Garcia-Castrillo L, et al. European Resuscitation Council guidelines 2000 for advanced paediatric life support. Resuscitation 2001; 48:231–324

60. Eisenberg M, Bergner L, Hallstrom A. Epidemiology of cardiac arrest and resuscitation in children. Ann Emerg Med 1983; 12:672–674.

61. Torphy DE, Minter MG, Thompson BM. Cardio-respiratory arrest and resuscitation of children. Am J Dis Child 1984; 138:1099–1102.

62. Phillips B, Zideman D, Wyllie J, et al. European Resuscitation Council guidelines 2000 for newly born life support. Resuscitation 2001; 48:235–239.

63. Carillo JA, Davis AL, Zaritsky A. Role of early fluid resuscitation in pediatric septic shock. JAMA 1991; 9:1242–1245.

64. Kallen RJ, Lonergan JM. Fluid resuscitation of acute hypovolemic hypoperfusion states in pediatrics. Pediatr Clin North Am 1990; 37:287.

65. Pollack CV. Prehospital fluid resuscitation of the trauma patient, an update on the controversies. Emerg Med Clin North Am 1993; 11:61–70.

66. Cochrane Injuries Group albumin reviewers. Br Med J 1998; 317:235–240.

67. Tobias JD. Shock in children: The first 60 minutes. Pedriatr Ann 1996; 25:330–338

68. Scheinkestel CD, Tuxen DV, Cade JF, et al. Fluid management of shock in critically ill patients. Med J Aust 1989; 150:508–517.

69. Lucking SE, Pollack MM, Fields AL. Shock following generalised hypoxic–ischaemic injury in previously healthy infants and children. J Pediatr 1986; 108:359–364.

70. Kern KB, Hilwig RW, Rhee KH, et al. Myocardial dysfunction after resuscitation from cardiac arrest: an example of global myocardial stunning. J Am Coll Cardiol 1996; 28:232–240.

71. Ushay MH, Notterman DA. Pharmacology of pediatric resuscitation. Pediatr Clin North Am 1997; 44(1):207–233.

72. Perkin RM, Levin DL, Webb R. Dobutamine: a hemodynamic evaluation in children with shock. J Pediatr 1982; 100:977.
73. Kern KB, Hilwig RW, Berg RA, et al. Postresuscitation left verntricular systolic and diastolic dysfunction. Treatment with dobutamine. Circulation 1997; 95:2610–2613.
74. Habib DM, Padbury JF, Anas NG et al. Dobutamine pharmacokinetics and pharmacodynamics in pediatric intensive care patients. Crit Care Med 1992; 20:601–608.
75. Martinez AM, Padbury JF, Thio S. Dobutamine pharmacokinetics and cardiovascular responses in critically ill neonates. Pediatrics 1992; 89:47–51.
76. Pollack MM, Fields AL, Ruttimann UE. Sequential cardiopulmonary variables of infants and children in septic shock. Crit Care Med 1984; 12(7):554.
77. Pollack MM, Fields AL, Ruttiman UE. Distribution of cardiopulmonary variables in pediatric survivors and non survivors of septic shock. Crit Care Med 1985; 13(6):454.
78. Carroll GC, Snyder JV. Hyperdynamic severe intravascular sepsis depends on fluid administration in cynomolgus monkeys. Am J Physiol 1982; 243:R131.
79. Hazinskin MF, Alberti TJM, Macintyre NR, et al. Epidemiology, pathophysiology and clinical presentation of gram-sepsis. Am J Crit Care 1993; 2:224–335.
80. Marcier JC, Beaufils F, Hartmann JF, et al. Haemodynamic patterns of meningococcal septic shock in children. Crit Care Med 1988; 16(1):27.
81. Sinclair JF, Skeoch CR, Hallworth D. Prognosis of meningococcal septicaemia. Lancet 1987; ii:38.
82. Carillo JA, Cunnion RE. Septic shock. Crit Care Clin 1997; 13(3):553–574.
83. Parker MM, Shelhamer JH, Bachharach SL, et al. Profound but reversible myocardial depression in patients with septic shock. Ann Intern Med 1984; 100:483.
84. Parker MM, Shelhamer JH, Natanson C, et al. Serial cardiovascular variables in survivors and non survivors of human septic shock: heart rate as an early predictor of prognosis. Crit Care Med 1987; 15:923.
85. Parker MM, Ognibene FP, Parrillo JE. Peak systolic pressure/end-systolic volume ratio, a load-independent measure of ventricular function, is reversibly decreased in human septic shock. Crit Care Med 1995; 23:1791.
86. Morris LR, Murphy MB, Kitbachi AE. Bicarbonate therapy in severe diabetic ketoacidosis. Ann Intern Med 1986; 105:836.
87. Mel JM, Werther GA. Incidence and outcome of diabetic carebral oedema in childhood: are there predictors? J Pediatr Child Health 1995; 31(1):17–20.
88. Uleck BW. Risk factors for cerebral oedema associated with diabetic ketoacidosis. Ann Neurol 1986; 20:407.
89. Rosenbloom AL. Intracerebral crises during treatment of diabetic ketoacidosis. Diabetic Care 1990; 13:22–23.
90. Rother KL, Schwenk WF. Effect of rehydration fluid with 75 mmol/L of sodium on serum sodium concentration and serum osmolality in young patients with diabetic ketoacidosis. Mayo Clin Proc 1994; 69:1149–1153.
91. Rosenbloom AL, Riley WJ, Weber FT, et al. Cerebral edema complicating diabetic ketoacidosis in childhood. J Pediatr 1980; 96:357–361.
92. Carvajal HF. Fluid resuscitation of pediatric burn victims: a critical appraisal. Paediatric Nephrology 1994; 8:357–366.
93. Harms BA, Bodai BI, Kramer GC, et al. Microvascular fluid and protein flux in pulmonary and systemic circulations after thermal injury. Microvasc Res 1982; 23:77.
94. Smith EL. Acute management of thermal burns in children. Surg Clin North Am 1970; 50:807–815.
95. Puffinbarger NK, Tuggle DW, Smith E. Rapid isotonic fluid resuscitation in pediatric thermal injury. J Paediatr Surg 1994; 29(2):339–342.
96. Browser-Wallace BH, Caldwell FT Jr. A prospective analysis of hypertonic lactated saline v Ringer's lactate-colloid for the resuscitation of severely burned children. Burns 1986; 12:402–409.
97. Mc Koy C, Bell MJ. Preventable traumatic deaths in children. J Pediatr Surg 1983; 18:505–508.
98. Cooper A, Barlow B, Davidson L, et al. Epidemiology of pediatric trauma: importance of population-based statistics. J Pediatr Surg 1992; 27:149–154.
99. Mayer T, Walker ML, Johnson DG, et al. Causes of morbidity and mortality in severe pediatric trauma. JAMA 1981; 245:719–721.
100. Garcia VF, Gotschall CS, Eichhelberger MR, et al. Rib fractures in children: a marker of severe trauma. J Trauma 1990; 30:695–700.
101. Giacomanotonio M, Filler RM, Rich RH. Blunt hepatic trauma in children: experience with operative and nonoperative management. J Pediatr Surg 1984; 19:519.
102. Barlow B, Niermirsky M, Gandhi R, et al. Response to injury in children with closed femur fractures. J Trauma 1987; 27:429–430.
103. Gentleman D, Dearden M, Midgley S, et al. Guidelines for resuscitation and transfer of patients with serious head injury. Br Med J 1993; 307:547–552.
104. Safe paediatric neurosurgery. London: Society of British Neurological Surgeons; 1997.

105. Williams RA. Injuries in infants and small children resulting from witnessed and corroborated free falls. J Trauma 1991; 31:1350–1352.
106. Standards document 2001. London: Paediatric Intensive Care Society; 2001.
107. High dependency care for children. London: Department of Health, 2001.
108. Scottish Office Department of Health. Working group on the transport of critically ill and injured children. Edinburgh: Scottish Office Department of Health; 2000.
109. Doyle E, Freeman J, Hallworth D, et al. Transport of the critically ill child. Br J Hosp Med 1992; 48:314–319.
110. Barry PW, Ralston C. Adverse events occurring during interhospital transfer of the critically ill. Arch Dis Child 1994; 71:8–11.
111. Britto J, Nadel S, Maconochie I, et al. Morbidity and severity of illness during interhospital transfer: impact of a specialised paediatric retrieval team. Br Med J 1995; 311:836–839.
112. Paediatric Intensive Care Society. Standards for transport of critically ill children. London: PICS; 1995.

FURTHER READING

Macnab A, Macrae D, Henning R. (2000) Care of the Critically Ill Child. Churchill Livingstone, London ISBN 0-4430-5394-4

CHAPTER 4

Consent issues in paediatric anaesthesia and critical care

Neil S Morton

LEGAL AND ETHICAL FRAMEWORK FOR GOOD CLINICAL PRACTICE

The legal framework within which paediatric anaesthesia and critical care are now conducted has changed in the last 10 years (Box 4.1). In addition, good practice guidelines are all relevant and helpful (Box 4.2).

These laws and guidelines have had direct effects on clinical practice and research in paediatric anaesthesia and critical care. It is important to note that there are differences between English and Scottish law which have direct relevance to the issue of consent. The full implications of recent constitutional changes in Northern Ireland and Wales are unclear at present.

PRINCIPLES OF CONSENT PROCEDURES

The legislation and guidelines are now child-centred and so the child has more individual rights.[1, 2] This means that the child must be assessed as to his or her competency to

---

Box 4.1 Relevant statutes and case law

Children Act 1989
Children (Scotland) Act 1995
Age of Legal Capacity (Scotland) Act 1991
Age of Majority Act 1969
Family Law Reform Act 1969
Gillick v West Norfolk and Wisbech AHA [1985], 3 ALL ER 402

Box 4.2 Useful guidelines (see references and useful addresses for full details)

Advisory Committee on Genetic Testing: Advice to ethics committees 1998

Association of Anaesthetists of Great Britain and Ireland: Consent for anaesthesia 1999

Association of British Pharmaceutical Industry: Guidance note: patient information and consents for clinical trials 1997

Declaration of Helsinki updated 1996

European Union: Good clinical practice guidelines 1993

General Medical Council: Seeking patients' consent: the ethical considerations 1998

General Medical Council: Good medical practice 1998

Human Fertilisation and Embryology Authority: Guidelines 1998

Medical Protection Society: Consent 1998

Medical Research Council: The ethical conduct of research on children 1993

Nuffield Council on Bioethics: Human tissue: ethical and legal issues 1995

Royal College of Paediatrics and Child Health: Guidelines for the ethical conduct of medical research involving children 1999

Royal College of Paediatrics and Child Health: Withholding or withdrawing life-saving treatment in children 1998

Royal College of Pathologists: Consensus statement of recommended policies for uses of human tissue in research, education and quality control 1999

Yorkhill Research Ethics Committee: Guidance on good practice for the conduct of research with children 1999

United Nations: Convention on the rights of the child 1997

---

understand what is proposed in terms of treatment or research. The United Nations Convention on the Rights of the Child[2a] states that children should be informed about decisions that affect them and they should be assured that they have the right to express their views freely, these views 'being given weight in accordance with the age and maturity of the child'. If deemed competent, the child's view of whether he or she wishes to give or withhold consent must be respected. At age 16 years, the decision has legal standing as if the patient is an adult. Under age 16 years, the child who is capable of understanding may give or withhold consent. In English law, the withholding of consent may be overridden by a parent, legal guardian or, in exceptional circumstances, by a court if it is in the child's best interests. This applies even when the child is held to be competent or over the age of 16 years. In Scotland, this is not possible.

The difficulty in these situations is in deciding whether children are able to understand what they are consenting to or the implications of withholding their consent. This implies that they must have an explanation in terms that they can understand in written and/or oral form.[1-7] It is good clinical practice to give an explanation concurrently to both parent/guardian and child about the procedure, benefits, risks, alternatives and implications of not proceeding.[1-3] The child's consent alone is legally acceptable if judged competent, but it is good practice to involve the parent/guardian unless issues of confidentiality preclude this. Documentation of all these steps and a summary of the discussions with parent and child in the clinical record are strongly recommended.[1, 2] So, if the child is judged capable of consenting, seek the consent of the child. In Scotland, the parents lose any right they may have had to consent on behalf of a capable child. It is the child's consent alone which is legally effective. This does not mean that those with parental responsibility should be excluded from any discussions and it is reasonable to involve parents in helping the child to reach a decision. In England, a person with parental responsibility or a court may overrule the views of a competent child when it is in the child's best interests. Parents have no right to insist on treatment which is not going to benefit the child.[1, 2, 4] These principles also apply to research with children.[1, 2, 6, 7]

Where a child of less than 16 years of age (and those aged 16–18 years in English law) is *not* competent to give or withhold informed consent, a person with parental responsibility may authorise investigations or treatment which are in the child's best interests. Interventions may also be refused by this individual if they do not feel the intervention is in the child's best interests but this is not binding upon the doctor and a court ruling may be sought. In an emergency, the child may be treated as long as treatment is limited to that which is reasonably needed.[1, 2]

PRACTICAL CONSENT PROBLEMS
Who can consent on behalf of an incapable child?[2, 5, 7, 8]

There may be a court order restricting parental rights and this should be checked. The following may give consent on behalf of an incapable child:

- the child's natural mother, whether married to the father or not;
- the child's natural father if married before or some time after conception. This includes fathers who are subsequently divorced;
- an unmarried father who has entered and registered a formal parental responsibilities and parental rights agreement with the mother;
- a legal guardian nominated in writing by a parent before the parent's death;
- a person holding a court order giving him or her the right to consent on the child's behalf;
- a person who has had delegated to him or her by a parent/legal guardian under a legal ruling the right to consent to medical procedures or treatment of the child. The court must have removed this right from parents. Parents may have full, shared or no parental responsibility if the child is subject to supervision from the local authority;
- a person aged 16 years or more who has been given care and control of the child (e.g. foster carers, grandparents, the local authority) except those involved in the setting of school and for procedures such as organ donation, non-therapeutic research or non-therapeutic treatment (e.g. cosmetic surgery).

When can a court dispense with the need for parental consent?

A court may grant authority for the medical examination and/or treatment of a child without the need for parental consent. This could be by means of a child protection or assessment order, a warrant for detention of a child in a place of safety or a supervision order from a children's hearing. However, it is important to realise that a child can still refuse and, if the child is adjudged capable by the attending doctor, the examination, procedure or treatment cannot proceed.

Consent for anaesthesia, anaesthetic procedures and analgesia techniques[5]

It is important that anaesthetists discuss the anaesthetic and analgesic techniques with children and their parents/guardians in terms that they can understand. General consent for anaesthesia is incorporated into the operation consent form but it is good practice to give a verbal explanation and to take verbal consent from the child and parent/guardian and to document these. This is particularly important for major cases, for invasive procedures and for analgesia techniques. Regional anaesthesia, central neuraxial block, patient-controlled analgesia (PCA) and analgesia in suppository form require specific explanation. At present, written consent documents for each anaesthetic or analgesic intervention are not required in the UK and the general consent process reinforced by verbal detail is acceptable. A note in the clinical record or on the anaesthetic chart about the explanation given is recommended. Many centres have both general and also specific written information sheets for parents and children about anaesthetic and analgesic procedures and recently the Royal College of Anaesthetists has produced downloadable templates on its website (www.rcoa.ac.uk). These may be included in the written information about the specific surgical procedure, about surgery in general (e.g. day surgery) or may be specifically about an analgesic technique such as epidurals or PCA. Most parents and children welcome this extra information.

What if the parents are not present when you visit the child to discuss anaesthesia and analgesia?

For elective work, it is wise to discuss the proposed anaesthetic and analgesic techniques with the child if competent and a person with parental responsibility face to face and to document this. Circumstances may prevent direct parental contact and a telephone contact is acceptable but should be witnessed and documented. If a parent/guardian is not contactable, this should be documented in the case record or on the anaesthetic chart and consideration given as to whether to proceed depending on the invasiveness and risks of the proposed techniques, the urgency of the clinical situation and the competence of the child. For emergency procedures, it would be reasonable to proceed without parental contact if it is in the best interests of the child that there should be no delay. In these situations, good documentation of the circumstances in the case record is essential.[1, 2, 5, 6]

What do you do if parents or those with parental responsibilities disagree?

This can be a difficult situation and may require detailed discussion, explanation and further investigation of the precise relationships of those with parental rights to each other and to the child. It is wise to try to negotiate agreement between family members but the natural parents do have priority in most situations if they are acting in the best interests of the child. As noted above, the parental responsibilities can be delegated in a variety of ways and this may add to the complexity of individual cases. In cases of dispute, it is wise to delay until a solution is agreed if this is possible.

What do you do if parent and child disagree?

The competent child has the right to consent or withhold consent as noted above. The parent may not overrule this in Scottish law but may in English law if he or she is found by legal ruling to be acting in the child's best interests. This applies up to age 18 years in the English jurisdiction.

What do you do in an emergency?

You must act in the best interests of the child with his or her consent or that of the parent or guardian where possible. Where time does not allow consent, life-saving treatment may be started and treatment given should be limited to that which is reasonably needed. An explanation to the parents should be given as soon as possible and the circumstances should be documented in the clinical record. If an apparently competent child refuses emergency treatment, it may be possible to proceed in England if you can demonstrate that you are acting in the child's best interests. If such a situation was challenged in court, the court will tend to support the doctor's actions and may also question the competence of the child.

What do you do if the child refuses anaesthesia?

For elective work, you should not proceed if the child is judged to be capable, as noted above. This may be inconvenient and upsetting to the child, parent and hospital but the child's view has to be accepted. Time may allow options to be explored, such as premedication, varying the method of induction of anaesthesia, involving the parent in the induction process and sometimes techniques such as hypnosis, guided imagery and distraction. The surgery may be rescheduled later on the same day or at a later date if agreement can be secured. It is important to state that the competent child must consent before premedication or other behavioural technique is embarked upon and may, even then, refuse!

For an incapable child who is demonstrating that he or she does not want you to proceed, the parent/guardian should be closely involved in the decision to proceed for elective work. Premedication and parental involvement in the induction are helpful, with the parent holding and gently restraining the child on his or her lap during the induction phase. With modern induction techniques this can usually be accomplished very quickly with the minimum of distress. For emergency work, refusal of a competent child is a difficult situation as the consequences of not proceeding could be detrimental to the child. Further explanation of the implications of refusal should be given to the child and to the parents and a resolution negotiated. In Scottish law, the child cannot be legally overruled if deemed competent. However, some would doubt whether the child could be deemed to be competent if refusing reasonable treatment. In such rare and difficult cases a second opinion and good documentation are recommended.

What do you do if the mother of the child is herself less than age 16 years?

This situation seems to be arising more often. Most recommend concurrent discussion with the natural mother and with her parent if confidentiality issues allow. A judgement about the capability of the natural mother would have to be made and consent documented appropriately. Some recommend countersignature by both the child's parent and grandparent and documentation of the circumstances in the clinical record as a sensible solution.

Is the parental wish for circumcision in a male infant acceptable?[4]

Circumcision raises difficult questions about the rights and freedoms of individuals. Many people maintain that individuals have a right to practise their religion unhindered. Others feel that it is unequivocally wrong to undertake a non-therapeutic surgical procedure, with its attendant risks, on an infant who is unable to consent. These are not solely medical matters and they cannot be resolved by the medical profession alone. They are matters for society as a whole to decide. Male circumcision is considered by many in the Jewish and Islamic faiths to be essential to the practice of their religion; they would regard any restriction or ban on male circumcision as an infringement of a fundamental human right. Many also believe that if doctors were prevented from carrying out the procedure, parents would turn in greater numbers to individuals who lack the skills and experience to perform it safely and competently. Others, including those who campaign against the practice of male circumcision, strongly believe that, because circumcision for non-therapeutic reasons carries risks, it is wrong to perform the procedure on children who are not old enough to give informed consent. In 1993 the Law Commission[4a] issued a consultation paper on consent in the criminal law. This paper argues that male circumcision is lawful in the UK, but this point has been challenged. Article 24.3 of the United Nations Convention on the Rights of the Child (ratified by the UK government in 1991) states that ratifying states should 'take all effective and appropriate measures with a view to abolishing traditional practices prejudicial to the health of children'. However, this must be balanced against Article 9.2 of the European Convention on Human Rights[4b] which protects the rights of individuals to practise their religion. The legal position is untested in the UK in the context of circumcision and therefore remains unclear.

There is also a wide variation of views on the role of the medical profession. Many believe that doctors have a duty to provide the public with objective information about circumcision; and that they should be obliged to provide counselling to parents before and after circumcising their child. Others believe that doctors should not put undue emphasis on the risks of the procedure, because there is insufficient evidence to justify worrying parents about them. Similarly, there is a body of opinion that because circumcision has very few medical benefits, and the potential dangers to the child far outweigh these, circumcision is inappropriate under any circumstances. Other people believe that circumcision causes no harm, and may be beneficial; some would recommend performing the procedure routinely.

The welfare of infants who are circumcised must be paramount, whatever the reason for undertaking the procedure. Any medical procedure must be undertaken in hygienic conditions, with appropriate pain relief and aftercare. If a doctor decides to circumcise a male child he or she must have the necessary skills and experience to perform the operation and use appropriate measures, including anaesthesia, to minimise pain and discomfort. The doctor must keep up to date with developments in the practice of male circumcision, including when the procedure is, and is not, necessary for medical reasons. The doctor must explain objectively to those with parental responsibility for the child any benefits or risks of the procedure, taking into account the age of the child. He or she must explain to those with parental responsibility that they may invite their religious advisor to be present at the circumcision to give advice on how the procedure should be performed to meet the requirements of their faith. The doctor must listen to those with parental responsibility and give careful consideration to their views. A doctor is not obliged to act on a request to circumcise a child, but an explanation should be given that you are opposed to circumcision other than for therapeutic reasons. Those with parental responsibility have a right to see another doctor. It is good practice to obtain the permission of both parents whenever possible, but in all cases obtain valid consent, in writing, from a person with parental responsibility before performing the procedure. Appropriate aftercare must be ensured (Box 4.3).

Can you refuse to anaesthetise a child?

You may be a conscientious objector to elective non-therapeutic procedures such as circumcision for religious or cultural reasons. You should be honest with the parents about your views but you should attempt to refer the case to a suitable qualified colleague prepared to undertake it. In an emergency, you are obliged to provide appropriate care.[1, 2, 4, 5]

Box 4.3 Summary of General Medical Council guidance on male circumcision 1998[4]

- Male circumcision is lawful with appropriate consent and information
- Ensure good clinical practice standards are met
- Consider each case as an individual
- Ensure written parental informed consent

How should you manage the child of Jehovah's Witnesses?[7]

The well-being of the child is overriding. In an emergency situation where the child is likely to succumb without the immediate administration of blood, then blood should be given without consulting a court and the court is likely to uphold the decision. In an elective situation, where parents refuse consent for transfusion, it may be necessary to apply to a court for a specific issue order but only after two consultants make a declaration in the case record that blood transfusion is essential to save life or prevent serious permanent harm. The parents should be told that this is to be done and should be properly represented in court. The Jehovah's Witness Hospital Liaison Committee can help come to a clear understanding about how individual situations can be resolved depending on the beliefs and wishes of the child and the parents.[7] The Children Acts in Scotland and England also apply in this situation in terms of competence of children to give their own consent and whether parents may override their wishes (see above). In the elective situation an individual anaesthetist may decline to take part in the care of a Jehovah's Witness and refer the case to a colleague but in an emergency is obliged to provide appropriate care.

Consent for medical imaging, video or audio recordings[9]

When photographs are to be taken as part of the confidential clinical record, it is acceptable to obtain verbal consent following discussion with a competent child supported by his or her parent or legal guardian, who may consent on behalf of a child who is not competent in his or her own right. When photographs are required for forensic, child protection or medicolegal reasons it may be inappropriate to seek consent. When photographs or videos are to be used for teaching of professional staff or students, written consent is necessary where patients are identifiable and is recommended even when patients are not identifiable. When photographs or videos are to be used for research, written informed consent *must* be obtained. The research protocol must have the approval of the Local Research Ethics Committee (LREC). The information and consent documentation should include specific mention of photographs, videos and electronic publishing where these are to be used. It must be explicitly stated whether the patient will be identifiable from these images or not and what type of publication will be used. Provided this is done, it will not be necessary to use a separate, additional consent form for photographs or videos for research. When photographs or videos are to be used for publication in journals, textbooks or electronic media, specific written informed consent will be needed if the patient is identifiable and is recommended if the patient is not identifiable. Consent should be taken by a suitably qualified member of staff and documented in the case record. It is recommended that both child and parent/guardian sign the form if this is possible.[8, 10]

INTENSIVE CARE ISSUES[1, 6, 11, 12]

The legal and ethical framework for decision-making in paediatric intensive care is more complex than in adult practice. Although the primary duty of care is to the child, the decisions usually involve parents or guardians acting as advocates for the child. It is important that good lines of communication are established as soon as possible between the paediatric intensive care unit staff and the parents or guardians because changes in the child's condition can happen very rapidly. The paediatric intensive care unit environment is complex and interventions must often be immediate before fully informed consent can be obtained. Each case must be considered individually, with the overriding principle of acting at all times in the best interests of the child within the prevailing locally determined medical, social and legal rules.

Parents can make decisions on behalf of an incapable child as long as this power is exercised reasonably and in the best interests of the child. It is good practice to keep parents fully informed about their child's condition and the level of life support required. Often in paediatric intensive care, life-saving measures have to be undertaken without specific consent because parents are not immediately available. Parents should be forewarned that this problem may occur during their child's stay in the unit. A good example is the need for emergency insertion of a chest drain for relief of a tension pneumothorax. The law will support such an intervention without specific written or verbal consent as it will assume that any reasonable parent would have given consent. Where it is not possible to gain consent in such a situation, the reasons should be noted in the case record and a confirmatory note from a second doctor is advisable. For non-life-saving interventions, parental consent should be sought. In most situations this is not a problem after risks and benefits are explained but what if the parent refuses? Parental refusal of life-saving treatment should be overruled by the child's right to live, but only in an emergency situation. Otherwise, the courts will have to decide.

Some invasive procedures are regarded as routine as opposed to extraordinary in paediatric intensive care (e.g. intubation, ventilatory support, insertion of intravascular monitoring lines). The list of conventional treatment interventions is expanding all the time to include new modes of ventilation, extracorporeal life support, nitric oxide and surfactant. Discussion with parents and information in both verbal and written form about risks and benefits of treatment are recommended. When techniques are part of a clinical trial, specific written informed consent is necessary. In such trials, control patients are usually offered conventional therapy and study patients receive the new treatment. If clear benefit is demonstrated, then it becomes ethically difficult to complete the study, i.e. the new treatment has become conventional. Parents may not be happy that their child is randomised to the group who will not receive the promising new treatment and may withhold consent. This is a difficult area as, unless well-conducted trials with sufficient patient numbers are performed, false clinical impressions of benefit may be gained and risks may not be revealed. The 'ethical window' for conducting such studies may only be open for a short time as new innovations are rapidly incorporated into clinical practice. It then becomes a problem not to use the technique if it is available and may be of benefit.

Beneficial treatment should be started and not withdrawn. Non-beneficial or futile treatment should not be started. Obtaining agreement that the situation is futile for an individual child may take some time to achieve, while the intervention needed is often urgent. To allow time for clarification that the situation is futile and to reach a consensus amongst staff and agreement with parents or guardians, treatment may have to be started but may be withdrawn later. However, difficulties can arise if agreement cannot be achieved. Disagreement between medical staff about the prognosis, disagreement between parents or between staff and parents may all lead to problems which can only be resolved with legal guidance or intervention. Parental pressure in favour of futile treatment or non-treatment should not be allowed to override the best interests of the child as determined by local medical, social and legal rules. It is best if an agreement between staff and parents can be achieved and documented but, for difficult cases, the courts should be involved.

Withdrawal of intensive care when it will not benefit the patient is acceptable ethically but must be fully discussed with relatives and staff and must be carried out tactfully and compassionately. A good unit will involve counsellors, religious advisors, support volunteers and support groups and will arrange follow-up contact with the family. Where withdrawal of intensive care is appropriate, the comfort of the child should be the first priority in the care given. Warmth, cleanliness, hygiene, oral feeds or fluids, human touch and pain relief are all essential components of comfort. These comforting measures may prolong the dying process but the quality of the process will be enhanced and the extra time for parents to adapt to the inevitable can be helpful. In some cases, parents may ask to take their child home to die and if possible this request should be accommodated. Recent well-publicised cases cannot be used as models for how to proceed in individual paediatric cases and each case must be considered separately with advice from the court if necessary.[12] This includes the problems of withdrawal of tube feeding and persistent vegetative state. A major difficulty in this field is the inaccuracy of paediatric neurological prognosis.

ORGAN RETRIEVAL AND DONATION IN CHILDREN[11]

Organ retrieval from children for donation is only possible if the child has been diagnosed as brainstem-dead. The criteria for establishing brainstem death are in principle the same in children over 2 months of age as in adults. Preconditions for applying the tests of brainstem death must be satisfied. In a patient who is comatose and mechanically ventilated for apnoea and in whom the diagnosis of structural brain damage has been established or in whom the immediate cause of coma is known, tests of brainstem function may be performed provided hypothermia, neuromuscular blockade, drug-induced coma, endocrine and metabolic disturbances have been excluded. Measurement of blood concentrations of sedatives and use of a nerve stimulator to exclude residual neuromuscular blockade are helpful in those children who have received sedatives and muscle relaxants. The tests of brainstem death should be performed by senior staff on two separate occasions. The pupillary response to light, corneal reflex, vestibulo-ocular reflex, doll's-eye reflex, motor response to pain in the distribution of the fifth cranial nerve, gag reflex in response to suctioning and apnoea in the presence of normal arterial oxygen and high arterial carbon dioxide levels are all checked.

It is rarely possible to diagnose brainstem death in infants less than 2 months of age and for babies less than 37 weeks' postconceptional age: the concept of brainstem death is probably inappropriate. Thus organ retrieval is unlikely to be achievable from children less than 2 months old. Harvesting of organs from anencephalic donors is also regarded as unacceptable in most countries because of the difficulty in defining brainstem death in these infants.

For healthy children to be allowed to act as donors of organs usually to siblings, the risks and benefits must be carefully discussed. The risk assessment depends upon the regenerative capacity of the tissue or organ being donated. Thus donating blood is less risky than donating bone marrow, skin, a lobe of liver or a kidney. These procedures are not therapeutic as far as the donor is concerned and are potentially harmful to the donor. The consideration that the donor may suffer some psychological harm if the donation does not proceed has also been taken into account in previous cases and the donor's level of understanding and ability to consent must also be considered. In the UK and some other countries, donation of non-regenerative organs from children is not regarded as being ethically acceptable and, with regard to partial liver donations, most authorities advise that the risks to a paediatric donor of the surgical resection outweigh the benefits.

CONSENT TO POSTMORTEM EXAMINATION

The difficult issue of consent for postmortem examination and the use of human tissues for diagnosis, research, education and quality control has been considered in detail in a number of recent reports.[13-18] Written information is helpful to parents to augment detailed verbal discussion.

RESEARCH ISSUES[1-7, 19-22]

For participation in research, it is good practice to seek consent from children and parents/guardians simultaneously unless issues of confidentiality are relevant and overriding. It is strongly recommended that recruitment should proceed only if both child and parent/guardian agree to inclusion, whatever the child's age and maturity. There is no lower age limit on the need to seek consent from the child but a judgement must be made about the child's ability to understand the information and consent documents and verbal explanations. The researcher alone should not make this judgement and the opinion of the lead consultant should be sought in cases of doubt.

There must be valid reasons why research involves vulnerable groups such as children – could this study be carried out in adults? Subjects should always be positively opting in to the research programme on the basis of fully informed written consent and should not be required to opt out of involvement in the research. For research in schools, it must be made clear whether research is therapeutic or non-therapeutic in nature, whether questionnaires or measurements are involved and the invasiveness of these. Consent must be of the opt-in type and opting-out consent is not acceptable. The child, parent, guardian, school authority and local education authority must be involved in the consent procedures. These principles apply to study subjects, controls and surveys for normative data. In general, to avoid multiple approaches for consent and to minimise risks and potential interactions, no subject should be enrolled in more than one research programme without careful consideration. It is the researcher's responsibility to check with the lead consultant, the general practitioner, case records, patient, parent/guardian and child as appropriate. Careful consideration must be given to the methods of recruitment, consent procedures and selection of control groups. Particular care is needed in assessing risks and benefits. Controls should get the best current standard of care or treatment and it is worth considering whether the subject could act as his or her own control, as this would involve fewer patients. If the study has a cross-over design, the consequences of discontinuation or changing of effective active treatment must be given due consideration. When placebo-controlled studies are proposed, the ethical aspects of study design must be given very careful thought, e.g. trials of analgesia. Information sheets must clearly explain the nature of random allocation, blinding and placebos if appropriate.

If research does not entail direct benefit to the subjects, the risks to them must be minimal. Minimal risk (the least possible risk) describes procedures such as questioning, observing and measuring children, provided that procedures are carried out in a sensitive way. Procedures with minimal risk include collecting a single urine sample (but not by aspiration), using blood from a sample that has been taken as part of investigation or treatment or taking an extra volume of blood from an indwelling line provided the total volume removed for research purposes is within the LREC guidelines.

Good clinical practice demands that obtaining blood samples from all children can and should be carried out without causing pain or distress to the child. Children should be given an explanation in words which they can understand. Local anaesthetic cream should be applied appropriately and venepuncture is preferable. The procedure should be carried out by an experienced person; extra blood for research purposes should only be obtained if the child and parents are willing and there are no signs of distress in the child or parents as observed by an independent observer. This approach balances the rights of the individual child, the need for the continuation of research in children, established custom and practice of research involving children and current legal opinion on consent by parents of an incapable child. Some LRECs will accept consent from a parent of a child who is incapable of giving his or her own consent to participate in non-therapeutic research if that research does not include procedures which are minimal-risk or less.

If a drug is to be tested on children there should usually be evidence of efficacy and safety in adults and the drug will usually have a licence for use in adults. It is recognised that this may not always be the case if children are likely to benefit from the drug more than adults (e.g. surfactant). It is the responsibility of researchers to ensure that they have the necessary trial certificates and they should communicate with the Medicines Control Agency if required. The pharmaceutical industry is moving towards concurrent evaluation of drugs in adults and children prior to licensing, as recently recommended by the US Food and Drug Administration. The information sheet should make explicit the current licence status of drugs. For new medical devices, the trial should be registered with Safety and

Efficacy Register of New Interventional Procedures (SERNIP), Academy of Medical Royal Colleges, 1 Wimpole Street, London W1M 8AE. Appropriate safety nets must be in place if things go wrong and so insurance/indemnity provisions such as recommended by the Association of the British Pharmaceutical Industry should be followed and details of the insurance arrangements must be incorporated into the patient information sheets.

Subjects' rights to privacy and confidentiality must be preserved. The terms of the Data Protection Act must be observed and subjects should be identified on documentation by a study number or hospital number only. If information is to be revealed, for example by drug company monitors, this must be explained in the information and consent documentation. If a child's affairs are to be discussed with a parent the child should be asked for permission to do so if confidentiality will otherwise be breached.

Participation must be voluntary and there must be no inducement or coercion to take part. Subjects and parents/guardians must have the right to decline to participate or withdraw at any stage without prejudice to care and without having to give a reason.

For use of surgical tissue that would otherwise be discarded, such as tonsils, foreskin and bone, consent should be obtained and the research detailed. In particular the duration of culture of cell lines should be defined.

For postmortem tissue such as pathological samples, aborted material and early pregnancy loss, termination of pregnancy, stillbirth, neonatal deaths and paediatric deaths, the guidelines from the Royal College of Pathologists, the Royal College of Obstetricians and Gynaecologists, the Human Fertilization and Embryology Authority and the Advisory Committee on Genetic Testing should be followed.[3, 13–17, 21]

There are often implications of positive results of genetic research for insurance, relatives and offspring and an adequate safety net of confidentiality and counselling must be ensured. Separate consent will be needed for testing family members, siblings and offspring.

Information and consent documents should be in plain English with a minimum of medical jargon. They should be distributed in advance, allowing a cooling-off period before a decision on consent is required. The parent and child should be given the opportunity to discuss the project with the researcher, have their questions answered and verbal explanations of the project given. The timing of the process of taking consent must be given careful thought (e.g. in day surgery). Written information which is to form the basis for gaining consent should include the following details:

- full title of study, investigators, department and hospital;
- an invitation to take part in the study;
- that it is a research study;
- the purpose of the study;
- a clear description of what it will involve;
- any trial treatment and whether there will be random assignment to each treatment;
- procedures to be followed, including all invasive procedures;
- the subject's responsibilities;
- those aspects of the trial that are experimental;
- the reasonably foreseeable risks or inconveniences to the subject;
- the reasonably expected benefits – where there is no intended (clinical) benefit to subjects, they should be made aware of this;
- the alternatives that may be available to the subject and their important potential benefits and risks;
- the compensation available to the subject in the event of trial-related injury;
- the treatment available to the subject in the event of trial-related injury;
- any anticipated expenses or payment to be refunded for participation;
- that participation is voluntary and that it is permissible to decline at any time without stating a reason and that this will not affect treatment

- that consent may be withdrawn at any time without giving a reason and that this will not affect care;
- that access may be required to confidential medical records;
- if the results are published, the subject's identity will remain confidential;
- any foreseeable circumstances and/or reasons under which the subject's participation in the research may be terminated;
- the expected duration of the subject's participation in the study;
- that the general practitioner will be informed of participation in the study;
- that the study has the approval of the LREC.

Recent problems faced by one LREC include genetic testing, use of staff blood samples for epidemiological research into hepatitis C, human immunodeficiecny virus testing as part of research protocols, extra non-therapeutic blood sampling from infants and ovarian storage prior to chemotherapy for later use for in vitro fertilisation in the surviving patient.

USEFUL ADDRESSES

- Advisory Committee on Genetic Testing (ACGT), ACGT Secretariat, Department of Health, Room 401, Wellington House, 133–135 Waterloo Road, London SE1 8UG
- Association of the British Pharmaceutical Industry (ABPI), 12 Whitehall, London SW1A 2DY
- General Medical Council, 178–202 Great Portland Street, London W1N 6JE http:\\www.gmc-uk.org
- Human Fertilization and Embryology Authority http:\\www.hfea.gov.uk
- Medical Research Council, 20 Park Crescent, London W1N 4AL
- Nuffield Council on Bioethics, 28 Bedford Square, London WC1B 3EG
- Royal College of Paediatrics and Child Health (RCPCH), 50 Hallam Street, London W1N 6DE http:\\www.rcpch.ac.uk
- Royal College of Pathologists, 2 Carlton House Terrace, London SW1Y 5AF http:\\www. rcpath.org

REFERENCES

1. General Medical Council. Good medical practice. London: General Medical Council; 1998.
2. General Medical Council. Seeking patients' consent: the ethical considerations. London: General Medical Council; 1998.
2a. United Nations Convention on the Rights of the Child. New York: UN; 2000.
3. Yorkhill Research Ethics Committee. Guidance on good practice for the conduct of research with children. Glasgow: Yorkhill Research Ethics Committee; 1999.
4. General Medical Council. Guidance on circumcision in children. London: General Medical Council; 1997.
4a. Law Commission: R v Brown [1993] 2 All ER 75, HL.
4b. European Convention on Human Rights. Strasbourg: Council of Europe; 1966.
5. Association of Anaesthetists of Great Britain and Ireland. Consent for anaesthesia. London: Association of Anaesthetists of Great Britain and Ireland; 1999.
6. Evans D, Evans M. What is this thing called consent? In: Evans EM, ed. a decent proposal: ethical review of clinical research. Chichester: Wiley; 1996:78–103.
7. Association of Anaesthetists of Great Britain and Ireland. Management of anaesthesia for Jehovah's Witnesses. London: Association of Anaesthetists of Great Britain and Ireland; 1999.
8. Anonymous. Videos, photographs and patient consent. Br Med J 1998; 316:1009–1011.
9. General Medical Council. Making and using visual and audio recordings of patients. London: General Medical Council; 1997.
10. Anonymous. Protection of patients' rights to privacy. Br Med J 1995; 311:1172.
11. Morton N. Paediatric issues. In: Pace NA, ed. Ethics and the law in intensive care. Oxford: Oxford University Press; 1996:125–133.
12. Royal College of Paediatrics and Child Health. Withholding or withdrawing life saving treatment in children. London: Royal College of Paediatrics and Child Health; 1997.
13. Confidential Enquiry into Stillbirths and Deaths in Infancy. The fetal and infant postmortem. London: Confidential Enquiry into Stillbirths and Deaths in Infancy (CESDI); 1999.

14. Scottish Office Department of Health. Code of practice on the use of fetuses and fetal material in research and treatment. Edinburgh: Scottish Office Department of Health; 1995.
15. Royal College of Pathologists. The retention and storage of pathological records and archives. London: Royal College of Pathologists and the Institute of Biomedical Science; 1999.
16. Royal College of Pathologists. Consensus statement of recommended policies for uses of human tissue in research, education and quality control. London: Royal College of Pathologists and the Institute of Biomedical Science; 1999.
17. Nuffield Council on Bioethics. Human tissue: ethical and legal issues. London: Nuffield Council on Bioethics; 1995.
18. HMSO. Review of the guidance on the research use of fetuses and fetal material (the Polkinghorne report). London: HMSO; 1989.
19. IFPMA. Guideline for good clinical practice. International conference on harmonisation of technical requirements for registration of pharmaceuticals for human use (ICH harmonised tripartite guidelines). Geneva: International Federation of Pharmaceutic Manufacturers Associations; 1997.
20. Royal College of Physicians. Guidelines on the practice of ethics committees involved in medical research involving human subjects, 3rd edn. London: Royal College of Physicians; 1996.
21. Royal College of Obstetricians and Gynaecologists. Ethical considerations relating to good practice in obstetrics and gynaecology. London: Royal College of Obstetricians and Gynaecologists; 1997.
22. Advisory Committee on Genetic Testing. ACGT advice to ethics committees. London: Advisory Committee on Genetic Testing; 1998.

FURTHER READING

Consent, rights and choices in health care for children and young people. London: British Medical Association; 2000.

CHAPTER 5

Day-case anaesthesia and pain control

Neil S Morton

STANDARDS

The multidisciplinary report *Just for the Day*[1] set out 12 quality standards for care of paediatric day cases (Box 5.1). These apply whether children are managed in a specialist paediatric unit or in an adult unit which has been adapted for children.

The important principles which can be drawn from these standards are that children should be managed by staff trained in their care, in appropriate child-friendly and child-safe facilities with free parental access to the conscious child. Preschool paediatric patients gain particular benefit from well-planned and conducted day care because separation from parents is reduced. For older children and parents the disruption to schooling and work is minimised.

PATIENT SELECTION[2, 3]

The range of procedures which can be carried out on a day-stay basis in children is quite broad (Table 5.1) but where there is a significant risk of postoperative haemorrhage (e.g. adenotonsillectomy), the likelihood of prolonged postoperative pain requiring complex pain control (e.g. many orthopaedic procedures) or operations involving opening of a body cavity, inpatient care is required. Even when a given procedure is technically feasible as a day case there may be other reasons for excluding this option related to the age, maturity, medical condition, anaesthetic risk factors or social circumstances of the child (Box 5.2).

Box 5.1 Twelve quality standards for paediatric day care[1]

1. Integrate the admission plan to include preadmission, day of admission and postadmission care with planned transfer of care to primary care and /or community services
2. Prepare the child and parents before and during the day of admission
3. Give specific written information to parents
4. Admit the child to an area designated for day cases and do not mix with acutely ill inpatients
5. Do not admit or treat children alongside adults
6. Specifically designated day-case staff should care for the child
7. Trained paediatric staff should be used
8. Organise care so that every child is likely to be discharged within the day
9. Ensure that the building, equipment and furnishings comply with paediatric safety standards
10. Ensure that the environment is child-friendly
11. Complete essential documents before each child goes home to ensure aftercare and follow-up are seamless
12. Establish paediatric nursing support for the child at home

Surgeons, paediatricians and anaesthetists may vary in their views about the suitability of individual procedures or patients. Some feel that bilateral procedures, orchidopexy, hypospadias correction, strabismus correction or prominent-ear correction are too difficult to manage as day cases but many units have developed techniques to manage all of these successfully. Attitudes are changing with regard to the management of adenoidectomy and adenotonsillectomy. More units in Europe and the UK are moving towards North American-style same-day care for adenoidectomy with a postoperative observation period of 4–12 h and short overnight stay for paediatric tonsillectomy ± adenoidectomy. The risks and benefits of this approach must be weighed for each individual child. Cases should be carefully selected according to the exclusion criteria in Box 5.2 and factors such as the experience of the

Table 5.1 Range of paediatric day-case procedures

Therapeutic	Diagnostic
SURGICAL	
General, e.g. herniotomy, hydrocele	Endoscopy ± biopsies
Urological,: e.g. circumcision, orchidopexy	Examinations under anaesthesia
Ear, nose and throat, e.g. myringotomy	Evoked-response audiometry
Dental, e.g. extractions	Measurement of intraocular pressure
Ophthalmology, e.g. squint correction	Biopsy: skin, bone, muscle, lymph node
Orthopaedics, e.g. change of plaster cast	Arthroscopy, arthrograms
Plastic surgery, e.g. prominent-ear surgery	
MEDICAL	
Venesection	Blood sampling
Intrathecal injection	Bone marrow sampling
Radiotherapy	Lumbar puncture
Change of urinary catheter	Needle aspiration cytology
Interventional radiology/cardiology	Metabolic/endocrine tests
	Computed tomography, magnetic resonance imaging and other scans

Box 5.2 Exclusion criteria for paediatric day-case anaesthesia

ANAESTHETIC AND SURGICAL FACTORS
- Prolonged surgery and anaesthesia (> 1 h)
- Junior unsupervised staff
- The occasional paediatric or neonatal case: surgeon and anaesthetist must be suitably trained and carrying out such cases regularly
- Opening of body cavity
- Significant risk of haemorrhage or body fluid loss requiring replacement
- Prolonged postoperative pain
- Difficult airway
- Sleep apnoea
- Malignant hyperthermia

AGE
- Preterm or ex-preterm baby of < 60 weeks' postconceptional age
- Significant ongoing problems related to prematurity
- Full-term neonate ≥ 37 weeks' postconceptional age where no inpatient neonatal care is available

MEDICAL FACTORS
- Poorly controlled systemic disease (e.g. epilepsy, asthma, cardiac disease)
- Uninvestigated heart murmur
- Metabolic disorders
- Diabetes mellitus
- Haemoglobinopathy
- Active infection (especially of respiratory tract, pertussis, respiratory syncytial virus, measles)

SOCIAL FACTORS
- Parent unwilling or unable to care for child at home
- The very anxious parent or child
- Single-parent family with many siblings and no help
- Poor housing conditions
- No telephone
- Inadequate personal transport
- Long distance or travelling time of > 1 h by car from hospital
- Sibling of victim of sudden infant death syndrome (SIDS)

surgeon, pain control, nausea and vomiting, bleeding, postextubation airway problems and re-establishment of oral fluid and dietary intake must be carefully dealt with to ensure success. Good follow-up after discharge and rapid access to help at home are particularly important for this patient group and the call-out rate to the general practitioner may be high.[2–4] Same-day paediatric tonsillectomy or adenotonsillectomy is not currently recommended in the UK.

The lower age limit for day-case surgery depends on the facilities available, the experience of staff and the workload. The healthy full-term neonate can safely undergo brief day-case surgery provided none of the other exclusion criteria apply and there is access to inpatient neonatal care if required. The preterm or ex-preterm neonate should not be considered for day care before 60 weeks' postconceptual age because of the risk of perioperative apnoea and, even beyond that age, other complications or sequelae of prematurity may preclude day-case management.

The child with an infection should have surgery postponed for at least 2 weeks after symptoms have resolved and if there is evidence of lower respiratory tract involvement, this delay should be extended to 4 weeks. If the child has measles, pertussis or respiratory syncytial virus infection, a delay of 6 weeks is recommended as respiratory tract irritability is so troublesome.[5] Beware the child with features such as purulent crusting around the nose, pyrexia, lethargy, productive cough and chest signs.[6] Chronic, non-purulent nasal discharge and non-productive cough are very common in children and there is no benefit in postponing their procedure provided they are otherwise suitable for day care.

Most paediatric day cases will be normal healthy children (American Society of Anesthesiology (ASA) 1) with a specific, often congenital problem requiring investigation or treatment. Those with mild systemic disease (ASA 2) and well-controlled more severe disease (ASA 3) can also be managed as day cases and this includes those with stable asthma, epilepsy and simple corrected congenital heart defects. Antibiotic prophylaxis is required for those in whom prosthetic material or pericardial patches have been used. The child with a heart murmur should not proceed to day surgery until further investigation has been carried out to determine its cause and paediatric cardiological advice should be sought. Clinical examination, ultrasound and electrocardiogram will elucidate the cause in most cases and those infants under age 1 year merit particular caution.[7] (See also p 114–116, Tables 6.2 A–C.)

PREPARATION OF CHILD AND PARENTS

Preparation for day care begins at the initial outpatient clinic visit. A clear verbal explanation to parents and child about what is to happen should be backed up by written information in the form of general instructions about day surgery and specific details about where to go, what time to arrive, what to expect for this particular surgical procedure and clear guidance about preoperative fasting. A preadmission programme is very useful for teaching the child and parents about the day-surgery unit's facilities, staff and ways of working.[1] A visit to the unit at an arranged 'Saturday club' or special introductory session can be used to great effect in allaying fears and anxieties. Toys, games, computer games, colouring books, videos and play therapy can all be employed depending on the child's age and maturity. Visits to the anaesthetic induction room and recovery area are very helpful and the types of anaesthesia, pain relief and postoperative care can be discussed with the parents and child. Badges and certificates of bravery or achievement are useful in young children. Preadmission clinics where physical examination, preoperative screening checks and blood tests are carried out can be useful in reducing cancellation of cases but the vast majority of paediatric day cases do not need preoperative investigations or tests. Telephone contact on the day before surgery is useful and gives an opportunity to re-emphasise preoperative instructions, to confirm attendance and to rule out last-minute reasons for postponement such as infections, travel difficulties or family problems. A reserve list can be held to replace these last-minute cancellations so that the operating session is used efficiently.

Fasting

The 643 fasting rules (Box 5.3) are easy to teach, although difficult to achieve in practice.[8, 9]

This scheme strikes a validated safe balance between prolonged fasting with the attendant risks of dehydration and hypoglycaemia and the risks of regurgitation and aspiration of gastric contents. Clear written instructions to parents with specific times may be helpful with a statement about encouraging clear fluid intake until a specified time. Those children listed for surgery in the morning should have different timed instructions from those whose

---

Box 5.3 Fasting rules

- 6 h for solids, milk or milky drinks
- 4 h for breast-fed infants
- 3 h for clear fluids, including fruit juices, fizzy drinks, water, tea and coffee without milk

> **Box 5.4** Examples of written fasting instructions
>
> **(A) FOR MORNING OPERATING LIST STARTING AT 0900 H**
>
> - _____ must have no food, milk or milky drinks after 0300 a.m. A drink of juice or water should be encouraged up to 0600 a.m. After that time, no food or drink should be taken
> - If your child is breast-fed, the last feed should be at 0500 a.m.
> - You should understand that for safety reasons the surgery will be postponed or cancelled if you do not follow these instructions
>
> **(B) FOR AFTERNOON OPERATING LIST STARTING AT 1330 H**
>
> - _____ must have no food, milk or milky drinks after 0730 a.m. A drink of juice or water should be encouraged up to 1030 a.m. After that time, no food or drink should be taken
> - If your child is breast-fed the last feed should be at 0930 a.m.
> - You should not starve your child from the night before his or her operation as this can cause dehydration and a low blood sugar level
> - You should understand that for safety reasons the surgery will be postponed or cancelled if you do not follow these instructions

surgery is to be in the afternoon. Examples are given in Box 5.4. The time of last intake of solids, milk or clear fluids should be noted on admission and if the child has been fasted for an excessively long time, and, especially if he or she weighs < 15 kg, consideration should be given to placing that child further down the operating list and giving a clear fluid drink under controlled circumstances on arrival. It must be stressed to parents that prolonged starvation can be harmful and children presenting for surgery in the afternoon should not be starved from the previous evening.[10]

The time of arrival in the day unit will depend on the time of surgery and, although staggered admission times are possible to minimise waiting time, it is usually easier to organise a set arrival time to allow adequate assessment by anaesthetist and re-examination by surgeon.

Parental involvement and premedication

Sedative premedication is unnecessary in the majority of paediatric day cases if children and parents are well prepared and particularly where there are good preoperative play facilities and child-friendly rooms for induction of anaesthesia. Parental involvement in the induction of anaesthesia can be very helpful, particularly for the preschool age group.[11, 12] Parents should not be forced to be present if they do not wish as there is evidence that many parents find this experience very stressful[13–15] and excessively anxious parents may transmit this anxiety to their child.[16] Intravenous induction is thought to be less psychologically disturbing to children than inhalational induction[17, 18] and many units in Europe use intravenous induction of anaesthesia as a routine, unless venous access is obviously going to be very difficult or where a child or parent has specifically requested an inhalational technique. The routine use of topical local anaesthesia of the skin with Emla cream[19] or tetracaine (amethocaine) gel[20] allows painless venous access after 60 and 40 min, respectively. Sedative premedication can be very helpful for selected cases where the child is very anxious, where the child has previously had a traumatic experience with the induction of anaesthesia, where the child has a needle phobia or for the inconsolable child. Oral midazolam 0.5 mg kg^{-1} is very effective when given 20–30 min prior to induction.[21–23] The standard formulation of midazolam is very acidic and tastes very bitter so must be disguised by a sweet liquid, either by preparation of a syrup in the pharmacy or by adding the midazolam to a small volume (1–2 ml kg⁻¹) of cola, lemonade or other sweet drink or by mixing with paracetamol syrup. This presupposes that the child will cooperate in drinking this solution. The same limitation applies to oral ketamine (up to 10 mg kg⁻¹). Other options such as intranasal midazolam, rectal induction or intramuscular ketamine are not very satisfactory as they involve a degree of restraint of the child to administer them, which many find unacceptable for elective day-case work. For the individual inconsolable child where the surgery is deemed to be essential (e.g. a dental abscess), then with parental consent a degree of restraint to administer an intramuscular premedicant may be justifiable and ketamine 5–10 mg kg⁻¹ or midazolam 0.1 mg kg⁻¹ can be used.

It is important that the child is carefully monitored after these premedicants as they act very quickly and can produce quite profound sedation. The available evidence suggests that oral midazolam does not delay discharge.[21–23]

Recently, fentanyl in the form of a lollipop has been described as a paediatric premedicant[24, 25] but many units try to avoid opioids in day cases due to the increased incidence of adverse effects such as nausea and vomiting.

SIMPLIFYING TECHNIQUES AND MINIMISING MORBIDITY

Minor sequelae of anaesthesia[26–28] become magnified in the day-surgery setting and many can be avoided by using the least invasive anaesthetic technique.

Induction

Intravenous induction with propofol 4 mg kg⁻¹ with added lidocaine (lignocaine) 0.2 mg kg⁻¹ is very effective and results in a slightly earlier recovery in older paediatric day cases than thiopentone induction.[29] The well-known clear-headed recovery and antiemetic effects are particularly useful in children. Where the laryngeal mask is to be used, insertion is facilitated by the use of propofol.[30] There has been a resurgence of interest in inhalational induction with the introduction of sevoflurane into clinical practice and a substantial body of evidence now attests to its efficacy and advantages over halothane, with the main drawback being cost.[31–35] The use of the Humphrey ADE circuit (able to operate in Mapleson A, D or E modes) and inspired-agent monitoring allows use of very low flows for spontaneous respiration techniques in children, with resultant economy of volatile agent consumption.

Maintenance

The laryngeal mask airway (LMA) has transformed the maintenance of anaesthesia for paediatric day cases[36] and tracheal intubation should only be needed in an emergency or for specific procedures such as upper gastrointestinal endoscopy. Head and neck procedures such as strabismus correction, tongue-tie release, correction of prominent ears and dental conservation or extraction can all be performed using the reinforced or conventional LMA with a spontaneous respiration technique.[37] Recovery after maintenance with sevoflurane and desflurane is more rapid and can be associated with restlessness and agitation but this will be minimised if good local or regional analgesia is also used.[31, 35] For certain procedures a total intravenous technique such as propofol infusion[30, 38, 39] can be beneficial, e.g. in minimising emesis after strabismus correction.

Analgesia

Good pain control is critical to the success of paediatric day-case surgery. Local analgesia should be used as a component of the anaesthetic technique in all paediatric day cases unless there is a specific reason not to, as it is so effective and safe.[2] Topical tetracaine (amethocaine) or oxybuprocaine for strabismus correction, topical lidocaine (lignocaine) gel after circumcision, wound instillation or wound infiltration with bupivacaine are all simple and highly effective.[40, 41] Topical diclofenac drops are also effective analgesics for strabismus surgery[37] and do not carry the risk of inadvertent trauma to the anaesthetised cornea. Peripheral nerve blocks are also highly effective. Single-injection techniques are preferred[40, 41] and the most useful are penile block, ilioinguinal/iliohypogastric block and great auricular nerve block. Caudal epidural block is also widely applicable in paediatric day surgery and motor block is seldom troublesome if bupivacaine 0.25% is used.[42] Recently, prolongation of analgesia from caudal bupivacaine single-injection techniques has been sought by the addition of opioids, α_2-adrenoceptor agonists and N-methyl-D-aspartate (NMDA) antagonists[42] and clonidine or ketamine looks particularly promising for paediatric day surgery, although clonidine can produce sedation and hypotension at higher dosage. Clonidine added to caudal bupivacaine is associated with a doubling of the duration of effective analgesia while ketamine quadruples the analgesia.[42]

Non-steroidal anti-inflammatory drugs should also be routinely used unless specifically contraindicated and several child-friendly formulations are available, e.g. ibuprofen syrup (10 mg kg^{-1}), diclofenac suppositories (1 mg kg^{-1}) and piroxicam melts (0.5 mg kg^{-1}), and these can be given after induction or as a component of the premedication. Ketorolac is available as an intravenous formulation and is widely used at a dose of 0.5 mg kg^{-1}. Paracetamol is also ubiquitous and can be given as a premedicant loading dose of 20 mg kg^{-1} or as a suppository after induction of anaesthesia. It is important to realise that the absorption of paracetamol suppositories is slow and poor so a higher loading dose of around 30–40 mg kg^{-1} must be given to achieve therapeutic plasma concentrations within 90 min.[40]

SEDATION OF CHILDREN FOR PROCEDURES

Children may attend on a day-case basis for diagnostic or therapeutic procedures. The current standards of selection, preparation, conduct and discharge are covered in detail by the evidence-based SIGN guideline, available at *www.sign.ac.uk*. The key recommendations are listed in Table 5.2.

POSTOPERATIVE CARE AND FOLLOW-UP
Recovery parameters and discharge criteria

Recovery milestones in children must be adjusted for the child's age, developmental stage, medical status, surgical procedure and social circumstances.[2, 3] The vital signs and conscious level should be normal for the child's age and preoperative level. There should be no respiratory distress or stridor, especially in those children who have been intubated. Swallowing, cough and gag reflexes should be fully regained and children should be able to move normally for their age. Motor blockade of the lower limbs after caudal or inguinal block can be troublesome in older children and may delay safe discharge.[9]

Reasons for hospital admission

Inevitably some children (around 1%) may require inpatient admission and parents should be aware of this possibility. Persistently abnormal vital signs or conscious level, any problem with the airway, motor blockade in an older child, persistent nausea and vomiting, bleeding, severe pain, unexpected surgical problems or unexpected intraoperative events (e.g. regurgitation, aspiration, bronchospasm, hypersensitivity reactions, suxamethonium apnoea, malignant hyperpyrexia) may all lead to admission for further care and investigations.

Postoperative nausea and vomiting

Strabismus surgery, orchidopexy, gastroscopy, a past history of postoperative nausea and vomiting (PONV) or motion sickness, tracheal intubation and opioids are the main risk factors.

Table 5.2 Recommendations of Scottish Intercollegiate Guidelines Network (SIGN) for safe paediatric sedation for procedures

QUICK REFERENCE GUIDE

Paediatric Safe Sedation

This Quick Reference Guide provides a summary of the main recommendations in the SIGN guideline on Paediatric Safe Sedation. This guideline is applicable to all children under 16 years of age undergoing painful or non-painful diagnostic or therapeutic procedures in the hospital, community, general medical or dental practice settings.

Sedation is defined as a drug-induced depression of consciousness during which patients respond purposefully to verbal commands, either alone or accompanied by light tactile stimulation. No interventions are required to maintain a patent airway and spontaneous ventilation is adequate. Cardiovascular function is usually maintained.

When using sedation in the primary care or outpatient setting, there should be no intention to progress to either deep sedation or general anaesthesia, even when sedation fails.

PREPARATION FOR SEDATION

It is essential that consent is obtained prior to the procedure and this should include an explanation of the procedure, the sedation technique proposed and possible adverse effects. Written informed consent should be obtained from the child (in the light of the Children (Scotland) Act 1995) where appropriate or from the parent or legal guardian.

Parental involvement

C Parental involvement in the preparation of the child and during the procedure has a sedative-sparing effect and may greatly reduce the distress caused by separation anxiety.

Facilities and personnel

D Sedation in children should only be performed in an environment where the facilities, personnel and equipment to manage paediatric emergency situations are immediately available.

☑ Sedation of children for diagnostic or therapeutic procedures should **not** be undertaken in general medical practice and out-of-hours centres.

D The roles and responsibilities of the 'operator' (the person carrying out the procedure) and the sedation practitioner may be merged to some extent but the guiding principle should always be that the operator should not be the person responsible for monitoring the child during the procedure.

☑ A medically or dentally qualified person should be identified to hold overall responsibility for the care of the sedated child until he or she is discharged.

Clinical assessment

D Children requiring sedation should receive a full preprocedure clinical assessment and only children who are normally healthy or have mild systemic disease should be considered suitable for sedation as outpatients.

D Children with contraindications to sedation should not be sedated.

D Extra caution should be exercised when sedating neonates and children under 5 years of age.

D Consideration should be given to the use of a general anaesthetic or anaesthetist-supervised sedation as an alternative.

Fasting

D The child should be fasted as for a general anaesthetic (6 h for solids or bottle milk, 4 h for breast milk, 2 h for clear fluids), except when nitrous oxide is the only sedative used.

Monitoring

C Observations from all children undergoing sedation should be recorded using a standardised template. All recordings, prescriptions and reactions should be documented on this chart and continued until discharge criteria are met.

Table 5.2 continued overleaf

Table 5.2 continued from previous page

SEDATION PRINCIPLES

B Sedative drug combinations should be avoided in children as they are often associated with deeper levels of sedation and with more adverse effects.

D If a child becomes disinhibited by sedative agents and becomes restless, uncooperative or unmanageable, elective or urgent procedures should be abandoned and rescheduling for general anaesthesia considered. For emergency procedures, arrangements to convert to a general anaesthetic should be considered when appropriate.

D The sedation practitioner must be able to manage and rescue a patient who enters a deeper level of sedation than intended.

☑ General anaesthetic agents should not be used to sedate children.

☑ An individualised dosing of sedative, based on age, weight, comorbidity, procedure and presence of other drugs should be devised for each child. Dosage of nitrous oxide inhalation sedation should be incrementally titrated according to the patient's response.

☑ The least distressing route of administration of the sedative agent should be used.

☑ The sedative prescription should always be double-checked by another person to ensure dosages are correct.

☑ For repeated procedures, consideration should be given to using sedation as part of a behaviour modification programme to sequentially reduce fear and anxiety with the aim of weaning the child from the need for sedation.

SEDATION TECHNIQUES

Sedation for painless procedures

D Non-pharmacological techniques should be used for painless procedures whenever possible.

Sedation for painful procedures

☑ For painful procedures, appropriate analgesia should be given first to prevent pain before considering sedation. Consideration should be given first to the use of analgesics that do not have sedative properties.

B Inhaled nitrous oxide produces the most rapid onset and offset of analgesia and may be appropriate for painful procedures in children who are able to cooperate.

☑ Opioids may be used for painful procedures but should not be used to sedate children undergoing painless procedures. Whenever opioids are given to children, the specific antagonist naloxone should be immediately available.

SEDATION FOR SPECIFIC PROCEDURES

Medical paediatrics: gastrointestinal endoscopy

A General anaesthesia should be the first choice for paediatric gastrointestinal endoscopy.

Medical paediatrics: oncology

B For brief, but painful or distressing oncology procedures, a combination of behavioural techniques and local anaesthesia is recommended. Systemic analgesia with inhaled nitrous oxide or opioids may be needed and some children may require a general anaesthetic depending on age and degree of distress.

B For repeated or prolonged oncology procedures, a general anaesthetic is recommended.

Medical paediatrics: cardiology

D For non-painful cardiology procedures, behavioural methods, sleep deprivation and scheduling postfeeding may be sufficient for many children.

D General anaesthesia is recommended for cardiac catheterisation procedures in children.

Medical paediatrics: nephrology

D Renal biopsy should be carried out under general anaesthesia or with an anaesthetist administering the sedation and monitoring the child.

Table 5.2 continued overleaf

Table 5.2 continued from previous page

Dentistry

D Attempts should be made to persuade the child to have dental treatment under local anaesthesia using the 'tell–show–do' technique, positive reinforcement and other acclimatisation methods before dental sedation is contemplated.

C Nitrous oxide/oxygen sedation (inhalation sedation), titrated to the individual child's needs, is recommended for use in all dental settings but particularly general dental practice and the community dental service.

D Children undergoing inhalational sedation in a dental surgery should be monitored visually until fully recovered.

D Single-agent sedation with midazolam is only recommended for intravenous dental sedation in patients over 16 years of age. Intravenous sedation should be avoided in younger children in primary or community dental practice.

B General anaesthetic drugs, combinations of sedative drugs or other routes of administration should not be used in general dental practice and the community dental service.

Radiology

D Children up to the age of 4 months should be imaged when asleep, postfeeding, and with no sedation.

C For painless imaging procedures lasting less than 60 min, children from 4 months to 5 years of age may be sedated using a single low-potency oral agent. Recovery may be slow, however.

D As failure of sedation is often due to only part of the dose being swallowed, the drug should be given in the radiology department by the sedation practitioner. Administration from a syringe is more successful than by spoon. The bitter taste of some agents should be partially disguised in a small volume of sweet juice.

D Interventional procedures under radiological control should be performed under general anaesthesia with topical and infiltration local anaesthesia for puncture sites.

D Oral benzodiazepines may be used to allay anxiety in individual children for distressing procedures.

Accident and Emergency

Children attending A&E departments for painful procedures can often be managed successfully with adequate sympathetic behavioural techniques (including play therapy, distraction, guided imagery) and local anaesthesia (topical, infiltration, nerve block).

☑ Nitrous oxide is very effective in school-age children who are able to cooperate and is particularly helpful as patients do not need to be fasted if nitrous oxide is used as the sole sedative/analgesic agent.

D For severe pain, opioids should be used by oral, intravenous or nasal routes.

☑ For repeated painful procedures, for more invasive procedures, for prolonged procedures and in the younger or distressed child, general anaesthesia is recommended.

CONTRAINDICATIONS

D *Children who have any of the following contraindications should not normally be sedated:*

- abnormal airway (including large tonsils and anatomical abnormalities of upper and lower airway)
- raised intracranial pressure
- depressed conscious level
- history of sleep apnoea
- respiratory failure
- cardiac failure
- neuromuscular disease
- bowel obstruction
- active respiratory tract infection
- known allergy to sedative drug/previous adverse reaction
- child too distressed despite adequate preparation

Table 5.2 continued overleaf

Table 5.2 continued from previous page

- older child with severe behavioural problems (as they have higher failure rate)
- informed refusal by the parent/guardian/child.

B *Children who have any of the following additional contraindications should not be sedated with nitrous oxide:*

- intracranial air (e.g. after skull fracture)
- pneumothorax, pneumopericardium
- bowel obstruction
- pneumoperitoneum
- pulmonary cysts or bullae
- lobar emphysema
- severe pulmonary hypertension
- nasal blockage (adenoid hypertrophy, common cold)
- pregnancy

RECOVERY AND DISCHARGE

☑ After the procedure, the patient may be discharged if the following criteria are met:

For a hospital setting

- airway patent and stable unsupported
- easily rousable
- oxygen saturation > 95% breathing air
- haemodynamically stable
- hydration adequate, no bleeding, urine output adequate
- returned to normal level of responsiveness and orientation for age and mental status, can walk unaided (if appropriate)
- no nausea and vomiting
- pain controlled

For non-hospital setting

- airway patent and stable unsupported
- easily rousable
- returned to normal level of responsiveness and orientation for age and mental status, can walk unaided (if appropriate)
- no nausea and vomiting
- pain controlled

The Scottish Intercollegiate Guidelines Network (SIGN) supports improvement in the quality of health care for patients in Scotland by developing and disseminating national clinical guidelines and facilitating their implementation into practice. SIGN guidelines provide recommendations for effective health care based on current evidence.

The recommendations are graded **A B C D** to indicate the strength of the supporting evidence. Good practice points ✓ are provided where the guideline development group wishes to highlight specific aspects of accepted clinical practice.

Details of the evidence supporting these recommendations and their application in practice can be found in the full guideline, available on the SIGN website: **www.sign.ac.uk**.

This guideline was issued in 2002 and will be considered for review in 2004.

For more information about the SIGN programme, contact the SIGN executive or see the website.

SIGN Executive
Royal College of Physicians
9 Queen Street
Edinburgh EH2 1JQ
www.sign.ac.uk

© Scottish Intercollegiate Guidelines Network, 2002

Reproduced with kind permission of SIGN (Scottish Intercollegiate Guidelines Network).

Propofol has a useful antiemetic effect and the use of laryngeal mask techniques with local analgesia and avoidance of opioids will minimise PONV. For those with a strong past history, the 5-hydroxytryptamine type 3 (5-HT$_3$) antagonists have the best efficacy and safety profile and do not produce sedation. Some units feel that too early or vigorous resumption of oral fluid intake increases the incidence of early PONV and adequately hydrated children need not necessarily have to take a drink as a prerequisite for being discharged home.[43, 44]

Postoperative instructions

The surgeon and anaesthetist should give clear verbal instructions about pain control, wound care, mobilisation and resumption of activities. This will be reinforced by nursing staff and by clear written instructions specific to each surgical procedure. These should explain the surgical procedure, type of incision, type of sutures and dressing. The measures to control postoperative pain, when to resume normal diet, restrictions on activities, when to allow bathing and washing, notes on wound care and what to do if problems arise should all be made clear. This should include a clear telephone contact either to the family doctor or to the day-surgery unit or hospital. Arrangements for follow-up by a district nurse, health visitor or family doctor and for review at the hospital outpatient clinic should be clearly documented. A discharge letter should be issued to the family doctor and either sent immediately or given to the family to deliver to the doctor.

Dressings

Care of the child at home can be facilitated by simplifying dressings and avoiding unnecessary dressings, e.g. after circumcision[45] and correction of prominent ears.[46]

Continuing pain control at home

Oral analgesics are the mainstay of continuing pain control at home after day surgery and it is vital to encourage parents to give analgesics pre-emptively and regularly for 24–48 h starting before any local anaesthetic block has worn off. Most hospitals dispense take-home medication to cover the analgesic needs for up to 72 h. Paracetamol 15–20 mg kg^{-1} orally 4–6-hourly is well tolerated and readily available in most households. Ibuprofen 10 mg kg^{-1} orally 6-hourly is suitable for moderate pain. An alternative is to combine oral paracetamol and codeine. After circumcision, parents can be taught to apply topical lidocaine (lignocaine) gel very successfully and after strabismus surgery diclofenac drops can be administered by parents.

Transport home

Children must have a responsible adult escort home after day surgery and this journey should be by private car or taxi, not public transport. Excessively long travelling time is a contraindication to day-case surgery.

Home visits/community liaison

A home visit is not required in all cases but it is well established that a trained paediatric nurse visiting selected cases is very reassuring to parents and children and reduces family doctor call-outs.[47–50] The nurse is involved in reinforcing advice to parents, assessing and giving pain relief, wound care, dressing removal, suture removal and audit.

CONCLUSION

Children can gain particular benefits from well-planned and carefully delivered day care with particular emphasis on pain control using local anaesthesia and simplification of anaesthetic techniques using modern agents.

REFERENCES

1. Thornes R. Just for the day. Children admitted to hospital for day treatment. Caring for children in the health services. London: 1991.
2. Morton NS, Raine PAM. Paediatric day case surgery. Oxford: Oxford Medical Publications; 1994.
3. Morton NS, Lord D. General principles of paediatric day case anaesthesia. In: Whitwam JG, ed. Day case anaesthesia and sedation. Oxford: Blackwell Scientific Publications; 1994:303.
4. Mackenzie K, Wilson JT. Personal communication. A prospective audit of recovery from tonsillectomy in children.
5. McEwan AI, Birch M, Bingham R. The preoperative management of the child with a heart murmur. Paediatr Anaesth 1995; 5:151–155.
6. Keneally JP. Day stay surgery in paediatrics. Clin Anesthesiol 1985; 3:679–696.
7. Vanderwalt J. Anaesthesia in children with viral respiratory tract infections. Paediatr Anaesth 1995; 5:257–260.
8. Phillips S, Daborn AK, Hatch DJ. Preoperative fasting for paediatric anaesthesia. Br J Anaesth 1994; 73:529–531.
9. Stuart JC, Morton NS. A clinical audit of day case surgery for children. J One Day Surg 1991; 1:15–18.
10. Miller DC. Why are children starved? Br J Anaesth 1990; 64:409–410.
11. McCormick ASM, Spargo PM. Parents in the anaesthetic room: a questionnaire survey of departments of anaesthesia. Paediatr Anaesth 1996; 6:183–186.
12. Kain ZN, Ferris CA, Mayes LC, et al. Parental presence during induction of anaesthesia: practice differences between the United States and Great Britain. Paediatr Anaesth 1996; 6:187–193.
13. Thompson N, Irwin MG, Gunawardene WMS, et al. Pre-operative parental anxiety. Anaesthesia 1996; 51:1008–1012.
14. Litman RS, Berger AA, Chibber A. An evaluation of preoperative anxiety in a population of parents of infants and children undergoing ambulatory surgery. Paediatr Anaesth 1996; 6:443–447.
15. Campbell IR, Scaife JM, Johnstone JMS. Psychological effects of day case surgery compared with inpatient surgery. Arch Dis Child 1988; 63:415–417.
16. Bevan JC, Johnston C, Haig MJ, et al. Preoperative parental anxiety predicts behavioural and emotional responses to induction of anaesthesia in children. Can J Anaesth 1990; 37:177–182.
17. Kotiniemi LH, Ryhanen PT. Behavioural changes and children's memories after intravenous, inhalation and rectal induction of anaesthesia. Paediatr Anaesth 1996; 6:201–207.
18. Kotiniemi LH, Ryhanen PT, Moilanen IK. Behavioural changes following routine ENT operations in two-to-ten-year-old children. Paediatr Anaesth 1996; 6:45–49.
19. Freeman JA, Doyle E, Ng TI, et al. Topical anaesthesia of the skin: a review. Paediatr Anaesth 1993; 3:129–138.
20. Lawson RA, Smart NG, Gudgeon AC, et al. Evaluation of an amethocaine gel preparation for percutaneous analgesia before venous cannulation in children. Br J Anaesth 1995; 75:282–285.
21. Cray SH, Dixon JL, Heard CMB, et al. Oral midazolam premedication for paediatric day case patients. Paediatr Anaesth 1996; 6:265–270.
22. McCluskey A, Meakin GH. Oral administration of midazolam as a premedicant for paediatric day-case anaesthesia. Anaesthesia 1994; 49:782–785.
23. McGraw T. Oral midazolam and postoperative behaviour in children. Can J Anaesth 1993; 40:682–683.
24. Friesen RH, Carpenter E, Madigan CK, et al. Oral transmucosal fentanyl citrate for preanaesthetic medication of paediatric cardiac surgery patients. Paediatr Anaesth 1995; 5:29–31.
25. Macaluso AD, Connelly AM, Hayes WB, et al. Oral transmucosal fentanyl citrate for premedication in adults. Anesth Analg 1996; 82:158–161.
26. Montenegro LM, Schreiner MS, Nicolson SC. Perioperative problems in pediatric anesthesia. Curr Opin Anesthesiol 1996; 9:221–224.
27. Patel RI, Hannallah RS. Anesthetic complications following pediatric ambulatory surgery: a 3 year study. Anesthesiology 1988; 69:1009–1012.
28. Selby IR, Rigg JD, Faragher B, et al. The incidence of minor sequelae following anaesthesia in children. Paediatr Anaesth 1996; 6:293–302.
29. Runcie CJ, MacKenzie S, Arthur DS, et al. Comparison of recovery from anaesthesia induced in children with either propofol or thiopentone. Br J Anaesth 1993; 70:192–195.
30. Morton NS, Johnston G, White M, et al. Propofol in paediatric anaesthesia. Paediatr Anaesth 1992; 2:89–97.
31. Murat I. New inhalational agents in paediatric anaesthesia: desflurane and sevoflurane. Curr Opin Anesthesiol 1996; 9:225–228.
32. Black A, Sury MRJ, Hemington L, et al. A comparison of the induction characteristics of sevoflurane and halothane in children. Anaesthesia 1996; 51:539–542.

33. Sury MRJ, Black A, Hemington L, et al. A comparison of the recovery characteristics of sevoflurane and halothane in children. Anaesthesia 1996; 51:543–546.

34. Kataria B, Epstein R, Bailey A, et al. A comparison of sevoflurane to halothane in paediatric surgical patients: results of a multicentre international study. Paediatr Anaesth 1996; 6:283–292.

35. Lerman J. Pharmacology of inhalational anaesthetics in infants and children. Paediatr Anaesth 1992; 2:191–203.

36. Haynes SR, Morton NS. The laryngeal mask airway: a review of its use in paediatric anaesthesia. Paediatr Anaesth 1993; 3:65–73.

37. Morton NS, Benham S, Lawson RA, et al. Diclofenac vs. oxybuprocaine eyedrops for analgesia after paediatric strabismus surgery. Paediatr Anaesth 1997; 7:221–226.

38. Doyle E, McFadzean W, Morton NS. IV anaesthesia with propofol using a target-controlled infusion system: comparison with inhalation anaesthesia for general surgical procedures in children. Br J Anaesth 1993; 70:542–545.

39. Watcha MF, Simeon RM, White PF, et al. Effect of propofol on the incidence of postoperative vomiting after strabismus surgery in pediatric outpatients. Anesthesiology 1991; 75:204–209.

40. Morton NS. (1994) Local anaesthesia for paediatric day-case surgery. In: Whitwam JG, ed. Day case anaesthesia and sedation. Oxford: Blackwell Scientific Publications; 1994:332.

41. McNicol LR. Local anaesthesia. In: Morton NS, Raine PAM, eds. Paediatric day case surgery. Oxford: Oxford Medical Publications; 1994.

42. Cook B, Doyle E. The use of additives to local anaesthetic solutions for caudal epidural blockade. Paediatr Anaesth 1996; 6:353–359.

43. Woods AM, Berry FA, Carter BJ. Strabismus surgery and post-operative vomiting: clinical observations and review of the current literature; a medical opinion. Paediatr Anaesth 1992; 2:223–229.

44. Baines D. Postoperative nausea and vomiting in children. Paediatr Anaesth 1996; 6:7–14.

45. Freeland AM. Evaluating the need for a Vaseline gauze dressing following circumcision in day surgery. Glasgow:Yorkhill NHS Trust Day Surgery Unit; 1996.

46. Ridings P, Gault D, Khan L. Reduction in postoperative vomiting after surgical correction of prominent ears. Br J Anaesth 1994; 72:592–593.

47. Anonymous. Following up day case anaesthesia in general practice. Drugs Ther Bull 1990; 28:81–82.

48. Postuma R, Ferguson CC, Stanwick RS, et al. Pediatric day-care surgery: a 30 year hospital experience. J Pediatr Surg 1987; 22:304–307.

49. Scaife JM, Campbell I. A comparison of the outcome of day-care and inpatient treatment of paediatric surgical cases. J Child Psychol Psychiatry 1988; 29:185–198.

50. Atwell JD, Gow MA. Paediatric trained district nurse in the community: expensive luxury or economic necessity? Br Med J 1985; 291:227–229.

CHAPTER 6

Anaesthesia: principles and techniques

Alison Carr, Ann Harvey

INTRODUCTION

Managing children in hospitals designed primarily for adults is very challenging. In the first section of this chapter, we will consider the general practical and organisational aspects of anaesthetising children in district general hospitals (DGHs). In the second section we will describe some important recent developments, and discuss anaesthetic techniques for common operations. We will include information from recent studies, if appropriate, to give an understanding of the important factors in selecting suitable techniques.

SECTION 1: General considerations

ORGANISATION

Of the many recommendations for the organisation of surgical and anaesthetic services for children discussed in Chapter 1, probably the most important are having trained staff with adequate ongoing experience, an environment and facilities appropriate for children, and scheduled paediatric operating lists.

Appropriate training and experience

All hospital staff involved in the perioperative care of children should be suitably trained and want to work with children. In particular, an anaesthetist in a DGH should have specific training in paediatric anaesthesia and manage enough children to comply with the recommendations for minimum case load (see Box 1.7). They should be supported always by skilled assistants (either operating department practitioners or anaesthetic nurses) who are trained and familiar with anaesthesia for children.

Environment and facilities

The environment in theatre must be suitable for children and should include a preoperative play area, a reception area designed for adolescents, an anaesthetic room with appropriate decorations and toys for distraction and a separate recovery area (see Ch. 8, Figs 8.3 & 8.4).

A full range of paediatric equipment should be immediately available wherever children are anaesthetised. Ideally, children should be anaesthetised in theatres designated *only* for paediatric surgery, to ensure that these are always adequately equipped and provide suitable environments. However, this arrangement is uncommon in DGHs and probably not an efficient use of expensive resources. Another good arrangement is to use only a few theatres for children and adapt them, for example, by stocking them with paediatric equipment, decorating anaesthetic rooms and providing toys. An alternative is to provide trolleys specifically for paediatric anaesthesia, ensuring appropriate equipment is available wherever children are anaesthetised. The trolleys should contain all necessary equipment organised in the drawers in a standard way. Examples are shown in Figures 6.1. and 8.2.

A list of contents, divided up by each drawer, should be attached. The inventory of equipment in the paediatric trolleys in Derriford Hospital, Plymouth is given in Table 6.1. Other useful information may be attached, including a drug formulary, resuscitation protocols and guidelines for analgesia in children.

Scheduled operating lists for children

Although several bodies recommend scheduling children on specific paediatric lists and not caring for them alongside adults,[1-3] these practices have not been widely implemented. A recent document from the Senate of Surgeons reinforcing the recommendations[4] may encourage their implementation.

PREOPERATIVE ASSESSMENT, PREPARATION AND PREMEDICATION
Assessment

The anaesthetist must see the parents and child preoperatively to make a thorough preoperative assessment, establish rapport, discuss anaesthetic techniques and obtain verbal consents when appropriate (e.g. for regional analgesia or suppositories). Details of previous anaesthetics and any family history of anaesthetic problems should be obtained. If the child had been distressed during induction previously, an alternative technique or sedative premedication may help, making the experience better for all concerned. The airway should be assessed and the presence of loose teeth, enamels, caps or crowns documented. Medication and drug allergies should be noted. The child should be weighed and his/her temperature and pulse recorded. It should also be confirmed that the child is adequately fasted. The assessment should include a detailed past medical history and systemic enquiry looking for conditions common in childhood, e.g. asthma, upper respiratory tract infections (URTIs) or heart murmurs.

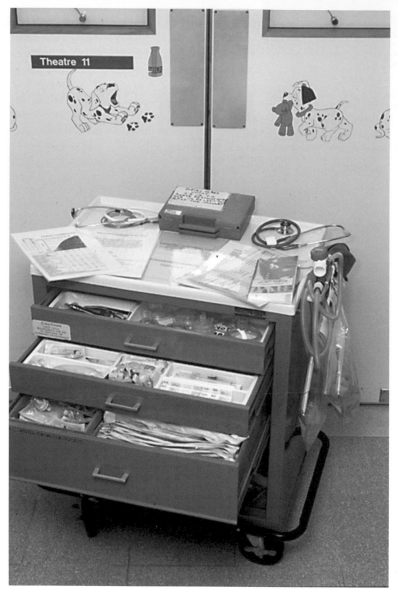

Fig 6.1 Paediatric equipment trolley used in theatres in Derriford Hospital. The trolley is wheeled into the anaesthetic room before a paediatric surgical list, providing the necessary anaesthetic equipment.

Asthma

Asthma is common and now affects 20% of children. The severity should be determined and may vary from mild (associated with exercise or respiratory tract infections) to severe (requiring frequent hospital admissions and oral steroids).

Upper respiratory tract infections

Children scheduled for surgery, particularly for ear, nose and throat (ENT) operations, often have 'runny noses'. A runny nose may have a benign and non-infectious cause (e.g. allergic or vasomotor rhinitis) or be the prodrome of a respiratory tract infection.

Table 6.1 Inventory of anaesthetic equipment in a paediatric trolley in Derriford Hospital, Plymouth

WORKTOP

Alder Hey ABC formulary.
Protocols for asystole, ventricular fibrillation, pulseless electrical activity and anaphylaxis in children
Guidelines for pain relief, infusions of sedatives and inotropes in children
Precordial stethoscope hanging on the side
Small blue box containing uncut tubes, out of packets: sizes 2.5–7.0 (×1 per size)

TOP DRAWER

Assorted plasters
Ribbon gauze
Spare laryngoscope batteries and bulbs
Guedel airways: sizes 000–3
Blood pressure cuffs: sizes from neonatal to small adult
Metal CO_2 sampling connector
Laryngoscopes with selection of blades (×2 each of neonatal, infant and small adult) and interchangeable handles (×2)
Clear masks, round (sizes 0, 1, 2), standard (size 3) (×2 of each)
Flexible introducers: small and medium
Vecafix
KY jelly
ECG stickers – paediatric
Magill forceps – adult and child
Connectors (15 mm with suction port)

MIDDLE DRAWER

Syringes: sizes 1–20 ml and 2 × 60 ml
Neoflons (24G)
Venflons: sizes 18G, 20G and 22G
Quick Caths: sizes 20G, 22G and 24G
Abbocaths (short): sizes 18G, 20G
Three-way taps
Padded splints
Alcohol swabs and wipes
Dental rolls
10 ml water, ×4 ampoules
10 ml normal saline, ×4 ampoules
Full range of intramuscular (IM)/intravenous (IV) needles
Drawing-up needles
Green gauze swabs
Connecta three-way taps
Venisystems with Luer-Lok
Additive labels

BOTTOM DRAWER

Full range of Portex Rae and armoured tracheal tubes (×2 of each)
Paediatric and child heat and moisture-exchanging filters
Suction catheters: sizes 6G and 8G (×4 of each), 10G and 12G (×2 of each)
Nasogastric tubes: sizes 6–14G (×2 of each)
Rectal and oesophageal temperature probes
Oesophageal stethoscopes and preformed ear pieces

Table 6.1 continued overleaf

Table 6.1 continued from previous page

Infant oximetry probes for ear and digits
Laryngeal mask airways (standard and armoured): sizes 1 and 3 (×1 of each), 1.5, 2 and 2.5 (×2 of each)

BOTTOM SHELF
Nuffield ventilator
Newton valve
Disconnect alarm
Complete T-piece breathing systems (×2) with long extension
Extension tubing for intermittent positive-pressure ventilation
Bubblewrap
Gamgee
Babies' bonnets
Emergency airway cannulation equipment
Emergency drugs
Intraosseous needles (infant and child)
100-ml burettes, with and without blood filters (×1 of each)
Triple and single lumen: one long + one short (×2 of each)
22G 6-cm Hydrocath™ (×2)
Laerdal™ self-inflating resuscitation bags, neonatal (250 ml), child (500 ml)
Child diathermy pads
Pressure gauge for T-piece breathing system

Several authors have attempted to assess the risks of anaesthetising a child with an URTI.[5, 6] In one study, cough, laryngospasm, bronchospasm and oxygen desaturation were two to seven times more likely in children with URTI during anaesthesia[5] and the likelihood of respiratory problems was 11 times greater than normal in these children if the trachea was intubated. Other authors report an increased incidence of transient oxygen desaturation perioperatively in children with URTIs.[7, 8] In another study[6] children undergoing minor surgery who had an asymptomatic or symptomatic URTI did not have an increase in respiratory complications. Complications occurred in children who had been recently infected with an URTI, particularly when tracheal intubation had been performed.

Since 20–30% of children have a runny nose for a significant part of the year, all children should be carefully assessed before proceeding with anaesthesia[9] by comparing their current with usual medical state (perhaps the child always has a runny nose) and determining the extent that surgery will improve them. Generally, a child with a runny nose may be anaesthetised if he/she is systemically well, apyrexial, has clear nasal secretions and no symptoms or signs of chest disease. Features suggesting infection include green nasal secretions, pyrexia, chest signs or an unwell child. Berry recommends postponing surgery for 1–2 weeks after an URTI and 4–6 weeks after a lower respiratory tract infection.[10]

Heart murmurs

A heart murmur may be 'innocent' or secondary to pathology in the heart or great vessels. 'Non-innocent' murmurs may be symptomatic or asymptomatic, as indicated by the clinical history. A classification of murmurs and guidelines for diagnosing an innocent murmur are shown in Table 6.2(A–C).

A child with a heart murmur should have an ECG and chest X-ray and paediatric advice sought (if possible) preoperatively. Generally, it is safe to proceed with anaesthesia in a child with an asymptomatic soft systolic murmur and no other features. The majority of these murmurs are innocent, and those caused by cardiac abnormalities are unlikely to produce haemodynamic disturbance during surgery. It is important, however, to give antibiotic

Table 6.2(A) Classification of heart murmurs

Heart murmurs may be classified simply into three categories:

Innocent/functional
Asymptomatic

- Usually ejection systolic
- Anaesthetic risk for children not increased during minor or intermediate non-cardiac surgery
- For example, clinically non-significant patent ductus arteriosus, atrial septal defect, ventricular septal defect
- Antibiotic prophylaxis for endocarditis required

Symptomatic

- Clinically significant patent ductus arteriosus, atrial septal defect, ventricular septal defect or more complicated cardiac malformations
- Antibiotic prophylaxis for endocarditis required
- Should be assessed preoperatively by a paediatric cardiologist

Table 6.2(B) When is a murmur innocent?

A murmur is innocent if:	*A murmur is not innocent if:*
● Early systolic	● End or pansystolic
● Quiet	● Diastolic
● No clicks	● Loud or long
● A continuous venous hum	● Associated with a click or a thrill
● Asymptomatic	● Associated with other cardiac signs or symptoms

Table 6.2(C) Characteristics of an innocent murmur

TYPES

Venous hum

- A blowing, continuous murmur, heard at the base of the heart, often just below the clavicles
- Due to blood flowing through the systemic great veins
- Varies with respiration and head position
- Disappears when lying down
- Is sometimes confused with a patent ductus arteriosus

Pulmonary flow murmur

- Soft, ejection systolic murmur heard in the pulmonary area
- Due to rapid flow of blood across a normal pulmonary valve
- Especially prominent when cardiac output is high (fever, exercise, anaemia)

Vibratory murmur

- Short, buzzing murmur heard in systole at the left sternal edge or apex
- Variable
- Changes with position

COMMON INVESTIGATIONS

Normal chest X-ray and ECG

MANAGEMENT

Reassure
No follow-up
No antibiotic prophylaxis

prophylaxis, if indicated, and scrupulously remove air bubbles from intravenous (IV) lines. A cardiological opinion can then be given later.

Preparation

Fasting guidelines

Preoperative fasting was introduced to reduce the risk and severity of aspiration pneumonitis. Although up to 76% of children have a sufficient volume of acidic gastric contents at induction to cause chemical pneumonitis, the clinical syndrome is rare.[11, 12]

Overwhelming evidence supports reducing the duration of fasting from clear fluids in children having elective surgery. The gastric contents of children allowed free clear fluids until 2 h before the scheduled time of anaesthesia are similar to those fasted for a long time. Although many have residual gastric volumes > 0.4 ml kg^{-1} with pH < 2.5, this is unaffected by prolonged fasting. To reduce regurgitation and aspiration, as much attention should be placed on identifying patients at risk and faultless airway management as on fasting.[13] However, it is imperative to fast children for at least 6 h after solid food to allow the stomach enough time to empty.[13]

Fasting times for breast- or bottle-fed babies are controversial. In term and preterm babies, breast milk has been shown to leave the stomach twice as rapidly as formula (emptying half-time for breast milk is approximately 25 min compared with 51 min for formula),[14, 15] although changes in the composition of formula milk over the years may make these results less applicable now. If aspirated, milk irritates the lung, leaving a residue in the alveoli. In addition, formula causes more pulmonary oedema than human or cows' milk because of its high carbohydrate content and hypertonicity.[16]

Recommendations for the duration of preoperative fasting have recently been revised in light of the extremely low incidence of aspiration pneumonitis during general anaesthesia in children. The guidelines used in Derriford Hospital are given in Table 6.3.

Children at risk of gastro-oesophageal reflux and aspiration (including those for emergency surgery) should be given special consideration. Fasting reduces gastric volumes in children presenting for emergency surgery but does not affect pH. Fifty per cent of children presenting for emergency surgery have a residual gastric volume > 0.4 ml kg^{-1} and pH < 2.5. Of children with trauma, those > 10 years of age with superficial injuries have the lowest risk of aspiration.[17] Children requiring emergency surgery should be fasted for food

Table 6.3 Current fasting guidelines in Derriford Hospital	
	Minimum period of fasting before anaesthesia
CHILDREN PRESENTING FOR ELECTIVE SURGERY	
● Solids	6 h
● Formula milk	4 h
● Breast milk	3 h
● Clear fluids	2 h
CHILDREN AT RISK OF GASTRO-OESOPHAGEAL REFLUX AND ASPIRATION PNEUMONITIS (INCLUDING THOSE PRESENTING FOR EMERGENCY SURGERY)[a]	
● Solids	6 h
● Formula milk	6 h
● Breast milk	6 h
● Clear fluids	6 h

[a]Non-urgent cases should be delayed overnight, if possible.

and drink preoperatively for at least 6 h, if possible, and anaesthetised using a rapid-sequence induction. Non-urgent surgery should be delayed overnight.[13]

Premedication

Topical anaesthetics

Ametop, a 4% tetracaine (amethocaine) gel, or Emla, a eutectic mixture of prilocaine and lidocaine (lignocaine) in an oily base, is widely used to provide topical local anaesthesia for cannulation in children scheduled for IV induction (Table 6.4).

Lawson and colleagues compared the efficacy of Ametop with 5% Emla cream applied for 40 min in 94 children having venepuncture.[18] Clinically acceptable conditions were obtained in 85% of children receiving tetracaine (amethocaine) gel compared with 66% given Emla. No significant adverse effects occurred in either group, although 37% of children given tetracaine (amethocaine) gel developed erythema at the application site. The authors concluded that Ametop had greater efficacy and faster onset than Emla and this supports anaesthetists' clinical experience. The effects of Ametop last several hours and vasodilatation, causing localised erythema, may aid IV cannulation. The manufacturers recommend removing it after an hour to avoid skin irritation. Compared with Emla, however, Ametop is expensive.

Emla must be applied for a minimum of 60 min and has an average duration of action of only 30–60 min[19, 20] and is less reliable than Ametop. Potential side-effects include toxicity from systemic absorption of lidocaine (lignocaine) and prilocaine, particularly if ingested. Emla cream is not recommended for babies < 1 month old or those < 12 months old receiving methaemoglobin-inducing agents (such as sulphonamides).[21]

Sedatives

Increasingly, children are admitted for surgery as day patients and the use of sedative premedication has consequently declined. Sedatives are, however, useful as anxiolytics (particularly for children requiring repeated operations) or as adjuncts to the anaesthetic technique.

Oral midazolam, 0.5–0.75 mg kg^{-1} (maximum 15–20 mg), is especially useful in day surgery because it has a rapid onset, producing reliable anxiolysis and sedation within 15–20 min. It lasts 45–60 min and prolongs neither recovery room nor discharge times.[22] The IV preparation is used because an oral formulation is unavailable in the UK. Its bitter taste can be disguised by mixing with neat orange cordial or Calpol (a paracetamol elixir).

Midazolam, 0.2–0.3 mg kg^{-1}, can be given intranasally and this route is used in some countries for premedicating less compliant children. It is rapidly absorbed (producing

Table 6.4 Premedication	
Drug and dose	**Interval before anaesthesia**
SEDATIVE PREMEDICATION	
Midazolam 0.50–0.75 mg kg^{-1}	20 min
Diazepam 0.1–0.3 mg kg^{-1}	1 h
Temazepam 0.5 mg kg^{-1}	1 h
Trimeprazine 3 mg kg^{-1}	2 h
TOPICAL LOCAL ANAESTHETIC GEL APPLIED TO THE BACKS OF BOTH HANDS	
Ametop™	45 min
Emla cream™	1 h

anxiolysis within 7.5–10 min and peak plasma concentrations at 10–30 min[23]) but is irritating to nasal mucosa and children frequently become upset immediately after application.[23]

Some common sedatives prescribed as premedication for children are listed in Table 6.4.

Analgesics

Oral paracetamol, 20 mg kg^{-1}, and/or non-steroidal inflammatory drugs (NSAIDs) (e.g. diclofenac 1–1.5 mg kg^{-1} or ibuprofen 5 mg kg^{-1}) are sometimes prescribed 1 h preoperatively by anaesthetists preferring the oral to rectal route.

Antiemetics

Oral antiemetics (e.g. metoclopramide 0.25 mg kg^{-1}) may be given preoperatively to children at particular risk of postoperative nausea and vomiting (PONV), but are more commonly given IV at induction. Some sedatives, such as trimeprazine or midazolam, also reduce postoperative vomiting (POV).[24] Midazolam may be more effective than trimeprazine. Nathwani et al reported no POV in 20 children given midazolam 0.5 mg kg^{-1} compared with 8/20 of those given trimeprazine 2 mg kg^{-1} for premedication before day surgery ($P = 0.003$).[25] Both were equally effective sedatives and anxiolytics.

Anticholinergic drugs

Atropine, 30 μg kg^{-1} orally or 20 μg kg^{-1} intramuscularly (IM), is sometimes prescribed as premedication. The effects are more reliable if given IM than orally.[26]

Are anticholinergic drugs actually necessary in modern practice? Historically, atropine was routinely given to children, either as premedication or IV at induction (20 μg kg^{-1}). Advocates claimed that dry mucous membranes reduced laryngospasm during gaseous induction and that preserving an adequate heart rate during vagal stimulation was vital to

Table 6.5(A) The advantages and disadvantages of atropine

Advantages	Disadvantages
	The side-effects of atropine are usually due to its vagolytic properties
● Dry mucous membranes may reduce the risks of laryngospasm and respiratory complications associated with inhalational anaesthetics	● Dry mucous membranes are more friable and uncomfortable for the child
	● There may be reduced mucociliary clearance for several hours after a single dose[379]
	● Thick, tenacious secretions are difficult to clear (do not give prophylactically to children with cystic fibrosis[27])
● Produces a dose-dependent tachycardia, maintaining cardiac output	● Dose-dependent tachycardia is detrimental in children with obstructive cardiac lesions
	● Reduces lower oesophageal sphincter pressure in infants and children, potentiating the risk of gastro-oesophageal reflux[380]
	● Interferes with temperature regulation (do not give prophylactically to pyrexial child)[27]
	● Overdosage and intoxication have been described
	● Transient cutaneous reactions may occur after intravenous injection

Table 6.5(B) Indications and contraindications for atropine

Indications	Contraindications
Few would support the *routine use* of atropine when anaesthetising infants and children.	The *routine use* of atropine should be avoided in
Pretreatment with atropine may be useful:	• children with cystic fibrosis
• to dry excessive secretions	• children with obstructive lesions of the heart, e.g. aortic stenosis, hypertrophic cardiomyopathy
• to dry mucous membranes before anaesthetising children with difficult airways	• children at increased risk of gastro-oesophageal reflux
• to prevent bradycardia	• febrile children
• during strabismus surgery	
• with high doses of opioids	
• with suxamethonium in infants	
Atropine is used to treat bradycardia *not induced* by hypoxaemia	

maintain cardiac output in small children. They also argued that atropine reduced critical incidents but had minimal side-effects.[27] However, others who had safely anaesthetised children without routinely using atropine for more than 10 years questioned its routine use, advocating it only for specific indications.[27] The advantages and disadvantages of pretreatment with atropine and the indications and contraindications for its use are given in Table 6.5(A and B).

Few argue that ether stimulated secretions but induction with halothane or sevoflurane is smooth and does not stimulate mucous secretions. Bradycardia related to anaesthesia has become less common because of the declining use of suxamethonium and the development of modern agents and it is usually caused by hypoxia (best treated with oxygen). Atropine does have some disadvantages if given indiscriminately (Table 6.5(A and B)). However, IV induction with propofol and alfentanil or remifentanil may provoke severe bradycardia and atropine (which should always be drawn up and available immediately) may be life-saving.[27]

ANAESTHESIA AND RECOVERY
Parents

Parents at induction

Several bodies have recommended allowing a parent to accompany a child for induction of anaesthesia if the parent wishes, providing it is in the interests of the child and acceptable to the anaesthetist.[1, 2, 28] This is usual practice in the UK and has potential benefits, some of which are illustrated in Figures 6.2 and 6.3. Studies have shown that having an intelligent, supportive parent or carer present during induction may be the best available substitute for premedication.[29]

A parent or carer:

1. is a familiar person who may allay anxiety and provide support and love;
2. may provide a lap for the child to sit on during a gaseous or IV induction (Fig 6.2);
3. can provide distraction during cannulation (Fig 6.3);
4. may be able to undertake necessary tasks the child may not allow the anaesthetist to do (e.g. preoxygenation or holding face mask during a gaseous induction);
5. may show, by example, that necessary procedures are not painful (e.g. attaching a pulse oximeter to his/her finger).

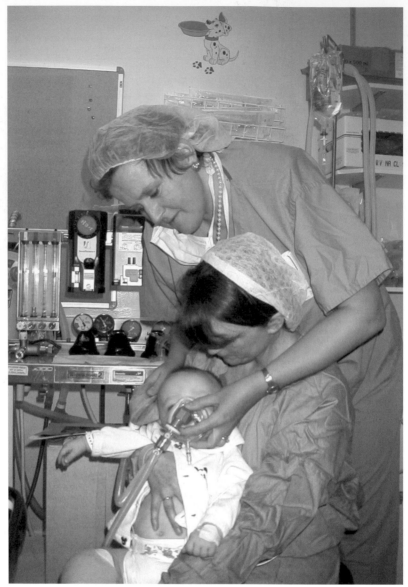

Fig 6.2 Eight-month old baby peacefully undergoing a gaseous induction sitting on his mother's knee.

However, there may be several disadvantages for the child, parent or anaesthetist. For example, extremely anxious parents seem to project anxiety on to their children.[30] Although the parent's role is to provide support, not all can do this successfully. They may become upset (particularly whilst managing their struggling child) or unnerved seeing their child motionless and limp; they may faint or refuse to leave after induction. Anaesthetists may initially find the presence of a parent uncomfortable but this often reflects their confidence and becomes less of a problem as they become more familiar managing children. This is supported by the favourable experiences of anaesthetists working in institutions where parents are commonly present during induction. In contrast, most negative reports come from centres where the practice is infrequent or does not occur at all.[31]

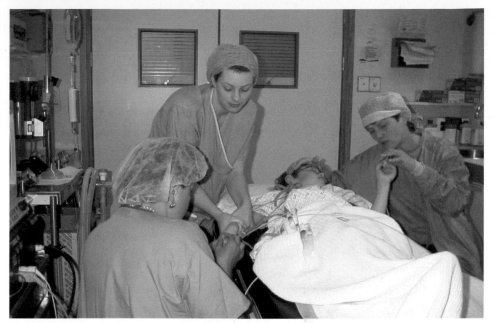

Fig 6.3 Mother comforting her son undergoing an intravenous induction.

Usually, everybody benefits if parents are present during induction if appropriate preparation, support and understanding are provided.[31] For the practice to succeed, parents should be told about their role (i.e. to provide distraction and comfort) and what to expect. The anaesthetist should explain the induction technique carefully and how the child is likely to respond. For example, during gaseous induction, a child (although unaware) may wriggle about during the excitation phase, whilst one given an IV induction will quickly become limp and apparently lifeless. The parent must also agree to leave immediately after induction and, in exceptional circumstances (i.e. if there is a complication), prematurely and that refusal will not be in the best interests of the child.

Although there is pressure today from society for parents to be present at induction, not all can cope. The anaesthetist must, therefore, assess the parent during the preoperative consultation, offering the chance to be absent if the anaesthetist doubts the parent's ability to cope. If this is dealt with sensitively, parents will not feel they have failed in their responsibilities. Another adult, either a suitable relative or a health-care worker who has established a rapport with the child, may be substituted.

Parents and rapid-sequence induction

A parent may accompany a child for a rapid-sequence induction if the anaesthetist thinks this appropriate. However, the anaesthetist should discuss the implications of emergency anaesthesia and the parent must understand the importance of leaving as soon as the child has lost consciousness.

Parents in recovery

Commonly, in the UK, a parent is called to the recovery room when their child has emerged from anaesthesia (Fig. 6.4). The benefits of a parent's presence at induction also apply to recovery. Who is better than a mother or father to console their child after surgery?

For this practice to succeed, a recovery area specifically for children, separate from the adult area, must be provided. It should be fully equipped, suitably decorated and staffed with

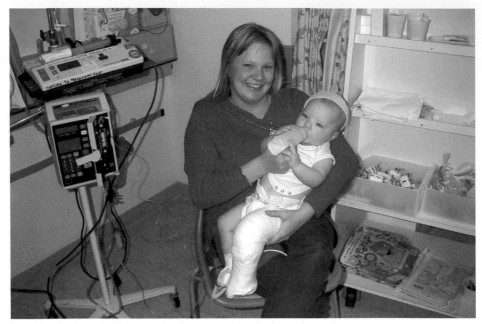

Fig 6.4 Infant being fed by his mother in recovery shortly after orthopaedic surgery.

recovery nurses with appropriate training and aptitude (Fig 8.4). Furthermore, it must allow children to be separated from the next child by curtains or a partition to maintain their dignity during a clinical procedure or allow mothers to breast-feed their babies, if appropriate, in privacy.

Action for Sick Children advocate having parents in recovery wards in their report, *Setting standards for children undergoing surgery*, and include guidelines for parents as an appendix.[28] They suggest telling parents in advance about the likely care given during recovery (e.g. recording pulse, blood pressure and respiratory rate frequently) and advising them of their role (i.e. to comfort and reassure their child by touching and talking gently to them). It should be stressed to parents that they must leave immediately if asked to, and that an explanation of the reason will be given at the first opportunity. Not all parents can cope with being with their child during recovery and they should be assessed individually.[32] Parents should know that they can leave at any time should they become distressed or uncomfortable.

In our hospital, children recover in a paediatric bay and curtains may be pulled around for privacy. One or both parents are brought in as soon as the child has regained consciousness. No additional staff are provided to look after parents. Sometimes, parents can be particularly helpful (e.g. for a child with special needs) and then we bring them in before the child has completely emerged from anaesthesia. In these circumstances, the anaesthetist describes very carefully what to expect and the potential problems that may necessitate them leaving the child early.

It is not always possible to predict the length of surgery. In Derriford Hospital, parents may borrow a bleep, giving them some freedom whilst allowing staff to contact them as soon as they are needed in recovery.

Induction

Gaseous or intravenous?

The choice of induction depends on several factors. For example, a gaseous induction is essential if there is airway obstruction, whereas a rapid-sequence induction is indicated if there is risk of aspirating gastric contents during anaesthesia (e.g. in a child with bowel obstruction, an acute abdomen or significant gastro-oesophageal reflux). Total intravenous anaesthesia (TIVA) is indicated for specific conditions (e.g. a family history of malignant hyperthermia) and may be a good choice for operations commonly associated with vomiting, such as middle-ear surgery. The wishes and previous experience of the child may influence the choice of technique (e.g. a gaseous induction will be difficult in a child with a fear of masks). When there is insufficient time available between admission and induction for topical anaesthetics to be effective, gaseous induction may be preferable.

New drugs in anaesthesia

VOLATILE AGENTS

Sevoflurane (a fluorinated methyl isopropyl ether) is a new volatile agent that is increasingly popular for induction in children and day-case anaesthesia.[33–35] In many hospitals it has replaced halothane as the agent of choice for gaseous induction. Its characteristics are excellent: it smells pleasant and produces smooth induction with less coughing, breath-holding or laryngospasm compared with other volatile agents.[36] Cost, however, often precludes its use for maintenance of anaesthesia. The incidence of PONV is lower than with halothane.[37]

Sevoflurane has a rapid onset of action during induction[38, 39] because of its low blood:gas partition coefficient (0.66) compared with halothane (2.26) or isoflurane (1.25). The minimum alveolar concentration (MAC) varies with age (< 6 months old, MAC is 3.3; > 6 months, 2.5; adults, 2.0).[40] Compared with halothane, sevoflurane is associated with more rapid emergence,[41–43] although increased excitement or delirium during recovery has been reported.[34]

In contrast to halothane, sevoflurane may increase heart rate and blood pressure during induction.[37, 44–46] Sevoflurane maintains heart rate and blood pressure more effectively than equianaesthetic concentrations of halothane and is associated with a lower incidence of cardiac arrhythmias.[47] At > 1 MAC, blood pressure may fall in children < 5 years, but not in older children. Heart rate is unchanged at 1 MAC in those < 3 years but may increase significantly in older children.[40]

Sevoflurane is particularly useful for inducing anaesthesia in children with airway difficulties. It is superior to halothane for bronchoscopy, endoscopy[48] or adenotonsillectomy, especially in children with URTIs.[49] Sevoflurane may be used as a sole agent for anaesthesia during insertion of a laryngeal mask[50, 51] or intubation (for which satisfactory conditions are obtained more rapidly than with halothane).[52] Sevoflurane can precipitate malignant hyperthermia in susceptible children.[53]

Sevoflurane is suitable for neuroanaesthesia. It decreases cerebral vascular resistance and oxygen consumption, but at 1 MAC does not change total cerebral or cortical blood flow. It may induce seizures in epileptic patients.[54]

The metabolism of sevoflurane has two potential problems:

1. Production of inorganic fluoride ions. Although sevoflurane is eliminated largely through the lungs, 5% is metabolised. Metabolic products include hexafluoroisopropanol (excreted renally) and inorganic fluoride ions. The metabolism of methoxyflurane (now no longer used) also produced an inorganic fluoride ion, which was associated with renal toxicity. Fluoride from sevoflurane, however, has not been shown to damage kidneys,[55, 56] probably because hepatic metabolism is thought to involve cytochrome P450 2E1, whereas methoxyflurane is metabolised via the cytochrome P450 31 system.[57]
2. Production of compound A. In combination with soda lime, sevoflurane may produce a toxic metabolite (compound A or olefin). Concentrations of compound A > 40 parts per million in rats produce renal toxicity, although even higher concentrations have not produced renal damage in humans.[58]

Desflurane is a fluorinated methyl ethyl ether differing structurally from isoflurane by the substitution of a fluorine atom for chlorine. It requires a different design of vaporiser because the saturated vapour pressure at 20°C is 669 mmHg, close to atmospheric pressure. Its most important characteristic is its extremely low blood:gas solubility coefficient (0.42). Tissue solubility is less than any other agent. MAC varies with age (9.16 for babies < 6 months; 9.92 for children > 6 months; 6 in adults) and falls by 24% when delivered in 60% nitrous oxide.[59]

Desflurane has a number of disadvantages:

1. Airway irritation. Desflurane is unsuitable for induction in children because it is very pungent and irritant, commonly causing severe coughing, laryngospasm or breath-holding.[60,61]
2. Cardiovascular effects. Desflurane may increase heart rate and systolic and pulmonary blood pressures in adults during induction or rapid increase in inspired concentration.[62] In children, heart rate and mean arterial pressure (MAP) increase during induction and heart rate remains high intraoperatively.[61]

Desflurane is, however, suitable for maintenance of anaesthesia in neonates, babies and children and maintains haemodynamic stability during surgery.[60] Recovery is rapid, but emergence delirium has been reported.[63] In ex-premature babies, desflurane is associated with a much lower incidence of postoperative complications (such as apnoea) compared with halothane or sevoflurane.[64]

TOTAL INTRAVENOUS ANAESTHESIA

Interest in TIVA in children has increased with better understanding of the pharmaco-kinetics and pharmacodynamics of the drugs used and the development of new drug delivery systems allowing closer titration of drugs. Propofol is most commonly used, often given concurrently with a powerful, short-acting opioid such as remifentil or alfentanil.

The benefits of TIVA include rapid wakening, less nausea or vomiting[65] and reduced pollution compared with inhalational anaesthesia. Disadvantages include the potential for awareness, less suppression of vagal responses and involuntary movements, but other side-effects (e.g. anaphylaxis, adrenal suppression, immune suppression or infection of infusion solutions) are rare.[66]

The dose of propofol for TIVA in children is twice that of adults (ED_{95} of 10.5 mg kg^{-1} h^{-1} compared with 5 mg kg^{-1} h^{-1} when combined with an alfentanil 50 μg kg^{-1} h^{-1}).[67]

OPIOIDS

Remifentanil is a potent synthetic μ-agonist derived from a phenylaminopiperidine propanoic acid. Analgesic potency is approximately 22 times greater than alfentanil.[68] Remifentanil has a very short half-life (making it suitable for infusion) because its methyl ester link is cleaved by tissue and blood esterases. The usual loading dose in adults is 1 μg kg^{-1} with a subsequent infusion of 0.25–1.0 μg kg^{-1} min^{-1}.[69] Offset of action is only 3–3.5 min and is independent of either the dose or duration of infusion. Consequently, another analgesic may be required very soon after stopping the infusion.

Pharmacokinetics are unaltered in liver or renal disease.[69] Side-effects are those common to all opioids (e.g. ventilatory depression, nausea and vomiting chest wall rigidity). Postoperative respiratory depression does not occur because of the rapid offset of action. However, the IV cannula should be flushed carefully at the end of infusion to prevent unintentional injection of this very potent opioid during recovery.

Remifentanil has been used successfully in babies (0.5 μ kg^{-1} min^{-1}, followed by 0.75 μg kg^{-1} min^{-1} at the onset of surgery)[70] although, in general, there is little information available on its use in children.

NON-DEPOLARISING MUSCLE RELAXANTS

Cisatracurium is an isomer of atracurium that also undergoes non-enzymatic (or Hoffman) degradation, making it suitable for patients with liver or renal disease. However, unlike atracurium, it does not release histamine (even up to a dose of $8 \times ED_{95}$) and is therefore associated with greater cardiovascular stability.[71] Cisatracurium has an onset time (from administration to maximal effect) of 2.2–2.3 min and an intermediate duration of action (27–34 min).[71] The usual dose in children ages 2–12 is 80–100 µg kg^{-1}.[71]

Rocuronium is an analogue of vecuronium with no reported side-effects.[72] It has a rapid onset and intermediate duration of action. Rocuronium 0.6 mg kg^{-1} produces good intubating conditions at 90 s and has a duration of action (defined as the time from administration to 25% electromyogram (EMG) recovery) of 24 min.[73] Increasing the dose to 0.8 mg kg^{-1} allows earlier intubation (at about 28 s) but prolongs the duration of block to 32 min.[73] Rocuronium has been used for rapid-sequence induction,[74] providing intubating conditions comparable to suxamethonium at 1 min.[72, 75]

The onset of action is more rapid in children compared with babies or adults and potency is reduced (ED_{95} in children is 409 µg kg^{-1} compared with 251 µg kg^{-1} in babies and 350 µg kg^{-1} in adults). Time to recovery, however, is unaffected by age.[74]

Mivacurium is a bisquaternary benzylisoquinolinium ester with a very short duration of action. Excretion is not dependent on liver metabolism or renal excretion because mivacurium is partly hydrolysed by plasma cholinesterase. However, patients with plasma cholinesterase deficiency may have prolonged block.[76] The ED_{95} is 90 µg kg^{-1}.[77]

The time taken to obtain good intubating conditions ranges from 90 to 120 s (depending on dose) and the block lasts 10–15 min. Onset is quicker[78] and potency slightly greater in infants compared with children.[79] Mivacurium may be infused at 10–16 µg kg^{-1} min^{-1} without prolonging recovery.[80] In the usual dose range, mivacurium is associated with cardiovascular stability but may cause histamine release at higher doses.

ANTIEMETICS

Serotonin/5-hydroxytryptamine type 3 (5-HT$_3$) receptor antagonists, found in the central nervous system and gastrointestinal tract, mediate afferent emetogenic stimuli. Selective antagonists, such as ondansetron or granisetron, are now widely used to reduce POV in children. They are as effective as, or better than, older drugs and have no significant side-effects.

Ondansetron prevents nausea and vomiting more effectively than placebo or droperidol.[81] The optimum dose in children is 100 µg kg^{-1};[82] 50 µg kg^{-1} is less effective and 150 µg kg^{-1} is no better.[83] Two doses have a greater effect than one.[84]

The minimum effective dose of granisetron to prevent emesis after paediatric surgery is 40 µg kg^{-1}.[85] Granisetron 40 µg kg^{-1} is more effective in children than droperidol 50 µg kg^{-1} or metoclopramide 0.25 mg kg^{-1}.[86] Its effectiveness is improved if given with dexamethasone (4 mg).[87]

Managing the airway

Tracheal intubation

The indications for tracheal intubation are similar to those in adults. Many anaesthetists intubate the tracheas of babies < 6 months of age, or weighing < 6 kg, to give continuous positive airway pressure (CPAP) or mechanically ventilate the lungs to try to decrease basal atelectasis. However, since the introduction of the laryngeal mask airway (LMA) and improved monitoring (particularly oximetry), this has become less common, particularly for short operations.

Extubation of the trachea with the child 'deep' or awake?

Advocates of 'deep extubation' state it allows the child to emerge from anaesthesia peacefully with minimal irritation to the trachea or pharynx, reducing coughing and laryngospasm. In contrast, advocates of 'awake extubation' claim this technique protects the airway until airway reflexes return when the child wakes. However, laryngeal incompetence after extubation is common and the risk of aspiration is not eliminated by consciousness.[88] Burgess and colleagues have suggested that laryngeal function is disturbed for at least 4 h after tracheal extubation.[89]

Any child at serious risk of aspirating gastric contents (e.g. one with a full stomach, acute abdomen or gastro-oesophageal reflux) should be fully awake before extubation to reduce the risk. The situation is less clear after nose or throat surgery where the airway remains completely unprotected until airway reflexes return if the tracheal tube is removed with the child asleep. Preventing tracheal soiling then depends on the patient's position (i.e. the lateral position with the head tilted down) and careful airway management (including suctioning) by the recovery nurse. Recent evidence, however, suggests that a tracheal tube protects the airway less effectively than previously thought, since blood can track below the vocal cords around the tube.[90]

Is there any evidence that one technique is superior? Patel and colleagues studied airway complications during emergence in otherwise healthy children having elective surgery (either correction of strabismus or adenotonsillectomy).[91] They found a higher SpO_2 during the first 5 min after extubation in children who were deep compared with those who were awake when the tube was removed, but no differences in the incidence of airway complications (e.g. excessive coughing, laryngospasm, stridor, sore throat or arrhythmias). The authors concluded that either the anaesthetist's preference or surgical requirements should determine the timing of extubation.

In another study, Pounder and colleagues compared the incidence of complications after awake or deep extubation in 100 children anaesthetised with either halothane or isoflurane for minor abdominal or urological surgery.[92] The authors reported that for both isoflurane and halothane, hypoxaemia ($SpO_2 < 90\%$) was more common in children extubated awake than deep. Isoflurane anaesthesia was associated with more coughing and airway obstruction after awake extubation than halothane.

The laryngeal mask airway

The LMA was introduced in the UK in 1985; since this time, indications for its use have increased exponentially. The LMA is inserted blindly into the pharynx to form a low-pressure seal around the laryngeal inlet without the need for muscle relaxants or deep anaesthesia, allowing administration of inhalational agents through an airway with minimal stimulation.[93]

LMAs have been developed for children by scaling down adult prototypes. The appropriate sizes for children of different ages, and their characteristics, are summarised in Table 6.6.

The airway of a baby or child differs from an adult's in that the glottis is more anterior and higher, and the epiglottis relatively larger and more floppy. Both factors account for the greater difficulty in positioning LMAs in babies or children. The epiglottis is prone to fold down into the bowl of the LMA, causing partial or total airway obstruction. Negotiating the posterior pharyngeal curvature is often the most difficult aspect of insertion. Various manoeuvres to facilitate this include repositioning the head, pulling the tongue forward, applying the mask firmly against the hard palate, inserting the LMA laterally, applying CPAP, using a laryngoscope,[94] inserting the LMA in the back-to-front position before rotating through 180°[95, 96] or partially inflating the cuff before insertion.[97]

Table 6.6 The laryngeal mask airway in children

Size	Child's weight (kg)	Cuff volume (ml)	Internal diameter (mm)
1	< 6.5	2–5	5.25
1.5	5–10 kg	5–7	6
2	6.5–20	7–10	7
2.5	20–30	14	8.4
3	30–70	15–20	10

The final position of the LMA in children is often imperfect despite usually providing a clinically acceptable airway. The epiglottis is frequently folded down, obscuring the laryngeal inlet in about half of children[98–101] and continued patency of the airway, particularly in babies, cannot be guaranteed. However, the results of a large prospective study of 1400 babies and children attest to the safety and efficacy of the LMA in paediatric anaesthesia.[102] The size 1 LMA, however, is associated with significantly more clinical problems ($P < 0.001$).

The indications for the LMA are numerous, although it will not protect the airway from soiling by gastrointestinal contents. Although several authors have described giving positive-pressure ventilation through the LMA in children,[103, 104] there is a greater danger of inflating the stomach than in adults, partly because the position of the LMA is often imperfect.

THE LMA AND THE 'DIFFICULT AIRWAY'

The LMA is particularly useful in children with abnormalities of the airway in whom intubation is difficult (e.g. Pierre Robin sequence or Treacher Collins syndrome). It can be used in place of a tracheal tube[105, 106] or to facilitate intubation by acting as a conduit for fibreoptic bronchoscopy and delivery of oxygen and volatile agents during cannulation of the trachea.[34, 107–112] Some authors have described inserting a tracheal tube blindly through the LMA in children[113] but others consider this inadvisable because of down-folding of the epiglottis into the bowl of the LMA.[98] Debreuil and Eccofey recommend assessing the position of the epiglottis fibrescopically first to reduce the risk of trauma.[114] Other techniques using an LMA to maintain a difficult airway in a child during intubation are described in Table 6.7.

The reinforced LMA was introduced into paediatric anaesthesia more recently.[115] It is used during surgery on the head or neck and, in many hospitals in the UK, during most ENT operations in children (including adenotonsillectomy) and for dental extractions.

Monitoring

General considerations

Except for specific circumstances (e.g. during rapid-sequence induction, or anaesthesia in babies, sick children or those with congenital heart disease), full monitoring is usually established after the child has lost consciousness in an attempt to reduce anxiety. Many children, however, may be persuaded to have the oximeter probe applied beforehand.

Monitoring should be consistent with the recommendations of the Association of Anaesthetists of Great Britain and Ireland.[116] Although precordial or oesophageal stethoscopes are not included in the Association's recommendations, these are cheap and safe, and provide continuous information about the cardiovascular and respiratory systems (e.g. loss of heart sounds may indicate hypovolaemia, breath sounds confirm ventilation). Moulded ear pieces may improve comfort when worn for more than a few minutes. Some oesophageal stethoscopes incorporate a thermistor for temperature monitoring. Systems are now available to transduce oesophageal stethoscopes.[117]

Table 6.7 Methods of tracheal intubation through the laryngeal mask airway (LMA)

Method	Reference
DESCRIBED IN INFANTS	
● A tube inserted into the trachea blindly through the LMA	Rabb et al[110]
● An oral preformed tracheal tube, size 3.5 or 4.0, passed through an LMA, size 1 or 2. An adult Portex intubating stylet is then inserted snugly into the endotracheal tube (with its connector removed) and the LMA removed. Subsequently, the stylet is removed and the connector inserted into the endotracheal tube	Osses et al[113]
● A fibreoptic laryngoscope (external diameter 3.5 mm) can be passed through the vocal cords via an LMA (size 1.5 or 2). A tracheal tube is then rail-roaded over the scope	Bandla et al[111]
● (In awake babies) two tracheal tubes without connectors (one pushed into the other to provide length) can be placed over a fibreoptic scope (external diameter 2 mm), which is then passed through the vocal cords via the LMA, which was removed. The trachea is then intubated with the serial tracheal tubes and the proximal one is removed	Theroux et al[112]
DESCRIBED IN CHILDREN	
● A gum elastic bougie can be advanced through an LMA (then removed) and used to guide a tracheal tube into the trachea.	Allison & McCrory[108]
● A fibreoptic bronchoscope can be inserted through an LMA and used to position a guidewire through the vocal cords under direct vision. The scope and LMA are then removed and the tube passed into the trachea over the guidewire	Heard et al[109]
● Alternatively, the guidewire can be stiffened with a urethral dilator before rail-roading the tracheal tube into the trachea	Walker et al[34]

Few anaesthetists would dispute the benefit of pulse oximetry as a continuous monitor during anaesthesia in babies or children. However, although oximetry may reduce the number and length of hypoxic events by giving an early warning, it does not reduce morbidity.[118] Similarly, extensive investigations in adults have failed to demonstrate that monitoring, especially pulse oximetry, improves outcome.[119, 120]

Monitoring the cardiovascular system

Continuous direct intra-arterial and central venous pressure monitoring is indicated for babies or children undergoing major surgery, particularly involving large blood loss or fluid shifts. Continuous direct intra-arterial pressure monitoring is useful where hypotensive anaesthetic techniques are employed.

ARTERIAL LINES

Arterial lines for children should have a small gauge, no taper, be non-pyrogenic, and be associated with a low risk of thrombosis. They are commonly made of Teflon, polypropylene or polyurethane. Appropriate sizes for children of different ages are given in Table 6.8(A).

An Allen's test[121] or finger plethysmography[122] should be performed, if possible, before insertion to assess collateral circulation. Arteries can be located by palpation, with a Doppler flow meter, or by transillumination with a cold light source (especially at peripheral sites). Cannulae can be inserted by direct arterial puncture, or using either the

Table 6.8(A) Sizes of arterial line for children of different weights

Weight of child	Gauge of peripheral arterial cannula
< 3 kg	24G
3–10 kg	22G
> 10 kg	20G

Table 6.8(B) Complications of arterial lines

All sites	Umbilical catheters
• Malfunction	Same as for all sites, plus:
• Thrombus formation	• Vascular spasm of lower legs
• Emboli	• Migration to renal arteries
• Paradoxical emboli	• Migration to coeliac trunk
• Ischaemia	• Renal hypertension
• Infection	• Necrotising enterocolitis
• Haemorrhage due to disconnection	• Paraplegia
• Sampling-related blood loss	
• Traumatic damage to related structures, e.g. nerves	

Seldinger technique[123] (with a 23G butterfly and a 15-cm wire of a 0.4-mm outer diameter) or a surgical cutdown. Once sited, the cannula should be securely fixed and the limb immobilised using splints and tapes.

Pressure transducers and lines can be kept patent by a continual flush system containing either normal saline or 5% glucose with added heparin (1 IU ml^{-1}) pressurised by either a bag or syringe driver and infused at 1–3 ml h^{-1}. Normal saline neither causes hypernatraemia[124] nor affects blood glucose measurements.

Fluid balance must be monitored carefully. Excessive blood loss can occur through disconnection (minimised by using Luer-Lok connectors) or frequent sampling and discarding of blood. Large volumes of fluid may also be given inadvertently.

Syringe drivers apply constant pressure and have a lower volume of fluid in the system compared with bags, but syringes must be changed more frequently. The tubing between the cannula and transducer should have a small internal volume to decrease wastage when sampling, and the volume required for flushing. Air bubbles must be fastidiously removed because these affect accuracy and increase the risk of emboli. Even 0.5 ml of flush can produce retrograde flow to cerebral vessels.

Complications associated with umbilical catheters depend on the tip position and the duration of use. Serious complications increase significantly if the tip lies within the thorax (T10 is probably optimum[125]). Complications associated with arterial lines are listed in Table 6.8(B).

CENTRAL VENOUS LINES

Central lines can be inserted into sites commonly used in adults. Catheters of 3.5 French gauge are recommended for neonates, 4 French gauge for children up to 10 kg, and 5–7 French gauge for older children and adolescents. In neonates, the umbilical vein can also be cannulated, usually with a 5 French gauge catheter.

COMPLEX MONITORS

Appropriate-sized equipment for more complex monitoring (e.g. measurement of pulmonary artery pressure or transoesophageal echocardiography) is increasingly available.

These techniques may be associated with significant morbidity or require expert interpretation and are not recommended for the occasional practitioner.

Temperature regulation and monitoring

Core temperature is most accurately monitored from a thermistor in the pulmonary artery. More commonly, however, temperature is recorded from other sites (such as the oesophagus, rectum, axilla or tympanic membrane) which give a reasonable approximation of core temperature.[126, 127] Urinary catheters incorporating thermistors have also been developed.

Heat loss is relatively greater in babies and children compared with adults because they have:

1. an increased body surface area to mass ratio;
2. increased thermal conductance from the core to the periphery (because of decreased insulation and increased cardiac output);
3. decreased radii of curvature, which increases radiation losses.[128]

Anaesthesia significantly impairs temperature homeostasis by a variety of mechanisms (Table 6.9).[128–133]

Mild hypothermia is not important intraoperatively[134] but postoperatively causes shivering (except neonates, who rely on non-shivering thermogenesis (NST)), increased oxygen demand, glucose utilisation and acidosis. These effects are not generally important in fit, healthy children but may be so in the critically ill.[135] Some of the consequences of hypothermia are listed in Table 6.10.

Heat loss can be eliminated by increasing ambient temperature and humidity. At theatre temperatures of 24°C or higher, all children remain normothermic providing general precautions are maintained, compared with only 70% at 21–24°C. However, all children lose heat at ambient temperatures below 21°C.[136] Other techniques for reducing heat loss and maintaining body temperature in babies and children are summarised in Table 6.11.

Active forced air-warming systems may be used over or under a child and are more effective than circulating water mattresses and Thermolite™ insulation.[137, 138] Risks associated with active heating systems include hyperthemia,[137] softening of the tracheal tube[139] and thermal burns.[140]

Table 6.9 The mechanisms by which anaesthetics impair temperature homeostasis

Anaesthetics decrease heat production by reducing:	Anaesthetics increase heat loss by:
● Behavioural responses	● Vasodilation, redistributing core heat (except ketamine)[378]
● Hypothalamic regulation	● Cooling with intravenous fluids/blood
● Metabolic rate	● Air flow circulation

Table 6.10 Consequences of postoperative hypothermia

Mild hypothermia causes:	Severe hypothermia causes:
● Prolonged drug metabolism	● Impaired platelet function and increased blood loss
● Shivering	● Delayed return of consciousness
● Wound infections	● Arrhythmias
● Prolonged hospital stay	

Table 6.11 Methods of reducing perioperative heat loss in babies and children

Passive techniques of heat conservation
- Insulating covers, including hat for the head
- Use of wrapping, e.g. polythene, to provide a microclimate
- Mattresses of low thermal conductance
- Covers with reflective surfaces
- Water-repellent drapes to prevent skin becoming wet causing heat loss via evaporation
- Bowel bags during surgery
- Heat and moisture exchangers (smallest dead space = 50 ml)
- Maintenance of high ambient temperature and humidity

Passive methods are generally safe and effective if used in combination (rather than alone)

Active techniques of temperature maintenance
- Fluid/blood warmers
- Forced-air warmers, e.g. Bair Hugger™, Warm Touch™
- Heated humidifiers, e.g. Fisher Paykell™
- Radiant overhead heaters (with or without servo control)
- Use of warm transport systems, e.g. incubators

SPECIAL CONSIDERATIONS IN BABIES

Neonates are even more likely to lose heat than older children and have limited ability to maintain normothermia, often only at considerable energy cost. NST (or brown-fat metabolism) occurs if skin temperature falls below 35°C and body temperature cannot be maintained by physical processes alone (such as changes in body position or vasoconstriction). Skin receptors (mainly in the face) stimulate the sympathetic nervous system causing noradrenaline (norepinephrine) release in brown fat (found around the scapulae, neck, adrenals and axillae), activating lipolysis and fatty acid oxidation, and increasing heat production and oxygen consumption by up to threefold. NST is principally an adaptation to the process of delivery and cannot be sustained indefinitely. Increased oxygen requirements will eventually cause hypoxia, acidosis, pulmonary vasoconstriction, respiratory distress, and even death. Oxygen consumption is minimised in clinical practice, therefore, by removing the need to activate additional intrinsic chemical heat production by providing a thermoneutral environment. The thermoneutral environment is a steady state in which metabolic rate is minimal and thermoregulation occurs by non-evaporative physical processes alone. It is determined both by temperature and humidity and depends on gestational and postnatal ages (Table 6.12). The thermoneutral temperature zone for adults is much wider (between 20 and 35°C).

Although NST is inactivated by anaesthetic agents, it is an important consideration during transport to and from theatre and in the immediate pre- and postoperative periods. Theatre should therefore be heated to as high a temperature as can be tolerated by the staff and babies transported in heated incubators.

Table 6.12 Thermoneutral environment for neonates (adapted from Steward)

Weight of baby	Thermoneutral temperature
1200 g	34–35.4°C
1500 g	34.4°C
2500 g	33.8°C, falling to 31°C at 2 weeks

THE RECOVERY WARD
Staffing

The ratio of recovery nurses to children should be high and these nurses should have particular experience of the problems children may present.[141] The American Society of Postanesthesia Nurses have made recommendations for staffing in the recovery ward (Table 6.13).[141]

Monitoring and resuscitation equipment

The level of monitoring (both by human observation and technological methods) during transfer to, and within, the recovery room should be high.[142] Recovery facilities should comply with the recommendations of the Association of Anaesthetists of Great Britain and Ireland[116, 143] and 'monitoring should be appropriate to the condition of the patient with the full range of (recommended) monitoring devices available'.

A full range of paediatric resuscitation equipment (probably best provided in a trolley), high-flow oxygen and air (especially for premature or ex-premature babies), suction, and a defibrillator with appropriate paddles should also be available.

Discharge criteria

Length of stay in recovery should be determined by the clinical state of the child and criteria for discharge should be clear.[142] Suggested criteria are listed in Table 6.14.

PREVENTING POSTOPERATIVE NAUSEA OR VOMITING

Nausea or vomiting after surgery is uncommon in children < 2 years of age but frequently affects older children.[144] Risk factors include:

1. Age > 2 years[145] and increasing age;[146]
2. Opioid analgesia, especially morphine;[147, 148]
3. Strabismus or middle-ear surgery, adenotonsillectomy or appendicectomy.

The anaesthetist can reduce the incidence by choosing appropriate anaesthetic (e.g. propofol) and giving prophylactic antiemetics at induction or before starting morphine infusion

Table 6.13 Suggested nurse-to-patient ratio in the recovery ward[141]

Class	Suggested nurse-to-patient ratio	Description
1	1:3	Awake
2	1:2	Stable, unconscious, uncomplicated, paediatric
3	1:1	Admission period, life support care required
		A second nurse should be available to assist

Table 6.14 Criteria for discharge from the recovery ward[142]

- The clinical condition must be stable
- Airway/respiratory function should be returned to normal
- Pain/nausea and vomiting must be controlled
- Consciousness should be restored, as well as movement appropriate to age or level of development

Table 6.15 Suggested antiemetic regimen for perioperative use in children

Give prophylactic intravenous antiemetics at induction to children:	• scheduled for surgery associated with high incidence of POV, e.g. squint correction, major ear surgery, adenotonsillectomy or emergency abdominal surgery • at high risk of POV, e.g. history of motion sickness or previous POV
Give prophylactic antiemetics to children receiving perioperative opioids:	• a single dose of IV antiemetic to children commencing PCA or an IV morphine infusion

Suggested drugs

		Receptor antagonism site:
First-line therapy	Ondansetron 0.15 mg kg⁻¹ IV 8-hourly	• Serotonin (5-hydroxytryptamine)
Second-line therapy	Metoclopramide 0.15 mg kg⁻¹ IV 8-hourly	• Dopamine
	Droperidol 25–50 µg kg⁻¹ IV	• Dopamine
	Cyclizine 1 mg kg⁻¹ IV	• Histamine

POV, postoperative vomiting; IV, intravenous; PCA, patient-controlled analgesia

or patient-controlled analgesia (see anaesthetic considerations for specific operations in the next section). Suggested antiemetics for perioperative use in children are summarised in Table 6.15.

Side-effects of some of the more commonly used antiemetics are thought to occur more frequently in children. Metoclopramide[149] and cyclizine are associated with extrapyramidal effects. Cyclizine may also cause anticholinergic effects. Droperidol, particularly in large doses, may cause drowsiness,[150] sedation,[150] dysphoria, restlessness and extrapyramidal effects in children.[151] Ondansetron, which is comparatively free of side-effects, is often the first-line treatment for POV in children.

SECTION 2: Anaesthetic techniques for specific procedures

ANAESTHESIA FOR EAR, NOSE AND THROAT SURGERY
General considerations
Children having ENT surgery may have impaired hearing or associated abnormalities and often require multiple procedures. Great care should be taken to provide a good anaesthetic service to ensure they have as pleasant an experience as possible, so minimising anxiety associated with subsequent operations. Conditions commonly associated with the need for ENT surgery and their anaesthetic implications are summarised in Table 6.16.

The 'shared airway'
During many ENT operations, the anaesthetist and surgeon must share the airway. The anaesthetic technique must provide adequate oxygenation and anaesthesia, and ensure the airway remains patent and protected throughout surgery.

Tracheal intubation remains the gold standard during operations on the nose or pharynx. Preformed oral tubes (e.g. the RAE 'south-facing' tube), are usually used; their southerly direction and peripherally placed connector allow the surgeon easy access. The reinforced LMA, described previously, is gaining popularity for ENT anaesthesia and in some hospitals is now used more often than a tracheal tube in children. The two are compared in Table 6.17.

Table 6.16 Some associated medical conditions and their anaesthetic implications in children presenting for ear, nose and throat (ENT) surgery

Associated condition	ENT surgery usually required	Anaesthetic considerations and implications
Vasomotor rhinitis or allergic rhinitis	Diathermy to inferior turbinates Reduction of inferior turbinates	May have difficulty breathing through the nose
Recurrent tonsillitis	Tonsillectomy	Children may have large tonsils impeding the insertion of a laryngeal mask airway blindly (a laryngoscope may be helpful)
Chronic airway obstruction (sleep apnoea)	Adenotonsillectomy	Severe chronic hypertrophy of the adenoids and tonsils sometimes causes obstructive sleep apnoea, with oxygen desaturation and snoring during sleep, daytime somnolence, and, rarely, cor pulmonale. Assess severity with a preoperative sleep study. Affected children are sensitive to sedative premedication (therefore avoid) and opioids (use other analgesics in preference). Airway obstruction is not immediately relieved by surgery. Postoperative complications, including apnoea, are more common, therefore monitor on high-dependency unit after surgery
Recurrent ear infections	Myringotomy and insertion of grommets Myringoplasty Adenoidectomy	Children with adenoidal hypertrophy may have difficulty breathing through the nose
Trisomy 21 (Down's syndrome)	See Table 6.19	See Table 6.19
Cystic fibrosis	Nasal polypectomy Antral lavage	A genetic condition affecting exocrine glands characterised by abnormal composition of exocrine secretions Respiratory failure ● Recurrent chest infections with eventual bronchiectasis ● Respiratory tract colonised by bacterial pathogens (*Staphylococcus aureus*, *Haemophilus influenzae* and *Pseudomonas aeruginosa*) ● Copious viscous secretions in the respiratory tract cause increased airway resistance, gas trapping and increased functional residual capacity ● V:Q mismatch results in hypoxia ($PaCO_2$ usually normal) ● Reduced lung compliance

Table 6.16 continued overleaf

Table 6.16 continued from previous page

		● Optimise condition. Chest physiotherapy pre- and postoperatively. Avoid atropine, if possible Pancreatic insufficiency ● Malnourished ● Occasionally diabetic May have biliary fibrosis and cirrhosis
Oculoauriculovertebral spectrum	Myringotomy and grommet insertion, middle-ear surgery	See Table 6.26
Treacher Collins syndrome	External and middle-ear surgery	See Table 6.26
Mucopolysaccharidoses (Hurler's syndrome/ type I is the prototype)	Tonsillectomy and adenoidectomy Myringotomy and grommet insertion Mastoidectomy Airway surgery	Difficult airway and difficult intubation ● Macroglossia ● Large head ● Nose often blocked due to adenoidal hypertrophy ● Short, thick neck ● Mucopolysaccharide deposition in trachea and bronchi produces narrowing Coronary artery disease and valvular heart disease – even in young children Cardiomyopathy Restrictive lung disease ● Thoracolumbar kyphosis ● Recurrent chest infections Obstructive sleep apnoea ● May require tracheostomy Hydrocephalus

For surgery on the larynx, trachea or bronchi, the anaesthetic technique must ensure adequate oxygenation and anaesthesia whilst providing the surgeon with an unobstructed view.

Minor surgery

Many children having minor ENT surgery (e.g. myringotomy and insertion of grommets, manipulation of nasal fractures, diathermy to inferior turbinates) are admitted as day cases. The anaesthetic technique chosen should allow the child to recover rapidly from anaesthesia, free from pain, nausea and vomiting.

A volatile agent delivered through a face mask or LMA is usually used for maintenance of anaesthesia in children having myringotomy or insertion of grommets. An LMA, however, allows the surgeon better access compared with a face mask[93] with fewer interruptions from the anaesthetist re-establishing the airway.

For children undergoing short procedures to the nose (e.g. manipulation of nasal fractures or diathermy to inferior turbinates) the reinforced LMA provides excellent airway protection.[152]

Table 6.17 A comparison of the laryngeal mask airway (LMA) with the tracheal tube for paediatric ear, nose and throat anaesthesia

Characteristic	Laryngeal mask airway	Tracheal tube
Ease of insertion	Inserted blindly into the pharynx without IV muscle relaxant or deep anaesthesia	Requires IV muscle relaxant or deep anaesthesia; performed at laryngoscopy under direct vision
Airway protection ● From blood and debris from the airway above	Secures and protects airway better than TT[90, 152, 206]	Secures and protects airway less successfully than previously thought[206]
● From aspiration of gastric protection	No protection	Protects
Emergence characteristics	Smooth: lower incidence of laryngospasm, coughing on removal and oxygen desaturation in comparison with tracheal extubation deep or awake[90, 152, 206, 207]	Higher incidence of laryngospasm, coughing on removal and oxygen desaturation than the LMA[90, 152, 206, 207]

IV, intravenous; TT, tracheal tube.

Middle-ear surgery

There are a number of specific considerations for anaesthesia in children having operations on the middle ear.

Postoperative vomiting

Nausea and vomiting are very common after middle-ear surgery[144] and the anaesthetist should select techniques and drugs to minimise POV. Although propofol effectively reduces POV after many other operations in children, propofol anaesthesia alone does not prevent vomiting after middle-ear surgery.[153] In a study comparing different anaesthetics, the incidence of vomiting in children given a propofol infusion during myringoplasty was high (55% compared with 70% of those given a thiopental/isoflurane technique), possibly because of the use of nitrous oxide or morphine. The high incidence of vomiting after middle-ear surgery in children justifies the use of a prophylactic antiemetic at induction, e.g. ondansetron 0.06 mg kg^{-1} IV,[154] granisetron 40 µg kg^{-1} IV[155] or prochlorperazine 0.2 mg kg^{-1}.[154]

Reducing bleeding

The surgeon operates through a microscope and, for optimal conditions, requires a 'bloodless field'.

MAINTAINING CARDIOVASCULAR STABILITY

Bleeding is increased by hypertension or tachycardia. The goals of anaesthesia are to produce a relatively slow pulse and a slightly lower than normal blood pressure. These may be obtained with sedative premedication (allaying anxiety and providing sedation), a smooth induction (avoiding coughing, crying or straining), a gentle laryngoscopy and adequate anaesthesia and analgesia. A balanced anaesthetic technique probably provides optimal surgical conditions.

TIVA, using remifentanil (0.25–0.5 µg kg^{-1} min^{-1}) and propofol (3–5 mg kg^{-1} followed by an initial infusion of 6–9 mg kg^{-1} h^{-1}) is an alternative technique allowing rapid control of the blood pressure and heart rate, and prompt recovery.

A summary of anaesthetic techniques for middle-ear surgery is given in Table 6.18.

Table 6.18 Anaesthesia for middle-ear surgery

Preoperative considerations	Deafness Previous ear surgery Anxiety	
Premedication	**Typical technique** Oral midazolam 0.5 mg kg^{-1} Ametop™ or Emla™ cream	**Alternative technique** Other sedative premedication or no premedication
Monitoring	Standard + facial nerve stimulator	
Perioperative considerations	*A bloodless surgical field* ● Smooth anaesthesia (avoiding crying, coughing and straining; gentle laryngoscopy and lidocaine (lignocaine) spray; gentle intubation when adequately anaesthetised) ● Control of EtCO$_2$ (positive-pressure ventilation) ● Careful positioning during surgery (head-up position, avoid kinking of great veins in the neck) *High incidence of POV*	
Induction	IV propofol, 3–5 mg kg^{-1} in O$_2$ and air	Inhalation of sevoflurane 1- 8% (or other halogenated agent) in N$_2$0 and 0$_2$ IV droperidol 25 μg kg^{-1} IV ondansetron, 0.15 mg kg^{-1} ± IM prochlorperazine 0.25 mg kg^{-1}
Pain management	IV remifentanil infusion, 0.25– 0.5 μg kg^{-1} min^{-1} commenced at induction IV fentanyl, 1–2 μg kg^{-1} or IV morphine, 50 –100 μg kg^{-1} 20 mins before end of anaesthetic Pain management as for intermediate/major surgery (see Table 7.7)	IV fentanyl 1–2 μg kg^{-1} or IV morphine 50–100 μg kg^{-1} boluses at induction and PRN
Position	Supine, head up tilt	
Airway Protection	Tracheal tube	
Method of ventilation	Intermittent positive pressure ventilation	
Maintenance	IV propofol, 6–9 mg kg^{-1} hr^{-1} in O$_2$ and air and IV remifentanil, 0.25–0.5 μg kg^{-1} min^{-1}	Halogenated agent (isoflurane 0.5–1%)
Muscle relaxant	Short-acting IV non-depolarising muscle relaxant to facilitate intubation	

137

Table 6.18 continued overleaf

Table 6.18 continued from previous page

Decisive steps		Discontinue N₂0 before tympanic graft
Fluid requirements	Standard	
Blood loss	Usually minimal	
Emergence	Smooth	
Precautions	Facial nerve damage possible. (Allow muscle relaxation to wear off to enable use of stimulator during operation to locate the facial nerve.)	Local anaesthetic and vasoconstrictor infiltration may cause cardiac arrhythmias with halothane (maximum dose of adrenaline (epinephrine) 5 µg kg⁻¹)

Inducing hypotension

Using TIVA, a bolus of remifentanil ($1 \ \mu g \ kg^{-1}$) provides rapid control of blood pressure and usually eliminates the need for hypotensive agents. Labetalol IV, $0.2 \ mg \ kg^{-1}$ every 5 min as necessary, may be given if optimal haemodynamics are not obtained with anaesthetic agents alone. Although other hypotensive techniques may be used (e.g. infusions of glyceryltrinitrate or sodium nitroprusside, or boluses of hydralazine), these are seldom used for middle-ear surgery and rarely necessary since the introduction of TIVA.

Improving venous drainage

Positioning the child with his/her head-up by 15–20° improves venous drainage and reduces bleeding. The head should be turned to the side and positioned carefully to avoid venous obstruction.

TOPICAL ADRENALINE (EPINEPHRINE)

The surgeon usually infiltrates the skin with a local anaesthetic containing adrenaline (epinephrine) to provide analgesia and haemostasis. Bleeding may be reduced further during microscopic surgery by applying small swabs soaked in dilute adrenaline (epinephrine) to the operative site.

IDENTIFYING THE FACIAL NERVE

The facial nerve emerges from the stylomastoid foramen to lie superficially close to the surgical site. The surgeon often uses a nerve stimulator to locate it when operating through a postauricular incision. Any muscle relaxant used to facilitate intubation should have a short duration of action and residual effects must have worn off by the time the stimulator is used.

NITROUS OXIDE

Nitrous oxide increases middle-ear pressure[156] and, if used during tympanoplasty, should be discontinued about 15 min before placing the tympanic graft.

Operations on the nose

Operations on the nose, even minor procedures (e.g. manipulating a nasal fracture) often produce considerable bleeding. The anaesthetic considerations are to protect the airway and reduce bleeding to improve operating conditions (if necessary). Surgeons often insert packs into the nose at the end of surgery to improve haemostasis, which some children find distressing.

Protecting the airway

The airway may be protected from blood or debris with a tracheal tube and throat pack or a reinforced LMA.[157]

Vasoconstrictors

A vasoconstrictor is often applied topically (e.g. cocaine or local anaesthetic with adrenaline (epinephrine)) or injected into the nasal mucosa to reduce bleeding. Local infiltration results in marked and unpredictable systemic uptake.[158] Nasal packs, often soaked in adrenaline (epinephrine) or phenylephrine, are sometimes inserted at the end of surgery. Again, marked absorption may occur. Hypertension from systemic toxicity can be treated with IV alpha-adrenergic blockers, such as phentolamine 0.1 mg kg^{-1} or labetalol 0.25–0.5 mg kg^{-1}.

COCAINE

Topical cocaine has been used clinically for more than 100 years because of its availability, low cost and anaesthetic and vasoconstrictor properties.[159] Complications of therapeutic doses of topical cocaine have been reported only in adults and include arrhythmias, myocardial infarction and sudden death from heart failure.[160]

ADRENALINE (EPINEPHRINE)

Adrenaline (epinephrine), usually combined with a local anaesthetic, is generally injected submucosally. For children breathing halothane spontaneously at normocapnia, Karl and colleagues recommend a maximum dose submucosally of 10 μg kg^{-1}.[161]

Anaesthesia for functional endoscopic sinus surgery (FESS)

The common indications for FESS in children are acute or chronic sinusitis, or choanal or nasal polyposis (children with cystic fibrosis are particularly prone to nasal polyps). Endoscopic techniques may also be used for ethmoidectomies, sphenoidotomies, maxillary antrostomies or nasal polypectomies.[162]
The major considerations for anaesthesia are:

1. to protect the airway from blood or debris by using a tracheal tube and throat pack or LMA;
2. to provide a bloodless field to allow the surgeon to see through the endoscope.

Many of the techniques to reduce bleeding during surgery on the middle ear described above (e.g. modest hypotension, head-up position) may be used during FESS. Bleeding can be reduced further with topical or submucosal vasoconstrictors.

Adenotonsillectomy

Adenoidectomy is used to relieve obstruction of the nasopharynx (manifest as snoring and mouth-breathing) or eustachian tubes (presenting as recurrent otitis media). Tonsillectomy is usually indicated for recurrent tonsillitis and less commonly for peritonsillar abscess, or chronic upper airways obstruction and sleep apnoea.

Anaesthetic considerations

There are several important anaesthetic considerations in children having adenotonsillectomy.

COMORBIDITY

Obstructive sleep apnoea. Children presenting with obstructive sleep apnoea frequently have hypertrophied tonsils causing hypoventilation with hypoxaemia, hypercarbia, acidosis, pulmonary vasoconstriction and pulmonary hypertension. Cor pulmonale, cardiac arrhythmias and seizures secondary to hypoxia may also occur. Important clinical clues to obstructive sleep apnoea include intermittent cyanosis and difficulty in arousal during the day[163] and the diagnosis is made with a sleep study. Recognising tonsillar hypertrophy early and removing the tonsils (sometimes as an emergency[163]) relieves reversible pulmonary hypertension and cardiac enlargement.

Down's syndrome. Children with Down's syndrome (trisomy 21) often develop tonsillar and adenoidal hypertrophy requiring adenotonsillectomy. These children commonly have partial upper-airway obstruction (UAO) during sleep, increased susceptibility to infection (particularly of the upper airways and lungs) and chronic catarrh. Several authors have

Table 6.19 The considerations for anaesthetising a child with Down's syndrome (trisomy 21) for adenotonsillectomy

Feature	Anaesthetic implications
Learning difficulties, communication problems, sensory impairment (poor vision, conductive and sensorineural deafness) and neuropsychiatric problems	Communication difficulties The child may not understand what is happening to him/her perioperatively and may be very anxious
Airway/breathing abnormalities ● Large tongue ● Micrognathia ● Short, broad neck ● Pharyngeal muscle hypotonia ● Partial upper-airway obstruction during sleep ● Increased incidence of congenital subglottic stenosis ● Sleep-induced ventilatory dysfunction	Gaseous induction may be preferable Vocal cord visualisation may be difficult A smaller tracheal tube than predicted by age may be required May develop postoperative stridor Sleep-induced ventilatory dysfunction occurs that may be exacerbated by opioid sedation and residual anaesthetic levels postoperatively Close supervision in recovery is essential until awake and apnoea monitoring for 24 h
Congenital malformations in 30–60% cases ● 50% endocardial cushion defects ● 50% other defects (ASD, VSD, PDA, TOF) Cor pulmonale may develop Acquired valvular dysfunction may occur	Antibiotic prophylaxis against endocarditis Understand the anaesthetic implications of the cardiac anomaly Cardiac arrhythmias may occur
Pulmonary hypertension may occur with/without cardiovascular lesions due to: ● Obstructive sleep apnoea ● Hypoventilation due to muscular hypotonia ● Chronic hypoxia secondary to chest infections	Susceptible to postoperative pulmonary complications
Atlanto-occipital instability Many case reports of subluxation after intubation	Radiological investigations *essential* if symptomatic: ● Sensory deficits ● Neck pain, limited mobility, torticollis ● Gait disturbance ● Spasticity

Table 6.19 continued overleaf

Table 6.19 continued from previous page

	If asymptomatic – no tests required but: ● Limit movement of the neck as much as possible during tracheal intubation ● Evaluate carefully postoperatively
Incidence of gastro-oesophageal reflux may be increased	Trachea should be intubated Airway management with an LMA is not advised
Increased susceptibility to infection	Take great care to cannulate veins aseptically
Hypothyroidism commonly associated	Check thyroid function
Sensitive to anaesthetic agents	Reduce the doses of opioids and anaesthetic agents

ASD, atrial septal defect; VSD, ventricular septal defect; PDA, patent ductus arteriosus; TOF, tetralogy of Fallot; LMA, laryngeal mask airway.

described the management of children with Down's syndrome[164–166] and the anaesthetic considerations for adenotonsillectomy are summarised in Table 6.19.

POSTOPERATIVE VOMITING

POV affects 70–73% of children anaesthetised for adenotonsillectomy using older techniques (i.e. induction with either thiopental or halothane, maintenance with halothane in oxygen and nitrous oxide, analgesia with IV morphine) and not given prophylactic antiemetics.[167, 168] POV is the commonest cause of unscheduled overnight admission after day-case adenotonsillectomy.[169] It is influenced by several factors.

Sedative premedication. Oral premedication with trimeprazine 4 mg kg^{-1} reduces POV after adenotonsillectomy more effectively than diazepam 0.5 mg kg^{-1}.[170] Midazolam 75 µg kg^{-1} IV after induction also reduces POV and the number of unscheduled admissions to hospital.[171]

Anaesthetic agents. POV after adenotonsillectomy is common with modern anaesthetic agents. Fujii and colleagues found a 65% incidence of vomiting associated with sevoflurane and nitrous oxide.[172] Propofol seems to produce a lower incidence of POV after adenotonsillectomy in children. Barst and colleagues showed the incidence of POV in the first 24 h to be 21% using propofol infusion compared with 55% using isoflurane.[173] Ved and colleagues showed maintenance with a propofol infusion produced 3.5 times less POV than halothane.[174] POV in the first 8 h affected 27% of children given a propofol induction followed by maintenance with either isoflurane or halothane.[175]

Spontaneous or positive-pressure ventilation. There is no difference in the incidence of POV after anaesthesia with spontaneous or positive-pressure ventilation.[176]

Antiemetics. Antiemetics given preoperatively (e.g. oral ondansetron 0.15 mg kg^{-1} [177]; dexamethasone 150 µg kg^{-1} IV – maximum of 8 mg[178]) or at induction (e.g. metoclopramide 0.25 mg kg^{-1}, ondansetron 0.15 mg kg^{-1},[168, 179–182] granisetron 40 µg kg^{-1} [172] or droperidol 50 µg kg^{-1} [183]) reduce the incidence of POV after tonsillectomy or adenotonsillectomy in children. Metoclopramide 0.15 mg kg^{-1} IV immediately before emergence is also effective.[167]

Some practitioners are concerned that ondansetron given before adenotonsillectomy (particularly for day-case surgery) may mask bleeding.[184, 185] Children who have received IV ondansetron should be carefully observed postoperatively for signs of occult haemorrhage.

Analgesia. IV or IM morphine (usually 0.1 mg kg^{-1}) has long been the gold standard for perioperative analgesia for adenotonsillectomy. Its routine use has been questioned, however, because of its high association with POV, which to children is often as distressing as a sore throat.[147] Giving a full dose of morphine (0.1 mg kg^{-1}) to every child is probably not justified.[147] Codeine phosphate 0.1–0.15 mg kg^{-1} is an alternative,[186] although it may be argued that its mildly superior effect on POV does not compensate for its weaker analgesic effect. Pain after tonsillectomy is very variable and, while some children will require opioid analgesia, most may be managed with a combination of NSAIDs and paracetamol.[147]

Local anaesthetic techniques have also been described. Topical 1% lidocaine (lignocaine) 4 mg kg^{-1}, sprayed evenly over the tonsillar beds, improves pain control immediately after tonsillectomy compared with IM codeine 1.5 mg kg^{-1}.[187] Infiltrating the anterior tonsillar pilla with local anaesthetic before incision (e.g. bupivacaine 0.25% with adrenaline (epinephrine) 1 in 200 000) is an alternative technique. Some authors have shown peritonsillar infiltration provides pain relief well beyond the immediate postoperative period[188–190] whilst others have shown only a brief effect.[191, 192] The technique, although simple, has produced major complications including IV or carotid artery injection (producing cardiovascular or central nervous system toxicity), airway obstruction, haemorrhage, allergy, vocal cord paralysis or mucosal sloughing. Peritonsillar infiltration must be performed by a skilled clinician familiar with the technique.

POSTOPERATIVE HAEMORRHAGE

Bleeding after tonsillectomy affects about 1–2% of children during the first 24 h, and 0.06% require a second general anaesthetic for re-exploration.[193, 194] It is sometimes life-threatening and children still die each year as a result.[195, 196] The incidence may be linked to surgical technique[197, 198] and primary haemorrhage is more common in children with URTIs.[199] The influence of NSAIDS is widely debated, and some authors are concerned about increased perioperative bleeding.[200]

NSAIDs, such as diclofenac or ketorolac, reversibly inhibit prostaglandin synthetase, impairing platelet function. Ketorolac 0.1 mg kg^{-1} has been associated with increased perioperative[201, 202] and early posttonsillectomy haemorrhage.[203] However, diclofenac 1 mg kg^{-1} IM at induction had little, if any, effect on perioperative bleeding, or the rates of re-exploration for control of haemorrhage (1%).[204]

Proponents of the use of NSAIDs during adenotonsillectomy in children state, however, that these drugs provide excellent analgesia, are opioid-sparing, and associated with a low incidence of POV. Many practitioners in the UK have used them routinely for adenotonsillectomy for a number of years. The Royal College of Anaesthetists has recommended avoiding NSAIDs in children with increased risks of bleeding or reduced platelet function[205] (Table 7.9).

MAINTAINING THE AIRWAY

The airway may be maintained for tonsillectomy through a tracheal tube or LMA. Several authors have described the use of the LMA during paediatric ENT surgery,[152, 206–208] and the reinforced version has been used successfully during tonsillectomy in over 800 children.[152] The LMA secures and maintains a patent airway throughout the operation and allows adequate access for the surgeon[206, 207] (Figure 6.5).

The LMA also protects the lower airway from soiling with blood or debris from above. The authors of one study injected methylene blue into the pharynx and showed that the LMA effectively prevented aspiration of the dye into the trachea.[209] Compared with a tracheal tube, the LMA also allows aspiration of less blood during adenotonsillectomy.[90, 152, 206] Williams & Bailey showed that blood commonly tracks past a tracheal tube in children (21/39), but not past an LMA (0/34).[206]

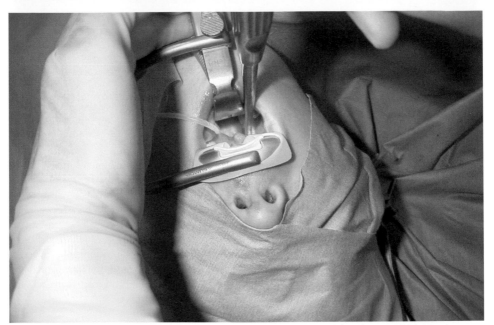

Fig 6.5 View of the oropharynx when a reinforced laryngeal mask airway is used for adenoidectomy in a child. The reinforced laryngeal mask airway tucks away beneath the Boyle-Davis gag allowing good access to the adenoidal bed.

The quality of recovery in children in whom LMAs have been used during tonsillectomy is superior to those who have been intubated (and extubated when either deep or awake)[90, 152] and postoperative laryngospasm or coughing is less common.[206, 207]

ANAESTHETIC TECHNIQUE
A suitable anaesthetic technique and alternatives are summarised in Table 6.20.

DAY-CASE ADENOTONSILLECTOMY
In many countries, fit children are admitted for adenotonsillectomy as day cases. These children must be selected carefully and have good overall medical health (particularly no central or obstructive sleep apnoea or history of abnormal bleeding), adequate social circumstances and live within 1 h of hospital.[210, 211] Complications (e.g. protracted vomiting, fever or haemorrhage) occur most frequently within the first 6 h after surgery, so it is imperative these children are observed in hospital for this period before discharge home.[194] Parents should be given information about possible complications and clear verbal and written guidelines for when, how and where to seek medical assistance, if needed.

ADENOTONSILLECTOMY FOR THE CHILD WITH OBSTRUCTIVE SLEEP APNOEA
Anaesthesia for children with UAO secondary to tonsillar hypertrophy requires special considerations because there is a risk of death if these children are not adequately assessed preoperatively.[163] Any cardiac decompensation should be treated medically before surgery. Premedication should be avoided because of the risks of ventilatory depression. Anaesthetists should anticipate a difficult intubation and an inhalational induction is indicated.[212] These children should be monitored for apnoea for 24 h postoperatively and those with pulmonary hypertension should be observed on the intensive care unit (ICU).

Table 6.20 Anaesthetic techniques for adenotonsillectomy

	Typical anaesthetic technique	Alternative technique
Perioperative considerations	Postoperative vomiting Perioperative bleeding Day-case procedure?	
Premedication	No sedative premedication Ametop™ or Emla™ cream	Oral midazolam 0.5 mg kg⁻¹
Monitoring	Standard	
Induction	IV propofol, 3–5 mg kg⁻¹ IV ondansetron, 0.15 mg kg⁻¹ N₂O/O₂	IV propofol 3–5 mg kg⁻¹ IV granisetron 40 µg kg⁻¹ or IV metoclopramide 0.25 mg kg⁻¹ O₂/air
Analgesia	*At induction,* IV fentanyl 1–2 µg kg⁻¹. Rectal diclofenac 1–1.5 mg kg⁻¹ and paracetamol 40 mg kg⁻¹ *In recovery,* IV fentanyl 1 µg kg⁻¹ or IV morphine 50 µg kg⁻¹ boluses PRN (For pain management for intermediate surgery, see Table 7.7)	IV fentanyl 1–2 µg kg⁻¹ or IV morphine 50–100 µg kg⁻¹ or IM codeine 1 mg kg⁻¹
Position	Supine, sandbag under shoulders ± head ring	
Airway protection	Reinforced LMA (contraindicated if there is a risk of aspiration of gastric contents)	Tracheal tube
Method of ventilation	Spontaneous	Intermittent positive-pressure ventilation
Maintenance	Halogenated agent (isoflurane 0.8–1.2%)	IV propofol 6–10 mg kg⁻¹ h⁻¹ in O₂ and air
Muscle relaxant	Not required	IV non-depolarising muscle relaxant, e.g. mivacurium 0.1 mg kg⁻¹ or atracurium 0.5 mg kg⁻¹ or suxamethonium 1–2 mg kg⁻¹ for intubation
Decisive steps	Insertion of Boyle-Davis gag may cause airway obstruction – check airway carefully by gentle ventilation manually to confirm ability to ventilate	
Fluid requirements	20 ml kg⁻¹ crystalloid during surgery and then maintenance fluids until drinking normally postoperatively	
Blood loss	Usually minimal	
Emergence	In the (left) lateral head-down position Remove LMA when awake	Reverse muscle relaxant if necessary Extubate 'deep' or awake

Table 6.20 continued overleaf

Table 6.20 continued from previous page

Oral intake	When tolerated
Postoperative observations	Risk of postoperative haemorrhage – observe for 6 h before discharge from hospital if day case and provide guidelines for parents and an emergency telephone contact

IV, intravenous; LMA, laryngeal mask airway; IM, intramuscular.

ANAESTHETIC TECHNIQUE IN THE CHILD WITH A BLEEDING TONSIL

Anaesthesia for re-exploration of a bleeding tonsil may be difficult, even in experienced hands. The most senior anaesthetist available and an experienced assistant should be present. All equipment should be checked and two suckers with wide-bore tubing available to remove blood clots.

Either a rapid-sequence or inhalational induction (with the child lying head-down in the left lateral position) may be used, depending on the familiarity and preference of the anaesthetist. The airway must be secured with a tracheal tube to prevent aspiration of blood from the stomach. A large-bore nasogastric tube should be inserted to remove gastric contents. At the end of the operation, the child should be woken up lying head-down on the left side and the trachea extubated when the child is awake.

There are several factors to consider when planning to reanaesthetise a child for surgical management of a bleeding tonsil.

Hypovolaemia. The volume of haemorrhage is often underestimated. There is often very little blood to see in the throat because much of it is swallowed and cannot be measured unless the child vomits. Vital signs in children, particularly blood pressure, are often well preserved because of high circulating catecholamines, and collapse occurs only when 40% of the circulating blood volume has been lost.

A full blood count, clotting screen (to exclude a coagulopathy) and cross-match should be taken and resuscitation started with warmed IV fluids. Blood loss is almost never so rapid that it cannot be compensated for by resuscitation and anaesthesia should be induced only when the child is haemodynamically stable.

Effects of previous anaesthesia. If the child has a primary tonsillar haemorrhage, the effects of the previous anaesthetic and any postoperative medication given may contribute to sedation and this must be considered when selecting the doses of drugs for the second anaesthetic.

Full stomach. The anaesthetist must assume the child has a full stomach and use an anaesthetic technique to protect the airway from aspiration of blood.

Upper-airway obstruction

UAO may present acutely or as part of a chronic illness. Anaesthetic management is often challenging and senior and experienced anaesthetic help is essential.

Ideally, all children with life-threatening UAO would present to a specialist centre with specially skilled staff and appropriate facilities. In reality, these children will usually be brought to the nearest hospital and immediate tracheal intubation (or a surgical airway, should this fail) will be required. Staff in all hospitals admitting children through an Accident and Emergency department must be competent to manage acute airway obstruction in children. Once the airway has been secured, however, children with airway pathology requiring surgery should be transferred to a specialist centre.

145

Children with partial airway obstruction often present with inspiratory or expiratory stridor. Inspiratory stridor is caused by airway obstruction at or above the vocal cords, whereas expiratory stridor results from subglottic obstruction. Hoarseness or weakness of the voice further suggests glottic involvement. Some causes of acute and chronic stridor are listed in Tables 6.21 and 6.22.

Causes of acute stridor

EPIGLOTTITIS

Epiglottitis has declined dramatically because of routine immunisation against *Haemophilus influenzae* B (HIB).[213, 214] It usually affects children aged 2–7 years, although it sometimes occurs in babies and adults. Children usually present with stridor, dysphagia, hoarseness and fever. Classically they sit up, leaning forward in a characteristic tripod position with their mouths open, drooling saliva, and look toxic. The onset of the illness is rapidly progressive and severe. Prompt anaesthetic intervention and tracheal intubation to prevent death from complete obstruction is essential.

Table 6.21 Causes of acute stridor

Infection	Epiglottitis
	Laryngotracheobronchitis (croup)
	Retropharyngeal abscess
	Bacterial tracheitis
	Acute laryngotracheitis
	Peritonsillar abscess
	Diphtheria
Inhaled foreign body	Peanut, watermelon seed
Laryngeal oedema	Posttracheal intubation
	Traumatic (inhalational injury, smoke or ingestion of corrosives)
Laryngeal spasm	Anaesthesia
Allergy	Angioneurotic oedema
Tumour	Benign or malignant

Table 6.22 Causes of chronic stridor

Supraglottic	Laryngomalacia
	Tonsillar hypertrophy
	Macroglossia
	Cyst (lingual, thyroglossal, aryepiglottic, laryngeal)
Glottic	Laryngeal papillomatosis, web or polyp
	Foreign body
	Vocal cord paralysis
	Dislocation of the cricothyroid or cricoarytenoid cartilage
Subglottic	Subglottic stenosis
	Foreign body
	Tracheobronchomalacia
	Vascular ring
	Haemangioma or tracheal cyst

It is imperative that a child with suspected epiglottitis is not upset because this may lead to total airway obstruction. For the same reason, the pharynx should not be examined, or IV access obtained whilst the child is awake.[215] If tolerated, oxygen given by a parent, either via a face-mask or by holding the end of the oxygen supply tubing near the child's face, is beneficial. The anaesthetic technique for laryngoscopy and tracheal intubation is described below. The epiglottitis is usually cherry red with a median groove, and the laryngeal inlet may also be obscured by oedema. Compressing the chest may produce bubbles at the laryngeal inlet which may guide intubation.

Once the trachea is intubated, the child should be sedated and transferred to the ICU. The child usually breathes spontaneously with CPAP of 2.5–5 cm H_2O. Sedation must be adequate to avoid accidental extubation. Children with epiglottitis usually respond quickly to therapy with IV ceftriaxone 100 mg kg^{-1} stat (maximum 4 g), followed by 50 mg kg^{-1} day^{-1} (maximum 2 g). Maintenance fluids are given either IV or nasogastrically (if early enteral feeding is the local policy). Extubation is usually possible within 1–2 days. Favourable signs suggesting diminished swelling of the epiglottis include resolution of fever and a leak around the tracheal tube. Before extubation, the epiglottis and larynx are usually examined, either fibreoptically or by formal laryngoscopy (under general anaesthesia).

Epiglottitis is rarely complicated by pulmonary oedema, classically developing after intubation. Possible causes include hypoxia, raised circulating catecholamines or a disturbed alveolar-capillary gradient. It resolves with intermittent positive-pressure ventilation (IPPV), positive end-expiratory pressure (PEEP) and diuretics.

ACUTE LARYNGOTRACHEOBRONCHITIS (CROUP)

Acute laryngotracheobronchitis is a common cause of stridor and a differential diagnosis of epiglottitis. Viral infection with parainfluenza, influenza or respiratory syncytial virus are the commonest causes.

Children with croup are usually aged 1–5 years, and boys are affected more than girls. Presenting signs are generally worse at night and include stridor, a barking cough and hoarse voice. The severity is more variable and the onset slower compared with epiglottitis, and the child is not usually toxic. Symptoms usually progress for 3–5 days before improving. Children with more severe illness develop respiratory distress with stridor, tachypnoea, nasal flaring and suprasternal and intercostal recession. Signs of progressing disease include worsening stridor at rest, increasing tachypnoea, cyanosis, sedation and worsening recession. As secretions accumulate and inflammation worsens, complete airway obstruction may occur.

As for epiglottitis, children should be disturbed as little as possible. Emergency treatment includes humidified oxygen, nebulised adrenaline (epinephrine) (5 ml kg^{-1} of 1:1000, maximum 5 ml), and intubation if the airway obstruction is severe. Respiratory compromise develops slowly and there is usually time to plan intubation under general anaesthesia, if necessary. Since the lower airways are also usually involved, IPPV is usually required after intubation. Recovery is slower than from epiglottitis and children who have required tracheal intubation usually remain intubated for several days. Maintenance fluids are given IV or nasogastrically.

Steroids. Although there have been conflicting reports of the benefits of corticosteroids in children with mild or moderate croup (i.e. not requiring intubation), recent reports suggest oral dexamethasone or nebulised budesonide is useful.[216, 217] Children requiring intubation should receive prednisolone 1 mg kg^{-1} 12-hourly, because this reduces the duration of intubation and the incidence of reintubation.[218]

OTHER INFECTIVE CAUSES OF ACUTE UPPER-AIRWAY OBSTRUCTION

A retropharyngeal abscess may complicate bacterial pharyngitis or pharyngeal trauma. Symptoms include neck stiffness, fever, dysphagia, drooling or progressive airway obstruction.

If the abscess bursts, pus may be aspirated into the lung. A retropharyngeal abscess may be diagnosed with a lateral neck X-ray, on which the larynx and trachea are displaced anteriorly.

The symptoms of a peritonsillar abscess (or quinsy) include a sore throat, fever, trismus or drooling. Marked tonsillar hypertrophy may develop with the risk of total airway obstruction and continuous observation is essential. Treatment includes antibiotics, needle aspiration and surgical exploration.

Bacterial tracheitis, usually due to staphylococcal infection, often follows croup. Treatment with IV flucloxacillin and prolonged intubation may be required. The tracheal tube may become blocked by sloughed tracheal mucosa.

TUMOUR

An airway tumour may present with acute airway obstruction. Malignant airway tumours are, fortunately, rare.

Causes of chronic stridor

LARYNGOMALACIA

In laryngomalacia, the laryngeal cartilages are incompletely mature and the epiglottis (or one of the arytenoids) tends to prolapse into the glottis during inspiration, producing stridor and suprasternal and intercostal recession. Laryngomalacia is the commonest cause of congenital stridor. Endoscopy is useful for diagnosis, during which the laryngeal wall may be seen in-drawing on inspiration. The condition is self-limiting and disappears as the child grows. Aryepiglottiplasty is only needed for babies with severe obstruction. Two-thirds of children with severe laryngomalacia also have gastro-oesophageal reflux.[219]

TRACHEOBRONCHOMALACIA

Tracheobronchomalacia is caused by either an absent or a defective cartilaginous ring producing a 'floppy' segment of the trachea or bronchus. During expiration, the central airways may narrow by more than 75%, causing stridor.[220] It is an important cause of airway distress in babies but usually resolves as the airway enlarges. It is particularly common after repair of a tracheo-oesophageal fistula and in babies born preterm.

Presentation varies from 'dying spells', wheezing, cyanotic spells or intermittent airway obstruction, to recurrent pneumonia or difficulty with extubation. Tracheobronchomalacia may be treated with long-term PEEP or CPAP via a tracheotomy. Surgical treatment includes tracheopexy, resection, external splinting, endobronchial stents or tracheobronchoplasty.

LARYNGOTRACHEAL STENOSIS

Laryngotracheal stenosis may be congenital or acquired. Long-term intubation is the commonest acquired cause, affecting 0.7–8% of intubated children,[221] and usually involving the subglottic area. There should be a high index of suspicion if dyspnoea or laryngeal stridor develops after prolonged intubation. Tracheotomy and tracheal reconstruction may be necessary.

LARYNGEAL PAPILLOMATOSIS

This is a rare condition, presenting with hoarseness, progressive dyspnoea and symptoms and signs of airway obstruction. It is the most frequent benign neoplasm of the larynx and biopsies are usually positive for human papillomavirus. Malignant transformation may occur and death by asphyxiation has been reported.[222] Lesions are cauliflower-shaped and frequently multiple and recurrent. Diagnosis is usually made before the child is 5 years old and the papillomas often regress around puberty.[223]

TRACHEOBRONCHIAL COMPRESSION

The trachea or bronchi may be compressed externally by a vascular ring or a mass such as a cystic hygroma (Figure 6.6A and B).

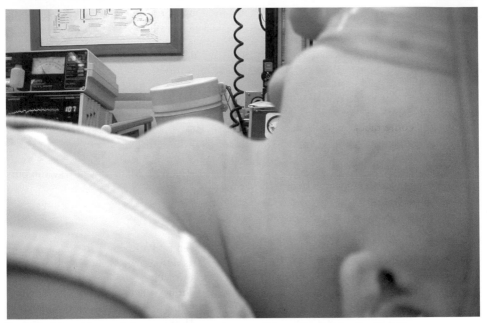

Fig 6.6A Baby with a cystic hygroma in the anterior part of the neck overlying the trachea.

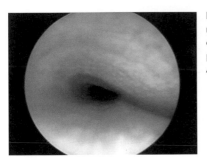

Fig 6.6B View of the trachea during microlaryngobronchoscopy. The cystic hygroma is causing compression of the trachea. (These figures were kindly provided by Dr Anna Johnson, Consultant Paediatric Anaesthetist, Derriford Hospital).

Anaesthetic management of acute UOA

The aim in managing acute UAO is to secure the airway safely with a tracheal tube. A senior anaesthetist, skilled anaesthetic assistant and an ENT surgeon capable of performing an emergency tracheotomy must be present throughout anaesthesia. Emergency drugs and anaesthetic equipment must be well prepared in advance. Equipment should include uncut tracheal tubes (down to the smallest size), several laryngoscopes, introducers and suction. Children with acute UAO may also have gastric distension and an increased risk of regurgitation and aspiration

Sedative premedication must not be used because it may precipitate total airway obstruction.

An inhalational technique (using either sevoflurane 1–8% in oxygen or halothane 1–5%) is the safest method of induction. The child may be unable to lie flat and anaesthesia should be induced in whatever position he/she finds easiest to breathe (usually sitting upright, leaning forwards). Oxygenation and gas exchange may be improved with CPAP, produced by partly occluding the bag of the T-piece circuit. Once the child is adequately anaesthetised, IV access should be obtained and atropine 10–20 µg kg^{-1} injected.

Induction will be slow and sufficient time should be allowed to obtain an adequate depth of anaesthesia before laryngoscopy to assess the airway. If a good view of the laryngeal inlet is obtained, the larynx and supraglottic structures can be sprayed with lidocaine (lignocaine) (maximum 4 mg kg^{-1}) to obtund the response to intubation. Occasionally, intubation is impossible and it will be necessary to continue the inhalational anaesthetic and proceed to tracheotomy. It is important that, throughout induction, the child breathes spontaneously because artificial ventilation of the lungs may be impossible. A muscle relaxant should never be given until the trachea has been intubated and the ease of artificial ventilation confirmed.

Inducing anaesthesia in a child with UAO is difficult and apnoea occurs easily. If this happens, the anaesthetist should try to ventilate the lungs manually with oxygen. Usually this is successful, but if not, the anaesthetist should attempt intubation. Intubation may be impossible, either because of difficulty visualising the larynx or inability to pass the tube through the narrowed lumen of the larynx or trachea. In these situations, an emergency cricothyroidotomy is indicated.

Once the airway has been secured, management depends on the cause of obstruction and the facilities available locally. Any surgery (e.g. resection of laryngeal papillomatosis) should be done in a specialist centre. If the obstruction does not resolve and cannot be corrected surgically, a tracheostomy may be required.

SEVOFLURANE OR HALOTHANE?

Sevoflurane has replaced halothane as first choice for inhalational induction in many countries. It induces anaesthesia more quickly, and is associated with fewer adverse cardiovascular effects or airway complications, and a more rapid recovery compared with halothane.[48, 224] However, many anaesthetists have concerns about using sevoflurane in children with UAO, particularly epiglottitis. Halothane has a longer duration of action, which may be enormously useful during a difficult laryngoscopy, whereas children anaesthetised with sevoflurane may lighten far too quickly.[224]

THE LMA

The LMA has been used successfully to maintain the airway in children with airway obstruction. For example, Asai and colleagues used an LMA in a child with tracheal stenosis in preference to a tracheal tube, which would have increased resistance to ventilation by narrowing the diameter of the airway further.[225] An LMA may also be less traumatic than a tracheal tube, which may cause oedema, worsening the stenosis.

The LMA is unsuitable for children with lesions of the oropharynx or epiglottis[226] since it is usually difficult to position and may worsen airway obstruction. As it cannot prevent tracheal collapse, it is unlikely to help those with tracheomalacia or external compression of the trachea.[227] If the abnormality lies within the larynx itself, attempts to insert an LMA correctly are unlikely to succeed.[228]

WHERE SHOULD SURGERY FOR SERIOUS AIRWAY PROBLEMS BE DONE?

Ideally, all airway surgery should be undertaken by a paediatric ENT surgeon (specialising in airway surgery) supported by a paediatric anaesthetist who routinely manages children with airway pathology, in a specialist centre providing neonatal and paediatric intensive care facilities and skilled anaesthetic and surgical assistance. Although this service is sometimes provided in the larger DGH (as in Plymouth), it is more usually confined to specialist children's hospitals.

Although children with life-threatening UAO often present acutely to their nearest hospital, they should be transferred to a specialist centre after immediate life-saving management is complete if they require surgery. Children with chronic airway pathology should be managed in a specialist centre from the outset.

Inhaled foreign body

Inhaling a foreign body is life-threatening, and the diagnosis must be considered in every small child presenting with respiratory symptoms of sudden onset. It usually occurs in boys aged 1–3 years[229, 230] and the material is generally organic,[229–231] most commonly peanuts.[230]

Clinical presentation

The child usually presents with cough, cyanosis, choking, wheeze, dyspnoea or fever.[230, 231] The most frequent clinical signs are depressed breath sounds, wheezing, retraction or rhonchi.[231] Normal breath sounds, however, do not exclude the diagnosis.

Foreign bodies most commonly lodge in the right main bronchus but may also be found in the left bronchus, larynx or oropharynx, depending on size and shape:[232] large foreign bodies (> 20 mm diameter) generally remain in the oropharynx (Figure 6.7A and B); irregular, pointed bodies of 8–15 mm diameter usually lodge in the larynx; and smaller, smoother or linear objects pass into the bronchi.

A foreign body in the oesophagus may also obstruct the airway, particularly if it compresses the trachea at a level where it is already narrow (e.g. at the cricoid or the level of the aortic arch).

LATE PRESENTATION

Diagnosing an inhaled foreign body is difficult if the history is unclear, the clinical features inconsistent and the foreign body radiolucent.[232] The possibility must always be considered, particularly in children < 3 years or those with a highly suspicious history, even without clinical signs or X-ray changes.[230] Early diagnosis and prompt endoscopic removal of the foreign body prevent serious complications, including death.

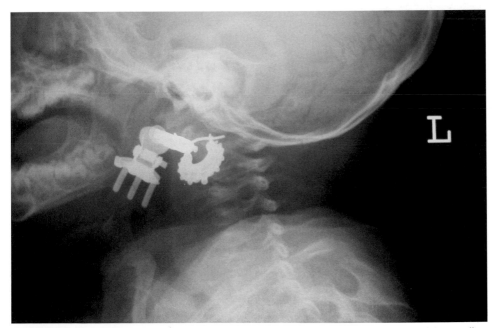

Fig 6.7A Lateral neck X-ray of an eleven-month old who had been playing with a hair slide while travelling in the car. The hair slide was inhaled and lodged in the oropharynx, causing the baby distress and inducing vomiting.

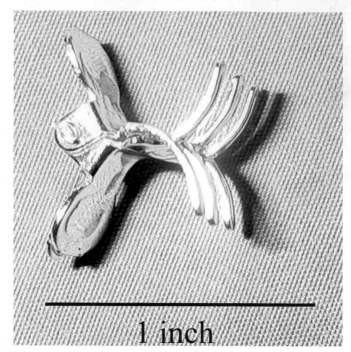

Fig 6.7B Hair slide, removed by direct laryngoscopy under inhalational anaesthesia.

X-ray features

A chest X-ray will confirm the diagnosis if the foreign body is radiopaque, but most are radiolucent and the diagnosis is then suggested by other changes that vary with time.[229] An X-ray within 24 h of inhalation is generally normal, whereas later films usually show abnormalities, commonly including atelectasis, emphysema, shift of the heart and mediastinum away from the aspirated body, or pneumonia. An end-expiratory film may show hyperexpansion of the ipsilateral lung caused by a 'ball-valve' effect. Pneumothorax is rare.

Anaesthesia

Successfully retrieving an inhaled body requires good team work between surgeon and anaesthetist. A child whose life is not immediately threatened should be transferred to a specialist centre, if this is possible without compromising his/her condition. If there is any risk that the foreign body may move, causing acute UAO during transfer, then it should be removed locally. Any hospitals accepting emergency paediatric admissions must have the resources to manage acute UAO or aspirated foreign body, including an ENT or thoracic surgeon able to bronchoscope a child and an anaesthetist competent in managing such a case.

There are several important considerations for anaesthesia. The clinical condition ranges from a few, relatively mild, respiratory symptoms and signs to pneumonia or acute respiratory failure.

1. An organic foreign body (especially a peanut) may induce airway hyperreactivity and inflammation and oedema of the bronchial mucosa. Reactivity often worsens with inhalational anaesthesia, which may cause laryngospasm or bronchospasm.
2. UAO slows induction of anaesthesia and the anaesthetist must take great care to ensure an adequate depth of anaesthesia before laryngoscopy.
3. Partial obstruction of a bronchus may produce a ball-valve effect, allowing air to enter the lung during inspiration but inhibiting deflation during expiration and causing hyper-

inflation of the obstructed lung. This may occur during either spontaneous breathing or IPPV, and can lead to either a simple or tension pneumothorax.

4. Total airway obstruction may occur at any time if the foreign body is mobile. The material may fragment or become impacted, making it difficulty to remove endo-scopically.

Sedative premedication may precipitate total (and sometimes fatal) airway obstruction and should be avoided. Anaesthesia should be induced and maintained with a volatile agent (either sevoflurane and halothane) in oxygen and the child should breathe sponta-neously throughout (unless respiratory failure is present) because this reduces the risks of hyperinflation of the lung and pneumothorax, and is less likely to disseminate the material distally.

A cannula can be sited before induction, if this is possible without upsetting the child, or immediately afterwards. IV atropine 10–20 μg kg^{-1} should then be injected to decrease secretions and prevent the dose-dependent bradycardia associated with high inspired con-centrations of halothane. Although sevoflurane is becoming increasingly popular, some anaesthetists still maintain anaesthesia with halothane because its slow offset allows an ade-quate depth of anaesthesia to be maintained during periods of uneven ventilation whilst the surgeon attempts to remove the foreign body. Cardiac arrhythmias, particularly in the presence of hypoxia and hypercarbia, may be a problem (see the section on sevoflurane or halothane, above).

Both adequate topical anaesthesia and a sufficient depth of general anaesthesia are essential for rigid bronchoscopy. When an adequate depth of anaesthesia is obtained, the larynx and trachea are sprayed at laryngoscopy with lidocaine (lignocaine) 4 mg kg^{-1}. Several minutes should then elapse.

A Storz paediatric bronchoscope, equipped with a Hopkins fibreoptic optical tele-scope, is usually used for rigid bronchoscopy in children (Fig. 6.8). It has excellent optics, a side-arm for attachment of a T-piece circuit (allowing spontaneous or assisted ventilation) and effectively acts in place of a tracheal tube. With the telescope in place, it is a closed system. When removed, the system should be closed with a window occluder.

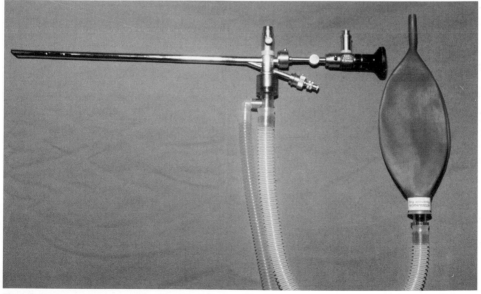

Fig 6.8 Storz bronchoscope with a Hopkins telescope. The T-piece circuit is connected to the side-arm.

The anaesthetist should observe chest expansion carefully. With the telescope in place, a large proportion of the internal diameter of the bronchoscope is occupied, increasing resistance to air flow, particularly with the smaller bronchoscope. This may impair ventilation, prolong exhalation and cause gas-trapping, barotrauma or pneumothorax. These risks may be avoided by frequently removing the telescope, allowing gas to escape.

It is essential to examine the airway endoscopically and remove any inhaled material before intubation with a tracheal tube because this may dislodge, impact or disperse the foreign body, causing total obstruction. Once the material has been removed, the airway may be maintained with a tracheal tube or LMA. The anaesthetic is then discontinued, 100% oxygen is given and the child observed closely until awake and extubated.

Early postoperative problems

Mucosal oedema of the subglottis, trachea or laryngeal inlet may occur after removal of an inhaled foreign body, particularly if it has become fragmented and dispersed or removal is difficult. Dispersed peanut oil in particular causes a chemical pneumonitis.

Corticosteroids given before and after bronchoscopy markedly decrease the incidence of postoperative subglottic oedema,[230] for example, IV dexamethasone 0.25 mg kg^{-1} preoperatively or at induction, followed by 0.1 mg kg^{-1} 6-hourly for 24 h. Other treatments include oxygen, and humidifying and warming inspired gases. Nebulised adrenaline (epinephrine) 1:1000 (0.5 ml kg^{-1} up to 5 ml) may produce dramatic, but short-lived, improvement and further nebulisers may be required regularly.

ANAESTHESIA FOR DENTAL SURGERY

Guidelines have recently been issued by the General Dental Council[233] and the Royal College of Anaesthetists[234] which will change the practice of anaesthesia in the dental chair, following concerns about the administration of general anaesthetic.[234] Firstly, the number of anaesthetics being administered in dental practice has increased rather than decreased since legislation to control the conditions for dental chair anaesthesia.[235] Secondly, death and critical incidents continue to occur in association with dental anaesthesia, usually in young, apparently healthy patients. Such deaths are usually associated with shortfalls in clinical practice which the General Dental Council, Royal College of Anaesthetists and the Department of Health[236] have taken steps to address.

The Royal College of Anaesthetists expects anaesthesia for dentistry to be of the same standard as anaesthesia for all other procedures in the UK. Patients undergoing dentistry should never be put at unnecessary risk. The decision to administer a dental anaesthetic should not be made unless there is no alternative method of treating the patient. The responsibility for recommending dental treatment under general anaesthesia rests on the referring dentist, the dentists performing the procedure and the anaesthetist administering the anaesthetic. All parties should be sure that the procedure is not possible without a general anaesthetic. The risks of general anaesthesia should be explained to the parents of a child scheduled for dentistry under general anaesthesia and alternatives must be offered where applicable.

Anaesthesia for children undergoing dental chair anaesthesia must be administered by an anaesthetist on the Specialist Register (Anaesthetics) or by a trainee working under supervision. Alternatively, non-consultant career grade doctors may anaesthetise children if they have an appointment within the NHS working under the line responsibility of a named consultant anaesthetist. All anaesthetists must have had appropriate experience of and training in dental anaesthesia. It is recommended that paediatric anaesthetists anaesthetise very young children.[234] Dentists can no longer provide general anaesthesia for dental surgery.

The report also states the requirements for dental anaesthesia.[234] The anaesthetist must have a dedicated assistant (operating department assistant or practitioner, dental nurse or nurse) who is suitably trained in this role and has no other duties. An unconscious child should be nursed with continuous monitoring and protected until fully awake in a suitably equipped recovery area. The child should be monitored by an anaesthetist or by an appropriately trained assistant, directly responsible to the anaesthetist.

All personnel working in a situation, where general anaesthesia is used for dental surgery, must be capable of basic life support. The anaesthetic team must have expertise in advanced life support and have regular updates in resuscitation.

Where should dental anaesthetics take place? Most general anaesthetics for dental procedures are uneventful. When a complication does arise however, it is imperative that emergency services are immediately at hand. Previous cases have shown that the further away the patient is from other clinical services the greater the risk of death should a complication occur. It is recommended that anaesthesia for dentistry be centralised to a dental anaesthetic facility in the district general hospital. In this setting, should a complication occur, emergency services are immediately available and there is direct access to intensive care beds. The dental department must be situated in a site allowing easy access for emergency services.

There are several reasons for children undergoing dental procedures under general anaesthesia. Very young children, who would not otherwise cooperate with treatment, may require dental extractions. Children in pain may require dental extractions. The tooth may be infected and extraction under local anaesthetic may not be possible. Older children may require orthodontic extractions, which may be preferable under general anaesthetic. Children with special needs may require a general anaesthetic for almost all dental procedures.

Paediatric dental surgery is usually performed as an outpatient service. Parents should be sent fasting guidelines and a preoperative questionnaire to complete about their child and accompany the child brought for dental extractions. Dental general anaesthetics should be provided on an inpatient basis to children with specific medical problems, for example, congenital heart disease, muscle diseases or cystic fibrosis, or to children with severe learning difficulties.

Paediatric dental anaesthesia is often more challenging than anaesthesia for day-case surgery. The children usually arrive for dental extraction about 15-20 minutes prior to general anaesthesia and leave the dental facility within 30 minutes of completing the procedure. There is seldom time to apply topical local anaesthetic gels prior to venepuncture and premedication is seldom used. The children arrive 'off the street', having been starved at home. Often the children have experienced failed attempts to extract the teeth under local anaesthetic and may be extremely uncooperative, occasionally confounded by the parents having concealed the purpose of the child's visit to the dental facility from the child. This may be an attempt to avoid the child distress or even just to ensure the child arrives at the dental facility.

Preoperative assessment of children arriving for dental extractions should confirm that fasting guidelines have been followed. An accurately completed preoperative questionnaire speeds up the preoperative assessment. The child should be examined as usual, but paying particular attention to excluding the presence of a heart murmur. Prophylactic antibiotics should be administered where appropriate. Consent for analgesia by rectal suppositories should be sought from the parent and child where appropriate if this is the anaesthetist's choice.

The choice of anaesthetic technique will depend on the anaesthetist. Any technique chosen should involve the use of short acting anaesthetic agents. Intravenous induction with propofol (3–4 mg kg^{-1}) and maintenance with isoflurane in nitrous oxide and oxygen is a suitable technique. Alternatively, gaseous induction with sevoflurane (1–8%) in nitrous oxide and oxygen, followed by the insertion of an intravenous cannula for safety, is another suitable technique. Maintenance may be with sevoflurane or isoflurane. Halothane may no longer be used for anaesthesia in remote sites due to the increased incidence of cardiac arrhythmias. Oral analgesia, for example paracetamol 20 mg kg^{-1} 1 hour before the anaesthetic or rectal suppositories of diclofenac 1–1.5 mg kg^{-1} or paracetamol 40 mg kg^{-1} at induction usually provide adequate postoperative analgesia. Infiltration of local anaesthetic into the gums is beneficial when adult molars are extracted. It is important to explain preoperatively to the child that their gums will be numb to avoid anxiety.

Monitoring is usually via pulse oximeter and capnograph. An electrocardiogram and blood pressure monitor should also be available. Dental anaesthesia involves sharing the airway with the dentist.

Anaesthesia is performed supine in most cases with the child lying on a trolley – the dental chair is becoming a rare commodity. The skill of the dentist and the anaesthetist are important in a successful outcome. Anaesthesia is usually maintained via inhalation through a nasal mask during the procedure. A laryngeal mask may be preferred if adult molar teeth or multiple teeth are being extracted. Before extracting the teeth, the dentist inserts a pack or some gauze swabs into the back of the mouth to protect the airway from blood and tooth fragments. Local anaesthesia infiltration improves postoperative recovery and comfort. At the end of the procedure, gauze swabs are placed over the tooth sockets for haemostasis and the child recovers in the left lateral head down position, receiving oxygen via a plastic mask. When the child is awake and able to stand and bleeding has stopped, the child may be discharged from the dental facility.

ANAESTHESIA FOR GENERAL SURGERY

General elective surgery in children

Penoscrotal or groin surgery

Penoscrotal or groin operations are often day-case procedures. A light general anaesthetic (using an LMA to maintain the airway) combined with a regional block (e.g. caudal, penile or iliac crest block) and diclofenac and paracetamol suppositories given at induction is a common technique. Caudal block provides good analgesia with few side-effects[237] and may even decrease the time to discharge because of smoother recovery and reduced requirements for supplemental analgesia.[238] It neither delays voiding of urine[239] nor produces clinically significant motor weakness at discharge (with dilute solutions of local anaesthetic).[240] Caudal analgesia may be safely prolonged in children older than 1 year by adding clonidine 1–2 μg kg^{-1},[241] ketamine 0.5 mg kg^{-1}, or adrenaline (epinephrine) 1:200 000 to the local anaesthetic solution[242, 243] (see Ch. 7). Caudal clonidine can be safely used for day surgery[241] but may cause marked sedation postoperatively.[244] However, any respiratory or cardiovascular effects are indistiguishable from those associated with plain solutions of local anaesthetics.[245] Ketamine produces no sedation and is preferable for day surgery.

Torsion of a testis

Torsion may cause testicular infarction and surgery should not be delayed to allow adequate fasting. The airway should be protected using a rapid-sequence induction. Muscle paralysis is unnecessary for surgery so, after intubation, the child may breathe spontaneously. A 'one-shot' caudal, combined with NSAIDs and paracetamol, provides good perioperative analgesia. Alternatives include opioids or infiltration with local anaesthetics.

Appendicectomy or perforated Meckel's diverticulum

Acute appendicitis usually presents in older children. The differential diagnosis includes a perforated Meckel's diverticulum, although anaesthetic management of both is similar. Some children are dehydrated on admission and fluid and electrolyte resuscitation must be completed before induction.

SCHEDULING OF SURGERY

Although a child with an acute appendicitis usually presents as an emergency, it is probably not necessary to operate during the night. Waiting until the next day, when the paediatric team is available, does not increase morbidity or mortality.[246]

ANAESTHESIA

A rapid-sequence induction is indicated to protect the airway. Rocuronium in high dose (0.9 mg kg^{-1})[247] has been used successfully as a alternative to suxamethonium, although muscle relaxation lasts 30–40 min.[248] If suxamethonium is used, a short-acting relaxant such as atracurium or vecuronium should be given subsequently. Anaesthesia is generally maintained using a volatile agent and nitrous oxide (or air) in oxygen. After reversal of muscle relaxation at the end of surgery, the child recovers head-down in the left lateral position and the trachea is extubated when the child is awake.

Intraoperative analgesia is usually provided by opioids (generally morphine), either as boluses or an infusion.[249] Some children will need opioids postoperatively for about 24 h, and these are best given as either IV infusions or patient-controlled analgesia. Opioid requirements are reduced by giving NSAIDs perioperatively[250, 251] or regularly after surgery,[252] or injecting local anaesthetic into the peritoneum and skin.[253]

LAPAROSCOPIC APPENDICECTOMY

Several authors report that laparoscopic appendicectomy in children increases the duration of surgery and the intraoperative requirements for opioids without significantly improving postoperative analgesia or allowing earlier discharge.[254–256] The high incidence of minor adverse events during surgery (such as hypercapnia, hypertension or hypotension) should be balanced against any potential, and as yet unknown, benefits.[257] With advances in the design of laparoscopic instruments for children and increasing experience of the technique, laparoscopic surgery may improve outcome measured by length of stay, analgesia requirements or infection rates.[256] Diagnostic laparoscopy may be useful for teenage girls in whom diagnosis may be unclear.[258, 259]

General surgery in babies

General considerations

The general considerations for providing a competent surgical service for babies is discussed in Chapters 1 and 2. If the recommended standards are not provided locally, then the baby should be transferred to another centre which does provide the recommended standards (usually the specialist centre).

WHAT GENERAL SURGERY SHOULD BE UNDERTAKEN IN THE DGH?

The range of operations undertaken within different age groups depends upon having appropriately trained staff with sufficient continuing experience and a reasonable throughput of cases (see Ch. 2). The Senate of Surgery recommends that all babies < 44 weeks postconceptional age requiring surgery (including pyelomyotomy, inguinal herniotomy or more complex procedures) are managed by specialist paediatric surgeons.[4] Whilst a few DGHs employ such surgeons and have the additional specific facilities to care for neonates, neonatal surgery is mainly confined to specialist children's hospitals. Very rare conditions may even need to be concentrated in a supraregional centre.

Common surgical conditions in babies > 44 weeks postconceptional age (such as pyelomyotomy, inguinal herniotomy, circumcision or intussusception) can be managed within a large, well-organised DGH admitting a reasonable number of babies for surgery if the service meet the recommended standards (see Ch. 2). In particular, Lunn advises that the anaesthetist should anaesthetise at least 12 babies aged < 6 months every year (see Ch. 1, Box 1.7).[260] There are no published standards for the minimum cases a surgeon requires to obtain adequate continuing experience managing babies.

Adequate paediatric support is another vital consideration in determining the type of surgery provided within a hospital. In most DGHs, paediatricians provide initial care and resuscitate sick babies. Some conditions, such as pyloric stenosis or intussusception, can produce considerable dehydration and hypovolaemia, which these clinicians must be able to recognise and competently treat.

PRINCIPLES OF ANAESTHESIA

Good preparation (particularly of equipment) in advance of the baby's arrival in theatre is essential. Equipment should include a range of tracheal tubes and laryngoscopes, and an introducer. Reducing heat loss (e.g. by increasing the ambient temperature to 25°C and relative humidity to 50%, using warm gamgee covers, an overhead heater and warming blanket, or a forced air-warming system and warming IV fluids) is particularly important.

The anaesthetic chosen should allow rapid recovery to avoid prolonged postoperative ventilation. Using a volatile agent with rapid offset (e.g. desflurane, sevoflurane), a short-acting muscle relaxant and giving no (or only small doses of) short-acting opioids is appropriate. Regional techniques, (e.g. caudal or nerve block, or infiltration with local anaesthetic) combined with general anaesthesia may eliminate or decrease requirements for postoperative opioids, probably reducing the risks of ventilatory depression.

Recommendations for perioperative IV fluids in babies and small children are summarised in Table 6.23.

Table 6.23 Perioperative intravenous fluid therapy for babies and small children	
Replacement of starvation deficit Depends on length of starvation	= hourly maintenance IV fluids (ml h^{-1}) × duration of starvation (h). Give deficit over 3 h in addition to hourly rate
	IV fluid used depends on age ● Use 5% dextrose half-strength Hartmann's solution (if < 6 months old) ● Lactated Ringer's solution is preferred by some anaesthetists in older babies
Maintenance IV fluids	● 4 ml kg^{-1} h^{-1} for first 10 kg body weight ● 2 ml kg^{-1} h^{-1} for next 10 kg body weight
	Use 5% dextrose half-strength Hartmann's solution
Replacement of third-space losses Depends on site of operation and extent of surgical exposure	Use lactated Ringer's solution
Suggestions	● Laparotomy: 6 ml kg^{-1} h^{-1} ● Femoral osteotomy: 2 ml kg^{-1} h^{-1}
Replacement of blood loss	Type of IV fluid used depends on Hb
● Calculate allowable blood loss	$= \dfrac{(\text{preoperative Hb–acceptable Hb})}{\text{mean of preoperative and acceptable Hb}} \times \text{CBV}$
Acceptable Hb ● Depends on age and clinical condition of baby	Suggest: ● Hb = 10 g dl^{-1} in a neonate ● Hb = 8 g/dl^{-1} in a healthy 3-month-old baby
Circulating blood volume	● 90 ml kg^{-1} for neonates ● 80 ml kg^{-1} for a 1-year-old baby
Replacement IV fluids	● Give 1 ml colloid/blood or 3 ml crystalloid for every ml blood loss ● Use colloid or crystalloid if Hb > acceptable for age ● Use blood if Hb = acceptable for age

IV, intravenous.

Pyloromyotomy

Congenital hypertrophic pyloric stenosis is the commonest surgical condition in small babies, affecting one in 400 live births,[261] usually boys aged 2–8 weeks. The pyloric muscles becomes thickened, obstructing the passage of gastric contents into the duodenum. Classically, the baby presents with projectile vomiting and a palpable 'pyloric tumour'. Sometimes gastric peristalsis is seen during feeding. An ultrasound scan may be necessary for an atypical history. These babies often have surgery in DGHs.

The baby may be severely dehydrated and a hypochloraemic alkalosis is usual. Although total body potassium is low, plasma concentrations are generally normal. Sodium concentrations also remain in the normal range because sodium is strongly conserved by aldosterone, released in response to hypovolaemia.

FLUID RESUSCITATION AND CORRECTION OF ELECTROLYTE ABNORMALITIES

Pyloric stenosis is not a surgical emergency and abnormalities of fluid balance, electrolytes and acid–base should be corrected over 24–48 h with IV fluids, usually 0.45% saline in glucose with KCl 20 mmol l^{-1}. The volumes required are calculated by adding the estimated fluid deficit due to dehydration (5, 10 or > 10% of body weight) to the daily requirements for maintenance and infusing this over 24 h. A baby is likely to be adequately resuscitated once the plasma chloride is 105 mmol l^{-1} and the bicarbonate > 38 mmol l^{-1}. A metabolic alkalosis must be corrected to reduce the risk of postoperative apnoea.

REDUCING THE RISK OF PULMONARY ASPIRATION OF GASTRIC CONTENTS

Reducing the volume of stomach contents preoperatively decreases the risk of aspiration during anaesthesia. The baby should be fasted and given IV fluids. A large-bore nasogastric tube should be inserted on admission and kept on free drainage and aspirated regularly. In many hospitals, the stomach is washed out via the nasogastric tube in an attempt to remove all traces of milk preoperatively. However, Cook-Sather and colleagues[262] found that the stomach often contained milk despite good preparation (including washouts) and large volumes of gastric fluid not substantially reduced by nasogastric suction preoperatively. Blind aspiration immediately before induction provides a reliable estimate of the volume of gastric fluid for most babies, but occasionally a small amount is retained, the clinical importance of which is uncertain.[262] Commonly in the UK, the nasogastric tube is aspirated with the baby in the right and left lateral and supine positions immediately before induction.

ANAESTHESIA

During a pyloromyotomy, the surgeon splits the pyloric muscles down to the mucosa through a small transverse incision in the right upper quadrant of the abdomen.

The anaesthetist should assume the baby has a full stomach and use a rapid-sequence induction (Fig. 6.9). Cricoid pressure effectively prevents aspiration in babies,[263] but may distort anatomy, making intubation difficult.

Many anaesthetists induce anaesthesia with atropine 10–20 μg kg^{-1}, thiopental 3–5 mg kg^{-1} or propofol 3–4 mg kg^{-1} and suxamethonium 2 mg kg^{-1}. Others facilitate intubation with atracurium 0.5 mg kg^{-1}, cisatracurium 0.1 mg kg^{-1}, or deep anaesthesia with sevoflurane to avoid suxamethonium because of the risk of undiagnosed myopathies. Mivacurium is an alternative, with a rapid onset in babies < 6 months.[264] Undiagnosed myopathy is rare, and the risks of not using a rapid-sequence induction must be balanced against those of aspiration when choosing the induction technique.

Anaesthesia is maintained with inhalational agents (e.g. sevoflurane 2–3% or desflurane 4–8% with either nitrous oxide or air in oxygen). A short-acting non-depolarising relaxant (e.g. atracurium or cisatracurium) may be given, if necessary. Sometimes the surgeon will

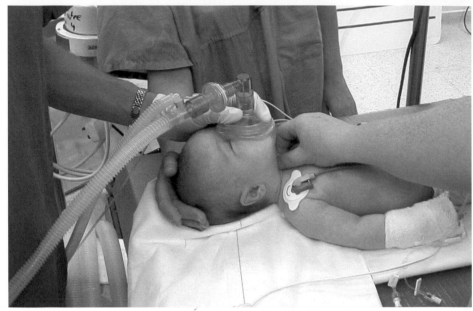

Fig 6.9 Rapid sequence induction with cricoid pressure in a 2 month-old baby scheduled for pyloromyotomy.

ask the anaesthetist to inject air through the nasogastric tube to check for leaks at the pylorus before closing the abdomen. At the end of surgery, muscle relaxation is reversed and the tracheal tube removed when the baby is fully awake.

A combination of rectal paracetamol (20–40 mg kg^{-1} initially and at regular intervals for 24 h, maximum 60 mg kg^{-1} day^{-1}) and wound infiltration with local anaesthetic provides adequate analgesia. Opioids are not required.

Surgeons usually allow feeding by about 12 h after surgery. Apnoea has been reported in term babies after pyloromyotomy and they should be monitored on the ward with an apnoea alarm for the first 12 h postoperatively.[265]

Inguinal herniotomy

Hernias commonly present at 6–12 weeks of age. If the viability of the bowel is in doubt, referring the baby to a tertiary centre should be considered.

The ideal timing is not defined but surgery should not be delayed unduly because of the risks of incarceration and gonadal ischaemia. There is an increasing tendency for early repair to decrease complication rates and the duration of surgery (which is technically easier when tissues are not distorted).[266] Most fit healthy babies can be managed as outpatients.

ANAESTHESIA

In fit healthy babies a light general anaesthetic (with or without a regional technique) is appropriate. Tracheal intubation and positive-pressure ventilation of the lungs are usual in small babies because the airway is difficult to control with a face mask, LMAs are often unreliable and gas exchange is easily compromised by general anaesthesia because of immaturity. Larger babies can breathe spontaneously through a face mask or LMA. If the bowel is incarcerated or obstructed, a rapid-sequence induction (as described for pyloromyotomy, above) is indicated.

Caudal block reduces the requirement for volatile agents (allowing prompt recovery) and provides postoperative analgesia, obviating the need for opioids and reducing respiratory depression.[267] Alternatively, the wound can be infiltrated with local anaesthetic. Paracetamol 20 mg kg^{-1} rectally at induction, and regularly 6-hourly for 24 h (maximum 60 mg kg^{-1} day^{-1}) improves analgesia. NSAIDs are inadvisable because of renal immaturity.

EX-PREMATURE BABIES

Inguinal hernias affect about 30% of babies with birth weights < 1000 g.[268] As more premature babies survive, so the rates for herniotomy will increase. Babies born prematurely (i.e. < 37 weeks postconception) are at risk of life-threatening apnoeas and bradycardia after general anaesthesia because of physiological immaturity.[269, 270] The risk is particularly high before 44 weeks' postconceptual age,[271] and considered significant until 60 weeks.[272] Risks are probably higher in those with a history of apnoea, necrotising enterocolitis, respiratory distress syndrome, bronchopulmonary dysplasia,[272] patent ductus arteriosus,[273] neurological disease[274] or anaemia.[270] All ex-premature babies < 60 weeks postconception should therefore be monitored for 12–18 h postoperatively.[274, 275] Hernias are often repaired whilst ex-premature babies are inpatients in the neonatal intensive care unit (NICU). If admitted from home, they should be observed postoperatively in a high-dependency unit (HDU) providing appropriate monitoring and staffed by nurses familiar with managing small babies. This is often most appropriately one associated with the NICU.

Preoperative methylxanthines, e.g. caffeine 10 mg/kg[276] or theophylline,[277] reduce postoperative apnoea and bradycardia in babies at risk. Caffeine is preferred because it is less toxic, with a higher therapeutic ratio and longer half-life.[277, 278]

For babies at risk of postoperative apnoea, spinal or caudal anaesthesia may obviate the need for general anaesthesia, reducing perioperative morbidity and mortality.[270, 279] However, these techniques are not completely reliable, failing in about 10% of babies, or need supplementing (e.g. with sedatives or other local techniques) in a further 10%.[281] They should not be undertaken by the occasional practitioner because of the potential for complications.[282] Although the incidence of postoperative apnoea is reduced compared with general anaesthesia using older agents, it is not completely eliminated.[281, 283]

With the introduction of desflurane and sevoflurane, regional techniques in awake babies may confer few, if any, advantages over light general anaesthesia.[284] For example, sevoflurane combined with caudal block provides a reliable, and possibly smoother, anaesthetic than a spinal alone but with comparable recovery.[285]

Intussusception

In intussesception, one segment of bowel invaginates into another and becomes ischaemic unless reduced promptly. Most can be reduced radiologically with an air enema, and < 10% of babies need surgery. In babies having surgery, reduction is often difficult, and the affected bowel is frequently ischaemic and requires resection. Intussusception is the commonest cause of bowel obstruction in babies under 1 year.

The operation is usually through a transverse right supraumbilical incision.

GENERAL CONSIDERATIONS

Any hospital admitting these babies must provide a radiologist proficient in reducing intussusception in babies using an air enema.

PREOPERATIVE PREPARATION

The baby may appear well in spite of losing large amounts of fluid into the bowel. IV fluids, often > 40 ml kg^{-1}, may be required to correct hypovolaemia.

PREOPERATIVE INVESTIGATIONS

A full blood count, urea and electrolytes and a group and save should be requested preoperatively.

ANAESTHESIA

Because of the risks of aspiration, the anaesthetist should use a rapid-sequence induction. Anaesthesia may be maintained with oxygen, air and a volatile agent. Nitrous oxide is best avoided because it worsens bowel distension.

BLEEDING

Blood loss, necessitating transfusion, may occur if bowel is resected.

ANALGESIA

Epidural analgesia through a caudal catheter is simple and effective for pain relief (see Ch. 7). In addition, paracetamol and diclofenac suppositories should be administered after induction and regularly postoperatively. NSAIDs should be withheld from babies resuscitated from hypovolaemia until adequate urine output has been established.

The baby usually remains fasted for 24–48 h postoperatively and maintenance IV fluids should be prescribed. Any baby requiring fluid resuscitation should be admitted to a HDU postoperatively. Fluid balance and urine output should be assessed hourly and IV fluids prescribed to maintain an adequate urine output ($1-2$ ml kg^{-1} h^{-1}).

Eye surgery

Extraocular surgery (e.g. syringing and probing of the lacrimal duct or correction of strabismus) or examination of the eyes under anaesthesia (e.g. for glaucoma or tumour) is common in DGHs.

Examination under anaesthesia

Babies and small children usually require general anaesthesia to examine their eyes and measure the intraocular pressure (IOP). Obtaining the 'real' IOP is difficult since anaesthetics affect IOP in a similar way to intracranial pressure (ICP) (see below). Intermittent IV ketamine or a light inhalational anaesthetic (to maintain normocapnia) is usual. Opioids are not required.

Cryotherapy and laser treatment in ex-premature babies

Retinopathy of prematurity occurs more frequently with increased survival of babies born weighing < 1000 g.[286]

Cryotherapy may be given on the NICU to babies still receiving mechanical ventilation. Small doses of opioids are often combined with a light inhalational anaesthetic.

Laser treatment normally takes place in theatre for safety reasons and because the electricity connections required are usually unavailable in the NICU. Laser surgery may be brief or take up to 2 h (depending on the severity of the retinopathy) and this influences the type of anaesthetic required. Often babies requiring treatment have chronic lung disease and oxygen dependence. A light inhalational anaesthetic (preferably using sevoflurane or desflurane) with tracheal intubation and mechanical ventilation is common. Paracetamol, given as a suppository at induction, provides adequate analgesia. At the end of surgery, the trachea is extubated only when the baby is breathing spontaneously and adequately. If the baby fails to breathe adequately, he/she may require IPPV postoperatively on the NICU.

Syringing and probing of the lacrimal duct

This minor procedure occurs most commonly in children > 6 months admitted for day surgery. Typically, the surgeon probes the nasolacrimal duct and then injects fluorescein (aspirated from the pharynx during injection) to check its patency. An LMA provides good protection of the airway and is preferable to a face mask. Tracheal intubation is generally unnecessary. An inhalational or intravenous induction and maintenance using a volatile agent in oxygen/nitrous oxide is appropriate. Diclofenac and/or paracetamol suppositories provide adequate postoperative analgesia.

Correction of strabismus

Correction of strabismus is the most common eye operation in children and usually a day-case procedure. Since the introduction of the LMA, tracheal intubation has become uncommon. There are several specific considerations for anaesthesia.

POSTOPERATIVE VOMITING

Vomiting is the most frequent complication after strabismus surgery in children,[146] affecting 16–88% of children > 2 years of age.[150, 287–290] Although rarely life-threatening, vomiting disturbs both children and parents and may delay discharge from hospital. Numerous authors have assessed the influence of different components of the anaesthetic techniques on its incidence.

PROPOFOL

Several authors have found that induction and maintenance of anaesthesia with propofol reduce POV after strabismus surgery,[248, 291–293] although this was not confirmed by others.[294] Propofol is less effective if opioids are given,[248] and similar rates of vomiting are obtained at less cost by giving prophylactic antiemetics with other anaesthetic drugs.[295]

ANTIEMETICS

Antiemetics, IV, at induction (e.g. metoclopramide 0.1–0.25 mg kg^{-1},[287, 296] ondansetron 0.1–0.15 mg kg^{-1},[297, 298] granisetron 40 µg kg^{-1} [172]) effectively reduce vomiting in children after strabismus repair. Droperidol 25–75 µg kg^{-1} is also effective,[150, 288] although larger doses are associated with delayed discharge home.

Perioperative analgesia influences POV and opioids have a particularly bad effect. Munro and colleagues found a 71% incidence of vomiting after strabismus surgery in children aged 2–12 years given IV morphine 0.1 mg kg^{-1} and metoclopramide 0.15 mg kg^{-1}, compared with only 19% in those given IV ketorolac 0.75 mg kg^{-1}. Pain scores and recovery times were similar.[299] Shorter-acting opioids (e.g. fentanyl 1 µg kg^{-1}) also increase vomiting compared with ketorolac or placebo after strabismus surgery in children and should be avoided.[300]

THE OCULOCARDIAC REFLEX

The oculocardiac reflex (or trigeminal–vagal reflex) produced by traction on the extraocular muscles commonly causes bradycardia, and sometimes chaotic arrhythmia or sinoatrial arrest. Serious complications may result.[301] Treatment is to stop traction and inject an anticholinergic drug IV (e.g. atropine 20 µg kg^{-1}). Many anaesthetists give either atropine 10 µg kg^{-1} or glycopyrollate 3–5 µg kg^{-1} IV at induction to prevent the reflex occurring.

POSTOPERATIVE PAIN

Pain is mostly conjunctival in origin. Topical analgesia with tetracaine (amethocaine),[302] oxybuprocaine or NSAIDs (e.g. diclofenac)[303] is effective and can be combined with oral or rectal NSAIDs and paracetamol. Opioids are usually unnecessary.

ASSOCIATED DISEASES

Squints may occur in children with generalised muscle disorders associated with malignant hyperthermia. However, the risk of malignant hyperthermia in others having strabismus surgery is no greater than in the general population.

NEUROSURGERY

Most neurosurgery in babies and children occurs in specialist paediatric centres, but some larger acute or single-specialty hospitals provide tertiary services for paediatric neurosurgery. The facilities and clinical standards should meet published recommendations (see Ch. 1).

Pathophysiology

Knowledge about intracranial physiology is incomplete because of the ethical problems of research in normal babies and children and is derived from clinical practice or extrapolated from adult studies.

The upper limit of normal for intracranial pressure (ICP) in each age group has been determined from measuring systems (e.g. the Cimino bolt) used for clinical monitoring in head injury, meningitis, near-drowning, intracranial haemorrhage or Reye's syndrome.[304, 305] The upper limit of normal is 3.5 mmHg in neonates, 5.8 mmHg in babies < 1 year, 6.4 mmHg in children < 3 years, and 6–13 mmHg at aged 7 years.[306]

Values for cerebral blood flow (CBF) are unknown in small children. In older children, CBF is twice that of adults (54–67 ml 100 g^{-1} min^{-1} in adults; 100 ml 100 g^{-1} min^{-1} in children)[307] and oxygen consumption one-third greater (3.3–3.7 ml 100 g^{-1} min^{-1} for adults; 5 ml 100 g^{-1} min^{-1} in children)[307, 308] The limits for autoregulation are assumed to relate to systolic blood pressure[309–311] but are not known precisely in children of different ages and normal blood pressure varies throughout childhood.[312] Carbon dioxide is thought to have the same effects on blood flow as in adults (hypercapnia causes vasodilatation, increasing CBF and ICP; hypocapnia causes vasoconstriction, decreasing CBF and ICP).[309, 313] Other causes of raised ICP include hypoxia[309] and raised venous or intrathoracic pressures (e.g. during coughing, CPAP or PEEP).

Clinical signs of intracranial hypertension

Below 18–24 months of age, the fontanelles are open because the skull sutures have not fused completely. Slow, chronic changes in the volume of cranial contents will expand the head without increasing ICP but acute changes in ICP (e.g. during induction of anaesthesia) cannot be accommodated so easily because the dura is relatively non-compliant.

Signs of raised ICP include a bulging fontanelle (not always reliable), irritability, depressed consciousness, apnoea, poor feeding, increased head circumference and distension of scalp veins. 'Sun-setting' develops over time, initially appearing intermittently, then continually, and indicating compensation for intracranial hypertension. The baby cannot look upwards (because of a fourth-nerve palsy) and only the upper halves of the pupil and iris are visible. Percutaneous subdural pressure monitoring via the fontanelle is safe and useful in neonates and infants.[314]

Children over 2 years old have a rigid non-compliant skull. Symptoms and signs of raised ICP include altered behaviour, headache, drowsiness, focal neurological signs (e.g. third- or fourth-nerve palsies), fits, spasticity, bradycardia and hypertension, and vomiting (sometimes causing dehydration or electrolyte abnormalities).

Insertion of ventriculoperitoneal (V-P) shunts

Causes of hydrocephalus

Non-communicating hydrocephalus may be congenital (e.g. Arnold–Chiari malformation, aqueduct stenosis, meningomyelocele, arachnoid cyst, porencephaly, Dandy–Walker syndrome) or acquired (e.g. arachnoiditis, infection, tumour, haemorrhage). Hydrocephalus is not always progressive but careful monitoring must continue to detect early signs of rising ICP.

Preoperative assessment

The anaesthetist must look carefully for clinical features suggesting raised ICP and conditions associated with hydrocephalus. A very high ICP should be lowered medically (see below) or by inserting a ventricular drain under local anaesthesia before induction of anaesthesia.

Babies born prematurely commonly develop hydrocephalus secondary to intraventricular haemorrhage. Anaesthetic implications of prematurity include bronchopulmonary dysplasia or oxygen dependence, increased risk of postoperative apnoea,[63] difficult venous access, subglottic stenosis or tracheomalacia and anaemia. Congenital hydrocephalus is sometimes associated with cardiac, renal, craniofacial or spinal malformations. Seventy-three per cent of patients with meningomyelocele have hydrocephalus caused by aqueductal stenosis.[315] A child with a long-standing infection of a V-P shunt may be poorly nourished or anaemic (sometimes disguised by dehydration).

Preoperative medical treatment of intracranial hypertension includes dexamethasone (0.25 mg kg^{-1}, followed by 0.1 mg kg^{-1} 6-hourly), mannitol 20% (1 mg kg^{-1}), or furosemide (frusemide) (0.5 mg kg^{-1}). Babies with posthaemorrhagic hydrocephalus may be given isosorbide, acetazolamide or furosemide (frusemide) to decrease the rate of cerebrospinal fluid production. Some of these can cause electrolyte disturbances.

Perioperative bleeding is uncommon but major bleeding may occur if a sinus is entered. Babies $<$ 3 months old should be cross-matched preoperatively.

Operation

Shunts for non-communicating (or obstructive) hydrocephalus are usually inserted into the peritoneum (V-P shunts). Less commonly, they drain into the atrium or pleura, but these are specialised procedures, not usually done in DGHs. Communicating hydrocephalus, caused by decreased brain substance (with secondary dilatation of the ventricles) or excessive cerebrospinal fluid production can be treated with a lumboperitoneal shunt.

Anaesthesia

GENERAL PRINCIPLES

The aims of anaesthesia are to prevent a rise in ICP and maintain cerebral perfusion pressure (CPP). CPP = MAP – ICP. Increased ICP or a fall in MAP decreases CPP.

PREMEDICATION

Sedative premedication should be avoided because it may further impair consciousness, producing hypoventilation or airway obstruction, hypoxia and hypercapnia, raising ICP. Topical local anaesthetics (Ametop or Emla) decrease the pain and distress of venous cannulation.

INDUCTION

Children scheduled for reinsertion of a V-P shunt may have had repeated anaesthetics, so it is important to make the experience as pleasant as possible and to consider anxieties related to previous experiences. Having a parent present during induction may reduce distress.

The ideal anaesthetic requires smooth cannulation and induction with fentanyl ($1–2$ µg kg^{-1}) or alfentanil (in increments of $10–40$ µg kg^{-1}),[316] thiopental or propofol, and a short-acting relaxant (e.g. atracurium 0.5 mg kg^{-1} or vecuronium 0.1 mg kg^{-1}) enables rapid intubation.

Fentanyl and morphine have little direct effect on ICP[317, 318] but alfentanil increases it[318] (although this finding has not been reproduced in children).[316] Sufentanil increases CBF in animals[319] and may be unsuitable for neuroanaesthesia. Care must be taken with opiates that depress breathing or promote vomiting postoperatively because these affect ICP indirectly.

Thiopental reduces ICP, CBF and cerebral metabolism, making it the ideal induction agent.[320] Propofol decreases CBF and metabolism, but can significantly cause MAP to fall, with an induction dose, reducing CPP.[321] At low concentration, halothane does not affect CBF, but at > 1 MAC obliterates the response to CO_2.[322] Sevoflurane has a similar effect on cerebral physiology as isoflurane, reducing cerebral metabolism but not affecting CBF (at up to 1 MAC), making them suitable for maintenance.[323–325] Enflurane is inappropriate because of its effects on the electroencephalogram,[326] and desflurane is unsuitable because it is a potent vasodilator.[327]

INTUBATION

Laryngoscopy and intubation increase MAP and ICP. These increases can be attenuated with IV lidocaine (lignocaine) 1.5 mg kg^{-1} given at induction[328, 329] or intraoperatively, if ICP unexpectedly increases.[330]

Sometimes, the theoretical ideal anaesthetic must be adapted. For example, it may be preferable to use a rapid gaseous induction with sevoflurane or halothane rather than struggle with a difficult cannulation (very sick babies tend to remain still, and may be easier to cannulate than less compromised children). Promptly taking over ventilation to control the $PaCO_2$ rapidly returns the cerebrovascular tone to normal.

If there is a risk of vomiting, a rapid-sequence induction using suxamethonium is appropriate, modified by giving an opioid or lidocaine (lignocaine) IV first to ameliorate the effects of laryngoscopy and intubation on ICP. Ventilation should be taken over quickly to prevent hypercapnia.

Intubating a baby with a large head may be difficult and the trunk should be raised (e.g. on layers of gamgee) to bring the head into the neutral position. Alternatively, the end of the trolley may be dropped (or a second assistant could support the head over the edge) during intubation.

Preformed tubes (e.g. RAE) are useful because ventilator tubing can be directed towards the feet, away from the surgical site. However, these have thicker walls than standard tubes (a half-size smaller than predicted is usual) and the distance between the line indicating the position for the lips and the tip of the tube is sometimes too long, especially for small babies. The anaesthetist must check and secure the tube carefully because he/she will have no access to the head during surgery.

INTRAOPERATIVE CARE AND MAINTENANCE OF ANAESTHESIA

The eyes should be taped and padded to avoid trauma. The head must be positioned carefully to avoid kinking neck veins; this may be difficult in babies or small children with large heads and short necks (padding and sandbags may help). The child is then tilted 15–30° head-up, to decrease ICP.[331]

Babies or small children with large heads are prone to considerable heat loss, particularly when wet with cerebrospinal fluid during surgery. General methods for conserving heat have been discussed previously (Table 6.11). The body core temperature (ideally 36–36.5°C) must be monitored carefully. Cooling reduces cerebral metabolic rate and is beneficial but also produces postoperative shivering, increased oxygen demand and delayed drug metabolism. The ideal temperature is, therefore, a balance between risks and benefits.

Maintenance is usually with a volatile agent (commonly isoflurane) in air and oxygen[332, 333] or TIVA. Nitrous oxide increases ICP, so is probably best avoided.[334] The lungs are usually ventilated to mild hypocarbia (3.5–4.0 kPa). Manual ventilation is less satisfactory than mechanical ventilation because high levels of PEEP result if insufficient time is allowed for expiration (i.e. breaths are 'stacked').

Cardiovascular instability may occur when raised ICP is suddenly relieved. Problems include arrhythmias and hypotension (particularly if preoperative hypertension was secondary to raised ICP and high-concentration volatile agents are used).[335] Blood loss is usually minimal.

Muscle relaxation is reversed at the end of surgery and the tracheal tube is removed only when the child is awake and breathing adequately.

ANALGESIA

Perioperative analgesia is usually provided by infiltrating local anaesthetic along the incision and course of the shunt, and giving IV fentanyl (1–2 µg kg^{-1}) or alfentanil (10–40 µg kg^{-1}). NSAIDs (except in babies) and paracetamol are usually adequate for postoperative analgesia.

POSTOPERATIVE CARE

Postoperatively, it is important to ensure adequate oxygenation and normal body temperature. Blood in the cerebrospinal fluid can cause cerebral irritability, which may respond to phenobarbital.[336] Children should be managed by staff who are familiar with the postoperative care of children with shunts and who are competent to monitor the neurological and conscious state. Children should lie flat, when possible, to prevent rapid collapse of the ventricular system, which occasionally causes a subdural haematoma. High-dependency care is required for those with a significant risk of postoperative apnoea (i.e. ex-premature babies), cardiovascular instability (from excessive cerebrospinal fluid drainage) or varying conscious state.[336]

ANAESTHESIA FOR ORTHOPAEDIC SURGERY

Anaesthesia for orthopaedic surgery is challenging because some children have complex medical problems and the regional techniques used are diverse. Children scheduled for orthopaedic surgery fall into one of two categories:

1. otherwise healthy children for correction of congenital deformities or treatment of an injury;
2. those with cerebral palsy or muscular disease scheduled for single or multiple procedures.

Orthopaedic operations in healthy children

Correction of talipes equinovarus ('club foot')

Babies with congenital club foot usually have surgery before they are weight-bearing, at about 5–7 months of age.

ASSOCIATED ANOMALIES

Most babies are healthy but some have associated orthopaedic disorders (e.g. arthrogryphosis multiplex or congenital dislocation of the hip (CDH)) or the talipes may form part of a syndrome.

ANAESTHESIA

The induction technique depends on the anaesthetist, and opioid analgesia (e.g. fentanyl 1 µg kg^{-1} IV) is often given. The baby usually lies supine for a posteromedial release, but prone for correction of equinovarus using the Cincinnati procedure (Fig. 6.10). Intubation (facilitated with a short-acting non-depolarising relaxant) and IPPV is usual for babies positioned prone or having long operations.

After tracheal intubation, the tracheal tube must be secured carefully and the eyes taped and padded. Anaesthesia is usually maintained with a volatile agent (e.g. isoflurane 0.75–1%) in nitrous oxide or air in oxygen.

During surgery, the lower leg is exsanguinated with a tourniquet. Tourniquets may be associated with mild hyperthermia in children.[337] Blood loss when the tourniquet is released is usually easily replaced with appropriate crystalloid or colloid and blood

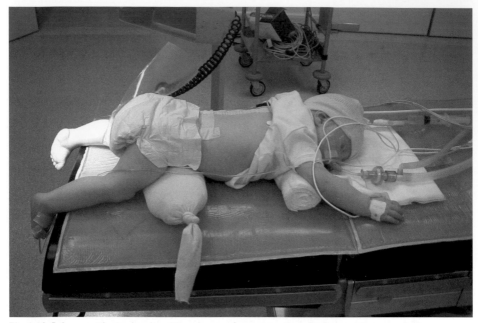

Fig 6.10 Baby anaesthetised and positioned prone for a correction of talipes equinovarus via the Cincinnati approach. Analgesia is provided via an epidural catheter inserted into the caudal space.

transfusion is almost never required for unilateral surgery. Significant leakage into the plaster may occur after major correction and it is our practice for bilateral club feet to do a major correction one side at a time and prescribe oral iron supplements (Sytron 0.5 ml kg^{-1} tds) postoperatively for two weeks. Surgery for the other foot is scheduled 2 weeks later.

At the end of the operation, the surgeon applies an above-knee plaster of Paris.

ANALGESIA

Regional techniques are ideal for operations on the foot.

1. A single caudal injection of local anaesthetic generally provides an inadequate duration of analgesia after correction of talipes equinovarus. A caudal epidural catheter may be inserted and local anaesthetic (e.g. 0.125% bupivacaine 0.25–0.4 ml kg^{-1} h^{-1}) infused continuously for 12–48 h.
2. Block of the sciatic (and femoral nerve at the groin or saphenous nerve at the knee, if necessary) using 0.5–0.75 ml kg^{-1} 0.25% bupivacaine with adrenaline (epinephrine) 1:200 000 may provide successful perioperative analgesia.

It is important that the colour and capillary refill of the toes on the side of operation are regularly checked postoperatively, particularly since the baby will initially have an anaesthetic leg.

In addition, paracetamol and NSAIDs (e.g. diclofenac) should be given at induction and regularly postoperatively.

REPEAT PROCEDURES

Short anaesthetics will be required a few weeks later for changing the plaster, making a cast for an ankle–foot orthosis, or removing any K-wires. Inhalational anaesthesia with sevoflurane in nitrous oxide and oxygen and analgesia with paracetamol and diclofenac suppositories allow rapid recovery and discharge home.

Open reduction of developmental dysplasia of the hip or femoral osteotomy

Open reduction for developmental dysplasia of the hip (DDH) is becoming rarer because of improved neonatal screening and the use of ultrasound. Surgery is indicated for late diagnosis (sometimes not made until aged 9–15 months) or if the hip is unstable in a spica.

Femoral osteotomy may take place from early childhood to adolescence. Children may be otherwise healthy (e.g. those with Perthes disease) or have associated medical problems (e.g. cerebral palsy or neuromuscular disease).

ANAESTHESIA FOR OPEN REDUCTION OF A CDH

Anaesthetic considerations are those for any major operation, with particular attention to maintaining normothermia. The baby usually lies supine. Tracheal intubation and positive-pressure ventilation are common because the child is usually < 12 months old and the operation may take several hours. Significant blood loss is possible (group and save preoperatively and site a large-bore cannula) but unusual, and blood can generally be replaced with crystalloid or colloid.

At the end, the surgeon applies a hip spica, for which the baby or child is raised on a box or special frame allowing access around the trunk and buttocks (Fig. 6.11).

ANAESTHESIA FOR FEMORAL OSTEOTOMY

Anaesthetic considerations are again as for major surgery. For bilateral or difficult osteotomies, tracheal intubation and positive-pressure ventilation are common because the procedure may take several hours. Spontaneous respiration via an LMA is appropriate for unilateral surgery in an older child. During surgery, the child is usually supine but occasionally the surgeon requests the prone position. Major bleeding is possible, particularly during bilateral surgery. Blood should therefore be cross-matched and a large-bore cannula inserted.

The surgeon stabilises the osteotomy with a blade plate and plaster of Paris is not usually applied. Children with cerebral palsy undergoing bilateral osteotomies usually have bilateral below-knee plasters applied at the end of surgery, joined by a 'broomstick'.

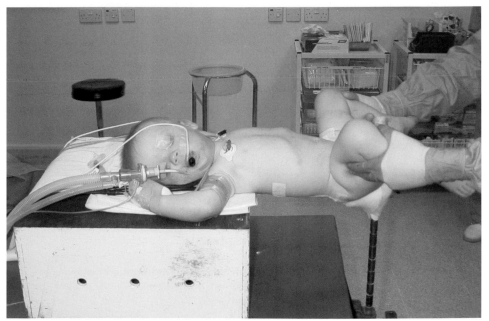

Fig 6.11 Eleven-month old baby with a congenital dislocation of the hip, placed on a box and post for application of a hip spica. The box supports the upper body and the post is placed between the legs.

ANALGESIA FOR OPEN REDUCTION OF A CDH OR FEMORAL OSTEOTOMY

Regional analgesic techniques are very appropriate, for example:

1. Lumbar epidural analgesia using local anaesthetics (e.g. 0.125% bupivacaine at 0.25–0.4 ml kg^{-1} h^{-1} for 24–48 h), opioid or a mixture of opioid and local anaesthetic. Clonidine 1–2 µg kg^{-1} may improve the quality of block obtained from local anaesthetics during the first 12 h, and may be used in children older than 12 months of age. Alternatively, preservative-free ketamine 0.5 mg kg^{-1} can be injected epidurally.
2. Fascia iliaca block using 0.5–0.75 ml kg^{-1} 0.25% bupivacaine with adrenaline (epinephrine) 1 in 200 000 (additional infiltration with local anaesthetic may be required for incisions above the greater trochanter). Some anaesthetists add clonidine 1–2 µg kg^{-1} to try to improve the quality of block. A lumbar plexus block using 0.5–0.75 ml kg^{-1} 0.25% bupivacaine with adrenaline (epinephrine) 1 in 200 000 is an alternative.

Some anaesthetists give a small dose of opioid (e.g. fentanyl 1 µg kg^{-1}) to provide intraoperative analgesia before the block is established. Analgesia is improved by giving coanalgesics (e.g. paracetamol and diclofenac suppositories) at induction and regularly after surgery.

Management of fractures

There are several anaesthetic considerations in children with fractures.

THE RISKS OF COMPARTMENT SYNDROME

Certain injuries and operations are associated with a higher risk of compartment syndrome than others. Compartment syndrome is particularly likely in distal limb injuries (e.g. fractured radius, ulna or tibia),[338] but less likely with fractures of the humerus or femur. It is also associated with leg-lengthening operations, tibial osteotomies and tendon transfers into the anterior compartment.[338]

Increasing pain and excessive sensory changes or motor weakness all suggest compartment compression and must be investigated promptly.[338] Any epidural infusion of local anaesthetic should be stopped. Sensory changes produced by epidural local anaesthetics should then resolve within 1–3 h.[338]

Analgesia when there is a high risk of compartment syndrome. Pain relief for children with fractures is often poor, partly because of the inexperience of junior surgeons and also because of concerns about masking the symptoms of compartment syndrome.[338]

For injuries or surgery associated with a high risk of compartment syndrome, dense regional block should be avoided and analgesia planned with the surgeon, taking into account the risks of early postoperative complications. Where these are high, Mubarak & Wilson suggest some preventive measures:[338]

1. prophylactic fasciotomies of at least the anterior compartment;
2. wide splitting of the cast postoperatively;
3. careful assessment and monitoring;
4. avoiding epidural local anaesthetics in favour of opioids epidurally or IV (patient-controlled analgesia or continuous infusion).

Analgesia when there is a low risk of compartment syndrome. For many injuries or operations the risks of compartment syndrome are very low and regional techniques (e.g. epidural infusions or nerve blocks) provide excellent analgesia.

When using a regional technique:

1. The anaesthetist must explain the side-effects (i.e. numbness and loss of power) adequately to the child preoperatively, stressing that these are temporary and unavoid-

able in order to provide good analgesia. Appreciating why his/her limb is numb may make the child less apprehensive, enabling him/her to tolerate the block better.
2. The child must be adequately assessed and monitored postoperatively to detect the early features suggesting compartment syndrome.

Reducing and immobilising a fracture in a plaster of Paris usually relieves much of the pain of simple fractures. Analgesics (e.g. diclofenac and paracetamol) should be given to all children at induction and regularly for at least 24 h and morphine prescribed PRN (IV or orally).

DELAYED GASTRIC EMPTYING

It is widely believed that all children with trauma should be considered unfasted regardless of fasting interval, but the evidence for this is inconclusive.[339] The volume of gastric residue at induction is > 0.4 ml kg^{-1} in 50% of children having emergency surgery, but is less than this in most older children and those with superficial injuries.[17] Bricker and colleagues showed some correlation between starvation time and gastric aspirate volume in children with acute trauma.[340] Although they found a closer correlation between this volume and the time between ingestion of food and injury, they were unable to predict a safe interval.[340] Phillips and colleagues, having reviewed relevant studies, suggest that children requiring surgery after trauma should be fasted for at least 6 h and their stomachs assumed to be full.[13] Pain or opioid analgesics further delay gastric emptying.

From a recent survey of current practice,[341] Marcus & Thompson conclude that not all anaesthetists believe that rapid-sequence induction is necessary for anaesthesia after trauma (forearm fractures) despite recent recommendations.[13, 17, 340] From their survey, rapid-sequence induction was usual for anaesthesia on the day of injury for children given clear fluids or food less than 3 and 6 h respectively before injury, but not for surgery scheduled later or in children fasted for longer periods.

Orthopaedic operations in children with cerebral palsy

Children with cerebral palsy may require minor surgery (e.g. injection of botulinum toxin or tendon releases) or complex multilevel surgery, simultaneously involving, for example, bilateral femoral and/or tibial osteotomies, and multiple tendon and soft-tissue releases.

General considerations

Cerebral palsy is a group of non-progressive disorders of motor function occurring in young children with brain injury. It has a spectrum of severity ranging from a child (often born prematurely) with spastic diplegia, who is often intellectually normal and seldom epileptic, to one with severe involvement of the whole body, who may be blind, deaf, epileptic and have severe learning and communication difficulties, quadraparesis, pseudobulbar palsy and feeding difficulties. Successful management requires a thorough understanding of all the anaesthetic implications (Table 6.24). Anaesthesia for these children was recently reviewed by Nolan and colleagues.[342]

Anaesthetic agents

Children with cerebral palsy have a reduced MAC compared with normal controls.[343] IV and inhalational anaesthetics must be titrated carefully.

Muscle relaxants

Sensitivity to depolarising muscle relaxants probably does not occur[344] and suxamethonium is safe for children with cerebral palsy. Resistance to non-depolarising muscle relaxants (probably not clinically significant) has been reported.[345]

Table 6.24 The anaesthetic implications of cerebral palsy

Feature	Anaesthetic implications
Learning difficulties, communication problems, sensory impairment (blindness, deafness)	Communication difficulties The child may not understand what is happening to him/her perioperatively and may be very anxious
Epilepsy	Avoid anaesthetic agents that may precipitate epilepsy Some children receiving anticonvulsants metabolise non-depolarising muscle relaxants rapidly
Respiratory insufficiency	Often associated with the development of scoliosis Positive-pressure ventilation may be preferred perioperatively Postoperative ventilation is seldom required
Gastro-oesophageal reflux, feeding disorders, drooling, malnutrition and growth impairment, constipation	An anaesthetic technique involving tracheal intubation must be used with a history of gastro-oesophageal reflux or when the clinical condition suggests its likelihood
Motor disability, deformity, spasticity, scoliosis, hip dislocation	Great care must be taken in positioning the child safely Contractures may make intravenous access difficult to find and nerve blocks difficult to perform

Analgesia

Regional analgesia is not contraindicated in cerebral palsy and may reduce muscle spasm after major surgery. IV morphine is less appropriate because of the associated 'morphine jerks' that may compound increased muscle tone, worsening pain.

Postoperative muscle spasm

Children with cerebral palsy often experience muscle spasm after major orthopaedic surgery on the legs, which may not be adequately controlled with epidural infusions of local anaesthetics. A low-dose benzodiazepine (e.g. midazolam 25–50 µg kg^{-1} h^{-1}, or oral or rectal diazepam 0.2 mg kg^{-1} every 3 h) effectively reduces tone, relieving spasm.

Injection of botulinum toxin

Botulinum toxin is sometimes injected into muscle to relieve spasticity temporarily.[346] This may be done in cooperative children awake after topical application of Ametop cream. A short general anaesthesia is often preferred for small children or those having several injections. Very rarely, generalised muscle weakness may occur a few days after injection.[346] Parents must be aware of this complication since urgent readmission to hospital is required in case respiratory muscle involvement results.

Orthopaedic operations in children with spina bifida

Myelomeningocele affects 2–5 per 1000 births. Children with spina bifida often have surgery to correct orthopaedic deformities, during which they should be positioned carefully to prevent pressure sores or injury. There are several specific anaesthetic considerations.

Latex allergy

The number of previous operations, rather than the diagnosis of spina bifida, determines the risk of latex allergy.[347]

Hydrocephalus

Most children develop hydrocephalus in infancy, usually associated with an Arnold–Chiari type II malformation,[348] and have a V-P shunt. Most of these children show a diminished response to hypoxia and may be more susceptible to postoperative apnoea.[349]

Respiratory complications

Many patients with myelomeningocele have short tracheas and an increased risk of endo-bronchial intubation.[350]

Orthopaedic operations in children with muscle disease

Muscular dystrophies

These are a group of progressive diseases ultimately producing muscle weakness and deformity.

Duchenne muscular dystrophy (DMD)

DMD is the commonest muscular dystrophy. It is X-linked, affecting about 1 in 3500 live male births. DMD is caused by a reduction or absence of dystrophin, a 427-kDa spectrin-like protein lying at the inner surface of the plasma membranes of skeletal and cardiac muscle fibres.[351]

Affected boys may present for surgery for leg deformities or stabilisation of progressive kyphoscoliosis. Cardiorespiratory function should be assessed carefully (with an ECG and echocardiograph) in those who are wheelchair-bound because they commonly develop cardiomyopathy and respiratory insufficiency with age.[352] Suxamethonium is contraindicated because it causes acute rhabdomyolysis and hyperkalaemic cardiac arrest.[353, 354] Although originally thought to be malignant hyperthermia (MH), this response is now considered more likely to represent an independent trait from MH in children with DMD.[352, 355] Similar concerns have also been expressed about the safety of volatile agents, although the evidence for this is less strong than for suxamethonium.[356] For general anaesthesia, many anaesthetists favour TIVA but this must be used carefully in boys with significantly impaired cardiac function. Propofol infusion combined with a lumbar epidural is also very suitable during surgery on the legs (Fig. 6.12). Regional or local techniques should be used, if appropriate, as alternatives to general anaesthesia or opioid analgesia. Boys with DMD are sensitive to opioids and non-depolarising relaxants, which must be titrated carefully to effect.

The detailed management of anaesthesia for boys with DMD was recently described in an editorial by Morris.[352]

Myotonic dystrophy (MD)

MD is a rare dystrophy (1 in 20 000 births) with autosomal dominant inheritance. It results from alterations in myotonin protein kinase that affect sodium channels in muscle, leading to hyperexcitability and preventing relaxation after contraction. Associated conditions include cardiac conduction disturbances and arrhythmias, ventilatory impairment, endocrine dysfunction (e.g. diabetes mellitus, hypothyroidism or adrenal insufficiency), dysphagia and decreased gastric motility.

Children with MD may require orthopaedic corrections of leg deformities. The condition has major implications for anaesthesia.

SUSTAINED MYOTONIC CONTRACTURES

Children with MD may develop sustained contractures affecting the jaw (making the airway difficult to manage) or respiratory muscles (making ventilation of the lungs impossible) in response to suxamethonium, cold, stress or pain. These children must be kept warm perioperatively and given adequate analgesia (e.g. with a regional block). A myotonic spasm, if

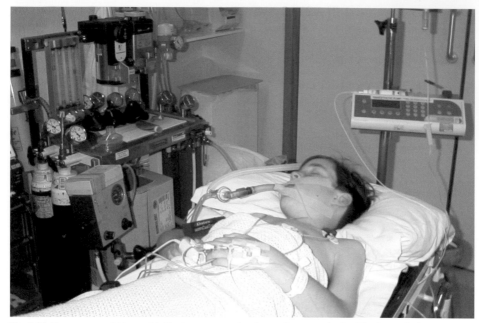

Fig 6.12 Eleven-year old boy with Duchenne muscular dystrophy, anaesthetised for lower limb orthopaedic surgery. An intravenous anaesthetic with a propofol infusion and a lumbar epidural is used. In the absence of gastro-oesophageal reflux, the airway is maintained with a laryngeal mask.

triggered, is frightening to clinicians, but usually self-limiting[357] and may respond to inhalational agents or procainamide.

SENSITIVITY TO ANAESTHETICS AND OPIOIDS

Children with DMD are very sensitive to opioids and anaesthetic drugs. They may become apnoeic after very small doses and recovery is often slow.

NON-DEPOLARISING MUSCLE RELAXANTS

The response to non-depolarising muscle relaxants is normal but a reduced dose is required due to muscle wasting.[358] Usually, the trachea can be intubated after IV induction followed by a volatile agent, without the need for muscle relaxants.

Local anaesthetic techniques should be encouraged, if appropriate, as alternatives to general anaesthesia. If general anaesthesia is necessary, either inhalational or IV agents may be used, cautiously titrated. If there is no risk of aspiration and respiratory function is good, spontaneous breathing through an LMA is acceptable. Alternatively, intubation and IPPV may be used and non-depolarising relaxants titrated carefully to ensure that the child breathes adequately at the end of anaesthesia.

MH AND MUSCLE DISEASE

The association between MH and neuromuscular disorders is controversial. DMD has been associated sporadically with MH, and a direct relationship is not proven.[359, 360] Neither halothane nor caffeine triggers abnormal contracture responses in skeletal muscle from dystrophin-deficient mdx mice (an animal model for human DMD), so dystrophin deficiency does not seem to be the primary cause of the MH-like crises reported in patients with DMD.[361] For further details on MH and muscle disease, please refer to the article by Wedel.[359]

ANAESTHESIA FOR PLASTIC SURGERY

Anaesthesia for elective plastic surgery (e.g. cleft lip or palate, syndactyly release or oto-plasty) is varied and interesting. Surgery for craniosynostosis is usually confined to specialist children's hospitals. The management of burns is described in Chapter 3.

Repair of cleft lip and palate

Cleft lip and palate are the commonest craniofacial anomalies (1 in 700 live births in the UK).[362] Cleft lip may occur alone, or with a cleft palate, and 25% are bilateral. Eighty-five per cent of babies with a bilateral cleft lip have an associated cleft palate.[363]

The primary aim in managing cleft lip and/or palate malformations is to produce a normal facial appearance and function, and normal hearing and speech.[362] Cleft lips are generally repaired at 6–12 weeks of age and palates by 18 months (although some surgeons repair the lip in neonates). Children with cleft lip and/or palate usually require at least three operations to the lip, palate and bone surrounding the upper teeth[362] and about 40% require surgery later to align the top jaw. A bone graft in the upper jaw may help the upper canine teeth erupt correctly and this is usually done at 8–10 years of age.

Recent recommendations on services for children with cleft lip and palate, from the Clinical Standards Advisory Group (CSAG),[362] will alter the delivery of cleft lip and/or palate services in the UK. Centres will be reduced to 8–15 regional centres (some of which are DGHs), with each cleft surgeon doing at least 30 primary closures of cleft lip and/or palate annually. However, this will impose greater distances for travel on affected children and their families. Details of the present and recommended services and the rationale behind the changes are summarised in Table 6.25.

General considerations

ASSOCIATED ANOMALIES

There are over 150 syndromes (many rare) that include cleft lip and/or palate. Several have significance for anaesthesia because of associated airway problems and difficulties with intubation. These include oculoauriculovertebral spectrum (Goldenhar syndrome or hemifacial microsomia), Treacher Collins syndrome and Pierre Robin sequence. Cleft palate may also be associated with cardiac or renal abnormalities, and these should be investigated before anaesthesia. The syndromes of anaesthetic importance are summarised in Table 6.26.

MANAGING THE DIFFICULT AIRWAY

The airway is often difficult to manage in babies with cleft lips and/or palate. Laryngoscopy is difficult (defined as Cormack and Lehane grade III or IV) in 3% of children with unilateral cleft lip, 46% with bilateral cleft lip and 35% with retrognathia (although intubation succeeds overall in 99%). It is more difficult in younger babies ($P < 0.01$), becoming straightforward in children > 5 years.[364]

Several authors have described methods for managing a difficult intubation in babies and other techniques used in older children may be adapted. Reported techniques include using a bougie,[365] displacing the larynx posteriorly by firm backward pressure on the thyroid or cricoid cartilage,[366] displacing the larynx by backward, upward and rightward pressure on the thyroid cartilage (a 'burp'),[367] fibreoptic laryngoscopy,[368] retrograde intubation,[369] digitally assisted intubation[370] and using a light wand.[371] The LMA has been used in place of a tracheal tube when intubation in a baby with Robin sequence was impossible[105] or as a guide to fibreoptic intubation (e.g. in Treacher Collins syndrome[372] (see also Table 6.7)).

ANAESTHESIA

Because of the potential for a difficult airway, anaesthesia should be induced with a volatile agent in oxygen. An oral airway or LMA may help maintain the airway during early

Table 6.25 Services for children with cleft lip and palate[a]

THE PRESENT SERVICE IN THE UK	THE SERVICE RECOMMENDED FOR THE UK BY CSAG
Approximately 1000 children are born with a cleft lip ± palate in the UK each year	The **key factor** in achieving successful care is a **first-class multidisciplinary team** with the right blend of specialties
57 units perform primary repair of cleft lip ± palate	• The team will be committed individuals working well together to agreed protocols
The teams include: • 75 surgeons (specialties include plastic surgery, oral and faciomaxillary surgery, ear, nose and throat surgery and paediatric surgery) • 70 speech and language therapists • 105 orthodontists	• Successful treatment includes surgery, orthodontic care, speech and language therapy, and depends on the skills of many allied health professionals
Outcomes of treatment of children with unilateral cleft lip and palate were studied by CSAG from 50 centres.	There should be 8–15 multidisciplinary cleft centres in the UK: • Each unit should have two cleft consultant surgeons, **each treating 40–50 cases per year** • Orthodontists and speech and language therapists will be similarly experienced.
The conclusions were: • Although there are excellent individual practitioners, many UK surgeons treat only one or two new cases per year • Although most parents believe their children receive excellent/good care, the general standard is well below that from the best European centres • Higher standards need to be achieved • Record-keeping is poor	Each centre must: • provide a cleft team for expert support and counselling to parents at diagnosis • initiate invasive treatment guided by protocols and after a multidisciplinary review • monitor patients for up to 20 years • undertake meticulous record-keeping so that audit and multicentred trials may be undertaken to improve standards

[a]Recommendations from *The Report on Services for Children with Cleft Lip and Palate*, from the Clinical Standards Advisory Group (CSAG).[358]

induction if there is a large cleft palate. Laryngoscopy should be done only once an adequate depth of anaesthesia has been obtained. The cords may be sprayed with topical local anaesthetic (usually lidocaine (lignocaine), 4 mg kg^{-1}) and a tracheal tube (commonly a south-facing RAE) is inserted into the trachea. A throat pack should be used during repair of cleft lip. For palate repair, this is generally inserted by the surgeon after positioning the tongue gag.

Before operating, the surgeon inserts a gag into the child's mouth, and it is essential to ensure that the tracheal tube remains patent by gently ventilating the lungs manually. A precordial stethoscope will help detect partial or total obstruction of the tube by a change in the character or an absence of breath sounds.

Anaesthesia is usually maintained with a volatile agent in air and oxygen. As the babies are generally young, and the duration of surgery is at least 1 h, relaxants are usually given and the lungs ventilated mechanically.

Maintenance fluids should be infused and blood loss replaced with appropriate crystalloid or colloid. Blood loss during a primary lip repair is minimal, and although greater during a primary palatoplasty, transfusion is rarely needed. Accurately assessing blood loss

Table 6.26 Syndromes of anaesthetic importance that may require cleft palate surgery

	Oculoauriculovertebral spectrum	Treacher Collins syndrome	Robin sequence
Also known as:	Goldenhar syndrome, hemifacial microsomia May represent gradations in severity of a similar error in morphogenesis		Pierre Robin syndrome
Aetiology	Abnormal morphogenesis of the first and second branchial arches ± vertebral anomalies ± ocular anomalies A non-random association of anomalies May represent the sequelae of a fetal vascular accident	Two cases described in 1900 by Treacher Collins, a British ophthalmologist Autosomal dominant Mostly fresh mutations Involved gene has been sequenced and probably plays a critical role in early embryonic craniofacial development	Primary anomaly is early mandibular hypoplasia prior to 9 weeks' gestation The tongue is placed posteriorly, preventing the palatal shelves from closing in midline, producing a cleft
Features	Usually unilateral, or at least asymmetrical. Bilateral disease (10%), barely indistinguishable from Treacher Collins syndrome, except by genetics	A great spectrum of severity	May occur as an isolated finding in an otherwise healthy infant Prognosis is good if neonatal airway problems are overcome May occur as a component of some multiple-malformation syndromes, such as trisomy 18 syndrome

Table 6.26 continued overleaf

Table 6.26 continued from previous page

	Oculoauriculovertebral spectrum	Treacher Collins syndrome	Robin sequence
Facial abnormalities may include:	Unilateral or asymmetric hypoplasia of malar, maxillary ± mandibular region	Down-sloping palpebral fissures	Micrognathia
		Hypoplasia of the malar bones ± cleft zygoma	
	Macrostomia	Mandibular hypoplasia	
	Hypoplasia of facial musculature	Auricular malformations	
	Epibulbar dermoids	Lower-lid coloboma	
	Extraocular muscle defects	Partial/total absence of lower lashes	
	Coloboma		
	Microtia	Low-set ears	
	Middle-ear anomaly with variable conductive hearing loss	Atresia of the external canal and conductive deafness	
Other anomalies/ difficulties	40% have vertebral anomalies (most commonly cervical) ● Hemivertebrae or hypoplasia of vertebrae ● Vertebral fusion and odontoid lengthening	Rarely, cardiac anomalies	Feeding difficulties common due to anatomical abnormalities
			Swallowing difficulties due to brainstem dysfunction
	Cardiac anomalies present in 35% ● VSD, PDA, tetralogy of Fallot, coarctation		Central apnoea may result from brainstem dysfunction

Table 6.26 continued overleaf

Table 6.26 continued from previous page

	Oculoauriculovertebral spectrum	Treacher Collins syndrome	Robin sequence
	Arnold–Chiari malformation or hydrocephalus Chest anomalies Renal abnormalities		
Airway abnormalities	Micrognathia Unilateral mandibular hypoplasia Cleft palate or high-arched palate Malfunction of soft palate Anomalies in function/structure of tongue May have sleep apnoea	Micrognathia, due to severe mandibular hypoplasia Small mouth ± Cleft palate or high-arched palate Incompetent soft palate Malocclusion of the teeth Narrow airway due to pharyngeal hypoplasia May have sleep apnoea	Micrognathia Cleft soft palate Glossoptosis Airway obstruction may cause sleep apnoea, hypoxia and cor pulmonale Intervening procedures (e.g. cleft palate repair) may make a once-uncomplicated laryngoscopy difficult by altering the visualisation of the larynx
Airway considerations	Difficult mask fit Difficult laryngoscopy and intubation	Difficult/impossible laryngoscopy and intubation	Difficult/impossible direct laryngoscopy and tracheal intubation

Table 6.26 continued overleaf

Table 6.26 continued from previous page

	Oculoauriculovertebral spectrum	Treacher Collins syndrome	Robin sequence
			Airway obstruction developing in the first 1–4 weeks of life may be relieved by: ● Nursing prone ● A nasopharyngeal airway ● Suturing the tongue to the lip ● Urgent tracheostomy
Alternative intubation techniques	Inserting the laryngoscope into the unaffected side provides room to displace the tongue LMA insertion under nebulised lidocaine (lignocaine) and intubation through the LMA Fibreoptic intubation	The Bullard laryngoscope LMA Placing the child prone may improve spontaneous respiration by preventing the tongue from falling back into the pharynx	LMA Digitally assisted intubation Fibreoptic nasal intubation Retrograde tracheal intubation Bullard laryngoscope Blind nasal intubation in the prone position with neck hyperextension
Prognosis	Airway often worsens with age	May require tracheostomy Growth during childhood may improve airway	Mandibular growth usually improves airway

VSD, ventricular septal defect; PDA, patent ductus arteriosus; LMA, laryngeal mask airway

during cleft-palate surgery is often difficult. In Plymouth, we put a mucus extractor in the suction line to collect and measure any aspirated blood. Swabs may also be weighed.

At the end of the operation, relaxation is reversed, the throat pack removed, the pharynx suctioned of blood and debris and the trachea extubated when the baby is fully awake.

In a baby with micrognathia, the surgeon may insert a suture into the tongue at the end of surgery. The suture is then pulled forward and taped to the lower jaw, so bringing the tongue forward and preventing airway obstruction. The suture is removed once the risk of obstruction has passed, usually at about 24 h.

ANALGESIA

Small babies are very sensitive to the respiratory-depressant effects of opioids and alternatives should be used, if possible. The surgeon usually infiltrates the palate or lip with local anaesthetics and vasoconstrictors (e.g. bupivacaine 0.25% with adrenaline (epinephrine) 1:200 000) to reduce blood loss and provide analgesia. The dose of adrenaline (epinephrine) should not exceed 5 µg kg^{-1}. Bösenberg & Kimble recommend infraorbital nerve blocks for analgesia for early repair of cleft lip to avoid opioid-induced respiratory depression.[373]

Some babies require opioids after palate repair and small doses (e.g. morphine 25 µg kg^{-1}) should be titrated carefully. Some anaesthetists give IM codeine 0.5–1 mg kg^{-1}. Additional analgesia should be provided by paracetamol (and in older babies NSAIDs) given at induction, and regularly thereafter.

Postoperative care

Babies may be nursed postoperatively on the ward after primary closure of a cleft lip. Babies should be assessed individually after palatoplasty to determine whether admission to the paediatric HDU/ICU is more appropriate. Babies with micrognathia or other significant anomalies should be admitted to a paediatric HDU/ICU for respiratory monitoring after palatoplasty.

Otoplasty

Otoplasty is a cosmetic operation in older children with prominent ears undertaken to avoid them being teased by their peers.[374] Otoplasty may be severely painful and has a high incidence of POV (48–85%).[375] Vomiting is a frequent reason for admitting children from the day-surgery unit after otoplasty.

Vomiting

Many factors contribute to vomiting after correction of prominent ears.

Stimulating a branch of the vagus nerve supplying the external auditory meatus and conchal hollow of the ear was used in Roman times to initiate vomiting after large meals.[376] Packing the ears after surgery seems to have a similar effect. Ridings and colleagues found that not packing the ears significantly reduced PONV compared with the usual practice of packing the external auditory meatus and concha (nausea 30% versus 83%, $P < 0.005$; vomiting 22% versus 63%; $P < 0.01$ respectively).[376]

Since POV is likely after otoplasty, a prophylactic antiemetic should be given at induction. POV is also influenced by the choice of analgesia and the quality of pain relief.

Analgesia

Using a regional nerve block or infiltrating with local anaesthetic are equally effective for perioperative analgesia and associated with similar rates of POV.[377] Sossai and colleagues found a mean duration of analgesia of 8.6 h for a nerve block with bupivacaine 0.5%, compared with 10.5 h for infiltration of the ear with local anaesthetic.[377] The incidences of POV were 43% and 36% respectively and were correlated with the use of opioids.[377]

Infiltration with local anaesthetic and adrenaline (epinephrine) improved the surgical field and provided haemostasis and the authors advocate this simpler technique.

Additional analgesia should be provided with NSAIDs and paracetamol given after induction and regularly after surgery.

Due to the high incidence of POV associated with otoplasty, opioids should be avoided.

Anaesthesia

Some older children tolerate otoplasty under local anaesthesia alone. General anaesthesia is used for the majority, with the airway maintained through an LMA or tracheal tube.

ANAESTHESIA FOR RADIOLOGICAL IMAGING

Imaging usually takes place in remote sites not designed for anaesthesia. The anaesthetist must ensure all appropriate equipment and drugs are available and should be assisted by a suitably trained, skilled individual, familiar with the location. Magnetic resonance imaging (MRI) and computed tomography (CT) are the commonest radiological investigations in children requiring general anaesthesia.

Considerations for MRI

Although MRI avoids the risks of exposing patients and staff to radiation, it provides several problems for anaesthesia[378] and other potential hazards to personnel in the scanner room.

1. Ferromagnetic materials are strongly attracted to the magnet and equipment containing these may act as a projectile, injuring personnel and damaging the scanner. A child with a metal foreign body (e.g. aneurysm clip, pacemaker, ferromagnetic artificial heart valve, or metal prosthesis or plate) may not enter the MRI scanner.

   Aluminium, stainless steel, brass and other alloys are MRI-compatible. A non-ferromagnetic anaesthetic machine is required for use in the scanner room and special trolleys, made from non-ferromagnetic materials, must be used instead of the standard patient trolleys.
2. A strong electrical current may be induced in a wire coil lying within the magnetic field and this may cause thermal injury. This is avoided by using special MRI-compatible monitor leads. The monitors themselves are usually located outside the scanner room and connected to the patient with long extensions.
3. Routine monitors and motorised equipment (e.g. syringe drivers) do not function reliably near the magnet.

MRI takes between 20 and 60 min in total, with the child having to remain still for individual episodes of 10 min each to avoid movement distorting the image. (CT using a new spiral scanner takes several minutes only.)

Anaesthesia

Several techniques have been described for sedating or anaesthetising children for imaging:

1. Hypnotic or anaesthetic drugs have been given orally or rectally (e.g. midazolam)[379] or IM (e.g. ketamine or methohexitone).[380] These methods of administration are associated with unpredictable onset of drug action, a variable depth of sedation/anaesthesia and prolonged recovery.[381] Rectal or IM administration may be unpleasant. For advice on sedation, see Ch. 5, p. 101–105.
2. General anaesthesia and tracheal intubation are sometimes used, although the depth of anaesthesia required for intubation is greater than needed for the investigation and recovery may be prolonged. Maintenance is usually with a volatile agent. Alternatively, the airway may be maintained with an LMA at a lighter plane of anaesthesia (Fig. 6.13).

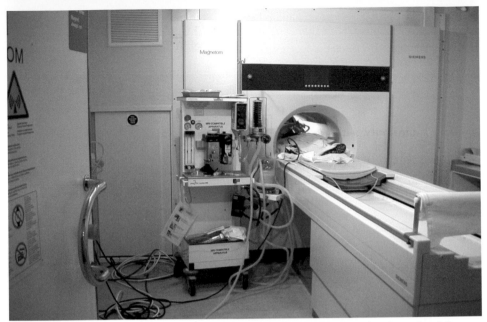

Fig 6.13 A boy anaesthetised for a MRI scan. An MRI-compatible anaesthetic machine is used to deliver an inhalational anaesthetic via a laryngeal mask airway. The pipelines for anaesthetic gases enter via a hole in the wall from manifolds in the room adjacent to the scanner. (This figure was kindly provided by Dr Anna Johnson, Consultant Paediatric Anaesthetist, Derriford Hospital).

3. A propofol infusion is an increasingly common technique for maintenance during MRI or CT scanning. Oxygen may be administered via nasal cannulae or a clear plastic mask.[378, 381] Frankville et al found that propofol 100 µg kg^{-1} min^{-1} (following halothane induction and propofol 2 mg kg^{-1}) prevented children moving during MRI.[381] SpO_2 transiently decreased in some children after the initial injection of propofol, but recovery was rapid and without POV.

TIVA without tracheal intubation during MRI scanning allows careful titration of sedatives and eliminates the need for a non-ferromagnetic anaesthetic machine or scavenging of waste gases. The child may be lightly sedated if left undisturbed, since there is no stimulation from the procedure or the airway. In addition, an infusion pump is more easily portable compared with an anaesthetic machine.[381] The pump should be housed outside the scanner room and the long lengths of IV tubing threaded through a hole in the wall to be attached to the child's IV cannula.

REFERENCES

1. Department of Health. Welfare of children and young people in hospital. London: HMSO; 1991.
2. Thornes R. Just for the day. Children admitted to hospital for day treatment. Caring for children in the health services. London: 1991.
3. Royal College of Paediatrics and Child Health. Accident and emergency services for children. Report of a multi-disciplinary working party. London: Royal College of Paediatrics and Child Health; 1999.
4. Senate of Surgery of Great Britain and Ireland. The provision of general surgical services for children. London: Senate of Surgery of Great Britain and Ireland; 1998.
5. Cohen MM, Cameron CB. Should you cancel the operation if the child has an upper respiratory tract infection? Anesth Analg 1991; 72:282–288.
6. Tait AR, Knight PR. The effects of general anaesthesia on upper respiratory complications in patients with upper respiratory tract infections. Can J Anaesth 1987; 34:300–303.

7. De Soto H, Patel RI, Soliman IE, et al. Changes in oxygen saturation following general anaesthesia in children with upper respiratory infection signs and symptoms undergoing otolaryngological procedures. Anesthesiology 1988; 68:276–279.

8. Levy L, Pandit UA, Rande GI, et al. Upper respiratory tract infections and general anaesthesia in children. Anaesthesia 1992; 47:678–682.

9. Hannallah RS. What's new in paediatrics? Problems Anaesth 1999; 11:95–105.

10. Berry FA. The child with a runny nose. Anesthetic management of difficult and routine pediatric patients. Churchill Livingstone, 1990.

11. Cote CJ, Goudsouzian NG, Liu LMP, et al. Assessment of risk factors related to the acid aspiration syndrome in pediatric patients – gastric pH and residual volume. Anesthesiology 1982; 56:70–72.

12. Manchikanti L, Colliver JA, Marrero TC, et al. Assessment of age-related acid aspiration risk factors in pediatric, adult and geriatric patients. Anesth Analg 1985; 64:11–17.

13. Phillips S, Daborn AK, Hatch DJ. Preoperative fasting for paediatric anaesthesia. Br J Anaesth 1994; 73:529–536.

14. Cavell B. Gastric emptying in preterm infants. Acta Paediatr Scand 1979; 68:527–531.

15. Cavell B. Gastric emptying in infants fed human milk or infant formula. Acta Paediatr Scand 1981; 70:639–641.

16. Moran TJ. Pulmonary edema produced by intratracheal injection of milk, feeding mixtures and sugars. Am J Dis Child 1953; 50:45–50.

17. Schurizek BA, Rybro L, Boggild–Madsen NB, et al. Gastric volume and pH in children for emergency surgery. Acta Anaesthesiol Scand 1986; 30:404–408.

18. Lawson RA, Smart NG, Morton NS. Evaluation of an amethocaine gel preparation for percutaneous analgesia before venous cannulation in children. Br J Anaesth 1995; 75:282–285.

19. McCafferty DF, Woolfson AD, Boston V. In vivo assessment of percutaneous local anaesthetic preparations. In vivo assessment of percutaneous local anaesthetic preparations. 1989; 62:17–21.

20. Hallen B, Olssen GL, Uppfeldt A. Pain-free venepuncture. Anaesthesia 1984; 39:969–972.

21. De Soto H. New pharmacologic agents and their use in pediatric anesthesia. Am J Anesthesiol 1995; 22:305–311.

22. Bensch CM, Strocel MC, Selley K. Preoperative medication for pediatric tympanotomy: necessary or not? J Am Assoc Nurse Anesth 1993; 61:424–425.

23. Greenberg JA, Davis PJ. Premedication and induction of anesthesia in pediatric surgical patients. Anesthesiol Clin North Am 1996; 14:781–802.

24. Parnis SJ, Foate JA, van der Walt JH, et al. Oral midazolam is an effective premedication for children having day-stay anaesthesia. Anaesth Intens Care 1992; 20:9–14.

25. Nathwani D, Rich P, Konieczko KM, et al. Midazolam vs trimeprazine premedication for children during day-care surgery. Br J Anaesth 1996; 76:589.

26. Gervais HW, El Gindi M, Radermacher PR, et al. Plasma concentration following oral and intramuscular atropine in children and their clinical effects. Paediatr Anaesth 1997; 7:13–18.

27. Johr M. Is it time to question the routine use of anticholinergic agents in paediatric anaesthesia? Paediatr Anaesth 1999; 9:99–101.

28. Action for Sick Children. Setting standards for children undergoing surgery. London: Action for Sick Children; 1994.

29. Hannallah RS, Rosales JK. Experience with parents' presence during anaesthesia induction in children. Can Anaesth Soc J 1983; 30:286–289.

30. Bevan J, Johnston C, Haig M, et al. Preoperative parental anxiety predicts behavioral and emotional responses to induction of anaesthesia in children. Can J Anaesth 1990; 37:177–182.

31. Hannallah RS. Who benefits when parents are present during anaesthesia induction in their children? Can J Anaesth 1994; 41:271–275.

32. Hall SC. Postanesthesia recovery care. J Clin Anesth 1995; 7:600–605.

33. Barker I. Is sevoflurane replacing halothane? Br J Anaesth 1998; 80:123.

34. Walker RWM, Allen DL, Rothera MR. A fibreoptic intubation technique for children with mucopolysaccharidoses using the laryngeal mask airway. Paediatr Anaesth 1997; 7:421–426.

35. Grounds RM, Newman PJ. Sevoflurane. Br J Hosp Med 1997; 57:43–46.

36. Scholz J, Tonner PH. Critical evaluation of the new inhalational anesthetics desflurane and sevoflurane. Anaesthesiol Reanim 1997; 22:15–20.

37. Kataria B, Epstein R, Bailey A, et al. A comparison of sevoflurane to halothane in paediatric surgical patients: results of a multicentre international study. Paediatr Anaesth 1996; 6:283–292.

38. Yurino M, Kimura H. Vital capacity rapid inhalation induction technique: comparison of sevoflurane and halothane. Can J Anaesth 1993; 40:440–443.

39. Patel SS, Goa KL. Sevoflurane. A review of its pharmacodynamic and pharmacokinetic properties and its clinical use in general anaesthesia. Drugs 1996; 51:658–700.

40. Lerman J, Sikich N, Kleinman S, et al. The pharmacology of sevoflurane in infants and children. Anesthesiology 1994; 80:814–824.

41. Sury MR, Black A, Hemington L, et al. A comparison of the recovery characteristics of sevoflurane and halothane in children. Anaesthesia 1996; 51:543–546.
42. Landais A, Saint-Maurice C, Hamza J, et al. Sevoflurane elimination kinetics in children. Paediatr Anaesth 1995; 5:297–301.
43. Muller CM, Krenn CG, Urak G, et al. Sevoflurane in paediatric anaesthesia. Acta Anaesthesiol Scand 1997; 111 (suppl):150–151.
44. Mori N, Suzuki M. Sevoflurane in paediatric anaesthesia: effects on respiration and circulation during induction and recovery. Paediatr Anaesth 1996; 6:95–102.
45. Kern C, Erb T, Frei FJ. Haemodynamic responses to sevoflurane compared with halothane during inhalational induction in children. Paediatr Anaesth 1997; 7:439–440.
46. Sarner JB, Levine M, Davis PJ, et al. Clinical characteristics of sevoflurane in children. A comparison with halothane. Anesthesiology 1995; 82:38–46.
47. Johannesson GP, Floren M, Lindahl SG. Sevoflurane for ENT surgery in children. A comparison with halothane. Acta Anaesthesiol Scand 1995; 39:546–550.
48. Meretoja OA, Taivainen T, Raiha L, et al. Sevoflurane–nitrous oxide or halothane–nitrous oxide for paediatric bronchoscopy and gastroscopy. Br J Anaesth 1996; 76:767–771.
49. Rieger A, Schroter G, Philippi W, et al. A comparison of sevoflurane with halothane in outpatient adenotonsillectomy in children with mild upper respiratory tract infections. J Clin Anesth 1996; 8:188–197.
50. Komatsu H, Chujo K, Morita J. Spontaneous breathing with the use of a laryngeal mask airway in children: comparison of sevoflurane and isoflurane. Paediatr Anaesth 1997; 7:111–115.
51. Kwek TK, Ng A. Laryngeal mask insertion following inhalational induction in children: a comparison between halothane and sevoflurane. Anaesth Intens Care 1997; 25:413–416.
52. Inomata S, Yamashita S, Toyooka H, et al. Anaesthetic induction time for tracheal intubation using sevoflurane or halothane in children. Anaesthesia 1998; 53:440–445.
53. Otsuka H, Komura Y, Mayumi T, et al. Malignant hyperthermia during sevoflurane anaesthesia in a child with central core disease. Anesthesiology 1994; 75:699–701.
54. Komatsu H, Taie DS, Endo S, et al. Electrical seizures during sevoflurane anesthesia in two pediatric patients with epilepsy. Anesthesiology 1994; 81:1535–1537.
55. Komatsu H, Ueki M, Morita J, et al. Clinical characteristics and biotransformation of sevoflurane in paediatric patients during antiepileptic drug therapy. Paediatr Anaesth 1996; 6:379–382.
56. Miguchi H, Arimura S, Sumikura H, et al. Urine concentrating ability after prolonged sevoflurane anaesthesia. Br J Anaesth 1994; 73:239–240.
57. Kharash ED, Hankins DC, Thimmel KE. Human kidney methoxyflurane and sevoflurane metabolism. Anesthesiology 1995; 82:689–699.
58. Bito H, Ikeda K. Closed circuit anaesthesia with sevoflurane in humans. Effects of renal and hepatic function and concentration of breakdown products with soda lime in children. Anesthesiology 1994; 81:366.
59. Fisher DM, Zwass MS. Desflurane in 60% nitrous oxide for infants and children . Anesthesiology 1992; 76:354–356.
60. Taylor RH, Lerman J. Induction, maintenance and recovery characteristics of desflurane in children and infants. Can J Anaesth 1992, 39.6–13.
61. Zwass MS, Fisher DM, Wellborn LG, et al. Induction and maintenance characteristics of anesthesia with desflurane and nitrous oxide in infants and children. Anesthesiology 1992; 76: 373–378.
62. Ebert TJ, Muzi M, Lapata CW. Neurocirculatory responses to sevoflurane in humans; a comparison with desflurane. Anesthesiology 1995; 83:88–95.
63. Welborn LG, Frazier LJ, Hannallah RS, et al. Comparison of emergence and recovery characteristics of sevoflurane, desflurane and halothane in paediatric patients. Anesth Analg 1995; 80:550.
64. O'Brien K, Robinson DN, Morton NS. Induction and emergence in infants less than 60 weeks post-conceptual age: comparison of thiopental, halothane, sevoflurane and desflurane. Br J Anaesth 1998; 80:456–459.
65. Weir PM, Munro HM, Reynolds PI, et al. Propofol infusion and the incidence of emesis in pediatric outpatient strabismus surgery. Anesth Analg 1993; 76:760–764.
66. Morton N. Total intravenous anaethesia (TIVA) in paediatrics: advantages and disadvantages. Paediatr Anaesth 1998; 8:189–194.
67. Browne BL, Prys Roberts C, Wolf AR. Propofol and alfentanil in children, infusion technique and dose requirements for total intravenous anaesthesia. Br J Anaesth 1992; 69:570–576.
68. Egan TD. Remifentanil pharmacokinetics and pharmacodynamics: a preliminary appraisal. Clin Pharmacokinet 1995; 29:80–94.
69. Lynn AM. Remifentanil: the paediatric anaesthetist's opiate? Paediatr Anaesth 1996; 6:433–435.
70. Eck JB, Lynn A. Use of remifentanil in infants. Paediatr Anaesth 1998; 8:437–439.
71. Meretoja OA, Taivainen T, Wirtavuori K. Cisatracurium during halothane and balanced anaesthesia in children. Paediatr Anaesth 1996; 6:373–378.

72. Vuksanaj D, Skjonsby B, Dunbar BS. Neuromuscular effects of rocuronium in children during halothane anaesthesia. Paediatr Anaesth 1996; 6:277–281.

73. Kelly O, Frossard J, Meistelman C, et al. Neuromuscular blockade following Org 9426 in children during nitrous oxide–halothane anaesthesia. Anesthesiology 1991; 75:A787.

74. Taivainen T, Meretoja OA, Erkola O, et al. Rocuronium in infants, children and adults during balanced anaesthesia. Paediatr Anaesth 1996; 6:271–275.

75. Stoddart PA, Mather SJ. Onset of neuromuscular blockade and intubating conditions one minute after the administration of rocuronium in children. Paediatr Anaesth 1998; 8:37–40.

76. Lejus C, Blanloeil Y, Le-Roux N, et al. Prolonged mivacurium neuromuscular block in children. Paediatr Anaesth 1998; 8:433–435.

77. Goudsouzian NG. Mivacurium in infants and children. Paediatr Anaesth 1997; 7:183–190.

78. Meretoja OA, Taivainen T. Mivacurium chloride in infants and children. Anaesthesiol Scand 1995; 106 (suppl):41–44.

79. Brandom BW, Meretoja OA, Simhi E, et al. Age related variability in the effects of mivacurium in paediatric surgical patients. Can J Anaesth 1998; 45:410–416.

80. Alifimoff AK, Goudsouzian NG. Continous infusion of mivacurium in children. Br J Anaesth 1989; 70:237–242.

81. Goodarzi M. A double blind comparison of droperidol and ondansetron for prevention of emesis in children undergoing orthopaedic surgery. Paediatr Anaesth 1998; 8:325–329.

82. Morton NS, Camu F, Dorman T, et al. Ondansetron reduces nausea and vomiting after paediatric adenotonsillectomy. Paediatr Anaesth 1997; 7:37–45.

83. Splinter WM, Rhine EJ. Prophylactic antiemetics in children undergoing tonsillectomy: high-dose vs low-dose ondansetron. Paediatr Anaesth 1997; 7:125–129.

84. Rose JB, Martin TM. Posttonsillectomy vomiting. Ondansetron or metoclopramide during paediatric tonsillectomy: are two doses better than one? Paediatr Anaesth 1996; 6:39–44.

85. Fujii Y, Tanaka H. Granisetron decreases postoperative vomiting in children. A dose-ranging study. Eur J Anaesth 1999; 16:62–65.

86. Fujii Y, Tanaka H. Prophylactic therapy with granisetron in the prevention of vomiting after paediatric surgery. A randomized, double-blind comparison with droperidol and metoclopramide. Paediatr Anaesth 1998; 8:149–153.

87. Fujii Y, Tanaka H, Toyooka H. Granisetron and dexamethasone provide more improved prevention of postoperative emesis than granisetron alone in children. Can J Anaesth 1996; 43:1229–1232.

88. Miller KA, Harkin CP, Bailey PL. Postoperative tracheal extubation. Anesth Analg 1995; 80:149–172.

89. Burgess GE, Cooper JR, Marino RJ, et al. Laryngeal incompetence after tracheal extubation. Anesthesiology 1979; 51:73–77.

90. Boisson-Bertrand D. Tonsillectomies and the reinforced laryngeal mask. Can J Anaesth 1995; 42:857–861.

91. Patel RI, Hannallah RS, Norden J, et al. Emergence airway complications in children: a comparison of tracheal extubation in awake and deeply anaesthetized patients. Anesth Analg 1991; 73: 266–270.

92. Pounder DR, Blackstock D, Steward DJ. Tracheal extubation in children: halothane versus isoflurane, anesthetized versus awake. Anesthesiology 1991; 74:653–655.

93. Ruby RRF, Webster AC, Morley-Forster PK, et al. Laryngeal mask airway in paediatric otolaryngological surgery. J Otolaryngol 1995; 24:288–291.

94. Elwood T, Cox RG. Laryngeal mask insertion with a laryngoscope in paediatric patients. Can J Anaesth 1996; 43:435–438.

95. McNicol LR. Insertion of laryngeal mask airway in children (letter). Anaesthesia 1991; 46:330.

96. Chow BFM, Lewis M, Jones SEF. Laryngeal mask airway in children: insertion technique (letter) Anaesthesia 1991; 46:590–591.

97. O'Neill B, Josephine J, Caramico L, et al. The laryngeal mask airway in pediatric patients: factors affecting ease of use during insertion and emergence. Anesth Analg 1994; 78:659–662.

98. Rowbottom SJ, Simpson DL, Grubb D. The laryngeal mask airway in children. A fibreoptic assessment of positioning. Anaesthesia 1991; 46:489–491.

99. Mizushima A, Wardall GJ, Simpson DL. The laryngeal mask airway in infants. Anaesthesia 1992; 47:849–851.

100. McLeod DH, Narang VPS. Functional and anatomical assessment of the laryngeal mask airway in infants and children. Anesth Analg 1992; 20:109.

101. Goudsouzian NG, Denman W, Cleveland R, et al. Radiologic localization of the laryngeal mask airway in children. Anesthesiology 1992; 77:1085–1089.

102. Lopez-Gil M, Brimacombe J. Safety and efficacy of the laryngeal mask airway. A prospective study of 1400 children. Anaesthesia 1996; 51:969–972.

103. Gursoy F, Algren JT, Skjonsby BS. Positive pressure ventilation with the laryngeal mask airway in children. Anesth Analg 1996; 82:33–38.

104. Vergese C, Smith TGC, Young E. Prospective survey on the use of the laryngeal mask airway in 2359 patients. Anaesthesia 1993; 48:58–60.
105. Beveridge ME. Laryngeal mask anesthesia for repair of cleft palate. Anaesthesia 1989; 44:656–657.
106. Ebata T, Nisiki S, Masuda A, et al. Anesthesia for Treacher Collins syndrome using a laryngeal mask airway. Can J Anaesth 1991; 38:1043–1045.
107. Hasan MA, Black AE. A new technique for fibreoptic intubation in children. Anaesthesia 1994; 49:1031–1034.
108. Allison A, McCrory J. Tracheal placement of a gum elastic bougie using the laryngeal mask. Anaesthesia 1990; 45:419–420.
109. Heard C, Caldicott LD, Fletcher JE, et al. Fiberoptic-guided endotracheal intubation via the laryngeal mask airway in pediatric patients: a report of a series of cases. Anesth Analg 1996; 82:1287–1289.
110. Rabb MF, Minkowitz HF, Hagberg CA. Blind intubation through the laryngeal mask airway for management of the difficult airway in infants. Anesthesiology 1996; 84:1510–1511.
111. Bandla HP, Smith DE, Kiernan MP. Laryngeal mask airway facilitated fibreoptic bronchoscopy in infants. Can J Anaesth 1997; 44:1242.
112. Theroux MC, Kettrick RG, Khine HH. Laryngeal mask airway and fiberoptic endoscopy in an infant with Schwartz–Jampel syndrome. Anesthesiology 1995; 82:605.
113. Osses H, Poblete M, Asenjo F. Laryngeal mask for difficult intubation in children. Paediatr Anaesth 1999; 9:399–401.
114. Dubreuil M, Ecoffey C. Laryngeal mask guided tracheal intubation in paediatric anaesthesia (letter). Paediatr Anaesth 1992; 2:344.
115. Goodwin APL, Ogg TW. An armored laryngeal mask airway. Anesthesiology 1992; 76:150.
116. Association of Anaesthetists of Great Britain and Northern Ireland. Recommendations for monitoring during anaesthesia and recovery (revised). Association of Anaesthetists of Great Britain and Ireland; 1994.
117. Barthram CN, Taylor L. The oesophageal and precordial stethoscope transduced as a monitor and teaching aid. Anaesthesia 1994; 49:713–714.
118. Cote CJ, Goldstein EA, Cote MA, et al. Single-blind study of pulse oximetry in children. Anesthesiology 1988; 68:184–188.
119. Moller JT, Pedersen T, Rasmussen LS, et al. Randomised evaluation of pulse oximetry in 20 802 patients I Design, demography, pulse oximetry failure rate, and overall complication rate. Anesthesiology 1993; 78:436–444.
120. Moller JT, Johannessen NW, Espersen K, et al. Randomised evaluation of pulse oximetry in 20 802 patients. II Perioperative events and postoperative complications. Anesthesiology 1993; 78:445–453.
121. Allen EV. Thromboangiitis obliterans: methods of diagnosis of chronic occlusive arterial lesions distal to the wrist with illustrative cases. Am J Med Soc 1929; 178:237.
122. Brodsky JB. A simple method to determine patency of the ulnar artery intraoperatively prior to radial artery cannulation. Anesthesiology 1975; 42:626.
123. Seldinger SI. Catheter replacement of the needle in percutaneous arteriography Acta Radiol Diagn 1953; 39:368.
124. Pais-Bahrami K, Karna P, Dolanski EA. Effect of fluids on the lifespan of peripheral arterial lines. Am J Perinatol 1990, 7:122.
125. Lowe SV, Deshpande JK, Tobias JD. Perioperative monitoring. In: Kamban J, ed. Cardiac anesthesia for infants and children. New York: Mosby Year-Book; 1994:92–108.
126. Robinson J, Charlton J, Seal R, et al. Oesophageal, rectal, axillary, tympanic and pulmonary artery temperatures during cardiac surgery. Can J Anaesth 1998; 445:317–323.
127. Harasawa K, Kemmotsu O, Mayumi J, et al. Comparison of tympanic, esophageal and blood temperature during mild hypothermic cardiopulmonary bypass: a study using an infrared emission detection tympanic thermometer. J Clin Monit 1997; 13:19–24.
128. Sessler DI. Perioperative heat balance. Anesthesiology 2000; 92:578–596.
129. Hervey GR. Thermoregulation. In: Emslie-Smith D, Paterson CR, Scratcherd T, et al, eds. Textbook of physiology, 11th edn. Edinburgh: Churchill Livingstone, 1988:510–533.
130. Imrie MM, Hall GM. Body temperature and anaesthesia. Br J Anaesth 1990; 64:346–354.
131. Annadata RS, Sessler DI, Tayefeh F, et al. Desflurane slightly increases the sweating threshold, but produces marked and non-linear decreases in the vasoconstriction and shivering thresholds. Anesthesiology 1995; 83:1205–1211.
132. Kurz A, Plattner O, Sessler DI, et al. The threshold for thermoregulatory vasoconstriction during nitrous oxide/isoflurane anesthesia is lower in elderly than young patients. Anesthesiology 1993; 79:465–469.
133. Matsukawa T, Kurz A, Sessler DI, et al. Propofol linearly reduces the vasoconstriction and shivering thresholds. Anesthesiology 1995; 82:1169–1180.
134. Morley-Forster PK. Unintentional hypothermia in the operating room. Can Anaesth Soc J 1986; 33:516–527.

135. Steward DJ. Manual of pediatric anesthesia, 2nd edn. Churchill Livingstone 1985:30–32, 67–68.

136. Imrie MM, Hall GM. Body temperature and anaesthesia. Br J Anaesth 1990; 64:346–354.

137. Kurz A, Kurz M, Poeschl G, et al. Forced-air warming maintains intraoperative normothermia better than circulating-water mattresses. Anesth Analg 1993; 77:89–95.

138. Borms SF, Engelen SL, Himpe DG, et al. Bair Hugger forced air warming maintains normothermia more effectively than Thermolite insulation. J Clin Anaesth 1994; 6:303–307.

139. Ayala JL, Coe A. Thermal softening of tracheal tubes: an unrecognised hazard of the Bair Hugger active patient warming system. Br J Anaesth 1997; 79:543–545.

140. Azzam FJ, Krock JL. Thermal burns in two infants associated with a forced air warming system. Anesth Analg 1995; 81:661.

141. Cullen DJ, Eichhorn JH, Cooper JB, et al. Postanesthesia care unit standards for anesthesiologists. J Post Anesth Nurs 1989; 4:141–146.

142. Bryant LD, Diersdorf SF. Postanesthesia recovery. Semin Pediatr Surg 1992; 1:45–54.

143. Association of Anaesthetists of Great Britain and Northern Ireland. Immediate post anaesthetic recovery. Association of Anaesthetists of Great Britain and Northern Ireland; 2002.

144. Kermode J, Walker S, Webb I. Postoperative vomiting in children. Anaesth Intens Care 1995; 23:196–199.

145. Karlsson E, Larrsson LE, Nilsson K. Postanaesthetic nausea in children. Acta Anaesthesiol Scand 1990; 34:515–518.

146. Lerman J. Surgical and patient factors involved in postoperative nausea and vomiting. Br J Anaesth 1992; 69 (suppl):24S–32S.

147. Mather S, Peutrell JM. Postoperative morphine requirements, nausea and vomiting following anaesthesia for tonsillectomy. Comparison of intravenous morphine and non-opioid analgesic techniques. Paediatr Anaesth 1995; 5:185–188.

148. Brennan LJ. Modern day-case anaesthesia for children. Br J Anaesth 1999; 83:91–103.

149. Casteels-van Daele M, Jaeken J, van der Schueren P, et al. Dystonic reactions in children caused by metoclopramide. Arch Dis Child 1970; 45:130–133.

150. Lerman J, Eustis E, Smith DR. Effect of droperidol pretreatment on postanesthetic vomiting in children undergoing strabismus surgery. Anesthesiology 1986; 65:322–325.

151. Dupre LJ, Stieglitz P. Extrapyramidal syndromes after premedication with droperidol in children. Br J Anaesth 1980; 52:831–833.

152. Nair I, Bailey PM. Review of uses of the laryngeal mask in ENT anaesthesia. Anaesthesia 1995; 50:898–900.

153. Habre W, Sims CL. Propofol anaesthesia and vomiting after myringoplasty in children. Anaesthesia 1997; 52 544–546.

154. Van den Berg AA. A comparison of ondansetron and prochlorperazine for the prevention of nausea and vomiting after tympanoplasty. Can J Anaesth 1996; 43:939–945.

155. Fujii Y, Toyooka H, Tanaka H. Granisetron reduces the incidence of nausea and vomiting after middle ear surgery. Br J Anaesth 1997; 79:539–540.

156. Chinn K, Brown OE, Manning SC, et al. Middle ear pressure variation: effect of nitrous oxide. Laryngoscope 1997; 107:357–363.

157. Williams PJ, Thompsett C, Bailey PM. Comparison of the reinforced laryngeal mask airway and tracheal intubation for nasal surgery. Anaesthesia 1995; 50:987–989.

158. John G, Low JM, Tan PE, et al. Plasma catecholamine levels during functional endoscopic sinus surgery. Clin Otolaryngol 1995; 20:213–215.

159. Verlander MJ, Johns ME. The clinical use of cocaine. Otolaryngol Clin North Am 1981; 14:521–531.

160. Chiu YC, Brecht K, DasGupta DS. Myocardial infarction with topical cocaine anesthesia for nasal surgery. Arch Otolaryngol Head Neck Surg 1986; 112:988–990.

161. Karl HW, Swedlow DB, Lee KW, et al. Epinephrine halothane interactions in children. Anesthesiology 1983; 58:142.

162. Stankiewicz JA. Pediatric endoscopic nasal and sinus surgery. Otolaryngol Head Neck Surg 1995; 113:204–210.

163. Mucklow ES. Obstructive sleep apnoea causing severe pulmonary hypertension reversed by emergency tonsillectomy. Br J Clin Pract 1989; 43:260–263.

164. Kobel M, Creighton RE, Steward DJ. Anaesthetic considerations in Down's syndrome: experience with 100 patients and a review of the literature. Can Anaesth Soc J 1982; 29:593–598.

165. Goldstein NA, Derek R, Armfield MD, et al. Postoperative complications after tonsillectomy and adenoidectomy in children with Down's syndrome. Arch Otolaryngol Head Neck Surg 1998; 124:171–176.

166. Mitchell V, Howard R, Facer E. Down's syndrome and anaesthesia. Paediatr Anaesth 1995; 5:379–384.

167. Ferrari LR, Donlon JV. Metoclopramide reduces the incidence of vomiting after tonsillectomy in children. Anesth Analg 1992; 75:351–354.

168. Litman RS, Wu CL, Catanzaro FA. Ondansetron decreases emesis after tonsillectomy in children. Anesth Analg 1994; 78:478–481.

169. Carithers JS, Gebhart DE, Williams JA. Postoperative risks of pediatric tonsilladenoidectomy. Laryngoscope 1987; 97:422–429.

170. van der Walt JH, Jacob R, Murrell D, et al. The perioperative effects of oral premedication in children. Anaesth Intens Care 1990; 18:5–10.

171. Splinter WM, MacNeill HB, Menard EA, et al. Midazolam reduces vomiting after tonsillectomy in children. Can J Anaesth 1995; 42:201–203

172. Fujii Y, Toyooka H, Tanaka H. Antiemetic efficacy of granisetron and metoclopramide in children undergoing ophthalmic or ENT surgery. Can J Anaesth 1996; 43:1095–1099.

173. Barst SM, Markowitz A, Yossefy Y, et al. Propofol reduces the incidence of vomiting after tonsillectomy in children. Paediatr Anaesth 1995; 5:249–252.

174. Ved SA, Walden TL, Montana J, et al. Vomiting and recovery after outpatient tonsillectomy and adenoidectomy in children. Comparison of four anaesthetic techniques using nitrous oxide with halothane or propofol. Anesthesiology 1996; 85:4–10.

175. Mendham JE, Mather SJ. Comparison of diclofenac and tenoxicam for postoperative analgesia with and without fentanyl in children undergoing adenotonsillectomy or tonsillectomy. Paediatr Anaesth 1996; 6:467–473.

176. Stow PJ, White JB. Anaesthesia for paediatric tonsillectomy. Comparison of spontaneous ventilation and intermittent positive pressure ventilation. Br J Anaesth 1987; 59:419–423.

177. Rose JB, Brenn BR, Corddry DH, et al. Preoperative oral ondansetron for pediatric tonsillectomy. Anesth Analg 1996; 82:558–562.

178. Splinter WM, Roberts DJ. Dexamethasone decreases vomiting by children after tonsillectomy. Anesth Analg 1996; 83:13–16.

179. Stene FN, Seay RE, Young LA, et al. Prospective, randomized, double-blind, placebo-controlled comparison of metoclopramide and ondansetron for prevention of posttonsillectomy or adenotonsillectomy emesis. J Anesth 1996; 8:540–544.

180. Lawhorn CD, Bower C, Brown RE Jr, et al. Ondansetron reduces posttonsillectomy vomiting in pediatric patients undergoing tonsillectomy and adenoidectomy. Int J Pediatr Otorhinolaryngol 1996; 36:99–108.

181. Splinter WM, Rhine EJ, Roberts DW, et al. Ondansetron is a better prophylactic antiemetic than droperidol for tonsillectomy in children. Can J Anaesth 1995; 42:48–51.

182. Furst SR, Rodarte A. Prophylactic antiemetic treatment with ondansetron in children undergoing tonsillectomy. Anesthesiology 1994; 81:799–803.

183. Grunwald Z, Schreiner MS, Parness J, et al. Droperidol decreases the incidence and the severity of vomiting after tonsillectomy and adenoidectomy in children. Paediatr Anaesth 1994; 4:163–167.

184. Hamid SK, Selby IR, Sikich N, et al. Vomiting after adenotonsillectomy in children: a comparison of ondansetron, dimenhydrinate and placebo. Anesth Analg 1998; 86:496–500.

185. Courtman SP, Rawlings E, Carr AS. Masked bleeding posttonsillectomy with ondansetron (letter). Paediatr Anaesth 1999; 9:467.

186. Zestos MM, Carr AS, McAuliffe G, et al. Subhypnotic propofol does not treat postoperative vomiting in children after adenotonsillectomy. Can J Anaesth 1997; 44: 401–404.

187. Bissonnette B. Lidocaine aerosol following tonsillectomy in children. Can J Anaesth 1990; 37:534–537.

188. Melchor MA, Villafruela MA, Munoz B, et al. Postoperative pain in tonsillectomy in general anaesthesia and local infiltration. Acta Otorrinolaringol Espanola 1994; 45:349–355.

189. Golsher M, Podoshin L, Fradis M, et al. Effect of peritonsillar infiltration on post–tonsillectomy pain: a double-blind study. Ann Otol Rhinol Laryngol 1996; 105:868–870.

190. Jebeles JA, Reilly JS, Gutierrez JF, et al. Tonsillectomy and adenoidectomy pain reduction by local bupivacaine infiltration in children. Int J Pediatr Otorhinolaryngol 1993; 25:149–154.

191. Stuart JC, MacGregor FB, Cairns, et al.Peritonsillar infiltration with bupivacaine for paediatric tonsillectomy. Anaesth Intens Care 1994; 22:679–682.

192. Wong AK, Bissonnette B, Braude BA, et al. Post-tonsillectomy infiltration of bupivacaine reduces immediate post-operative pain in children. Can J Anaesth 1995; 42:1–5.

193. Crysdale WS, Russel D. Complications of tonsillectomy and adenoidectomy in 9409 children observed overnight. Can Med Assoc J 1986; 135:1139–1142.

194. Guida RA, Mattucci KF. Tonsillectomy and adenoidectomy: an inpatient or outpatient procedure? Laryngoscope 1990; 100:491–493.

195. Rasmussen N. Complications of tonsillectomy and adenoidectomy. Otolaryngol Clin North Am 1987; 20:383–390.

196. Witucki J. Complications of tonsillectomy. Otolaryngol Polska 1992; 46:46–51.

197. Szeremeta W, Novelly NJ, Benninger M. Postoperative bleeding in tonsillectomy patients. Ear, Nose Throat 1996; 75:373–376.

198. Unlu Y, Tekalan SA, Cemiloglu R, et al. Guillotine and dissection tonsillectomy in children. J Laryngol Otol 1992; 106:817–820.
199. Tan AK, Rothstein J, Tewfik TL. Ambulatory tonsillectomy and adenoidectomy: complications and associated factors. J Otolaryngol 1993; 22:442–446.
200. Robinson PM, Ahmed I. Diclofenac and post-tonsillectomy haemorrhage. Clin Otolaryngol 1995; 19:483–484.
201. Rusy LM, Houck CS, Sullivan LJ, et al. A double-blind evaluation of ketorolac tromethamine versus acetaminophen in pediatric tonsillectomy: analgesia and bleeding. Anesth Analg 1995; 80:226–229.
202. Splinter WM, Rhine EJ, Roberts DW, et al. Preoperative ketorolac increases bleeding after tonsillectomy in children. Can J Anaesth 1996; 43:60–63.
203. Gunter JB, Varughese AM, Harrington JF, et al. Recovery and complications after tonsillectomy in children: a comparison of ketorolac and morphine. Anesth Analg 1995; 81:1136–1141.
204. Thiagarajan J, Bates S, Hitchcock M, et al. Blood loss following tonsillectomy in children: a blind comparison of diclofenac and papaveretum. Anaesthesia 1993; 47:132–135.
205. Royal College of Anaesthetists. Guidelines for the use of non-steroidal anti-inflamatory drugs in the perioperative period. London: Royal College of Anaesthetists; 1998.
206. Williams PJ, Bailey PM. Comparison of the reinforced laryngeal mask airway and tracheal intubation for adenotonsillectomy. Br J Anaesth 1993; 70:30–33.
207. Webster AC, Morley-Forster PK, Dain S, et al. Anaesthesia for adenotonsillectomy: a comparison between tracheal intubation and the armoured laryngeal mask airway. Can J Anaesth 1993; 40(12):1171–1177.
208. Wehrle HJ, Gottstein P. Experiences with use of the laryngeal mask with flexible, wire reinforced tube for ENT interventions in children. Anastesiol Intensivmed Notfallmed Schmerzther 1997; 32:151–154.
209. John RE, Hill S, Hughes TJ. Airway protection by the laryngeal mask: a barrier to dye in the pharynx. Anaesthesia 1991; 46:366–367.
210. Reiner SA, Sawyer WP, Clark KF, et al. Safety of outpatient tonsillectomy and adenoidectomy. Otolaryngol Head Neck Surg 1990; 102:161–168.
211. Shott SR, Myer CM 3rd, Cotton RT. Efficacy of tonsillectomy and adenoidectomy as an outpatient procedure: a preliminary report. Int J Pediatr Otorhinolaryngol 1987; 13:157–163.
212. Feilberg VL, Sorensen JN, Eriksen HO. Hypertrophic tonsils, upper airway obstruction and cardiac complications. A combined otological, medical and anesthesiological problem. Ugeskr Laeger 1993; 155:3003–3005.
213. Senior BA, Radowski D, MacArthur C, et al. Changing patterns of supraglottitis: a multi-institutional review. Laryngoscope 1994; 104:1314–1322.
214. Hoekelmen RA. Epiglottitis: another dying disease? Paediatr Ann 1994; 23:229–230.
215. Tarnow Mordi WO, Berrill AM, Darby C, et al. Precipitation of laryngeal obstruction in acute epiglottitis. Br Med J 1985; 290:629.
216. Landau L, Geehoed GC. Aerosolised steroids for croup. N Engl J Med 1994; 331:322–323.
217. MacDonald WBG, Geehoed GC. Management of childhood croup. Thorax 1997; 52:757–759.
218. Tibbals J, Martin LD, Wetzel RC. Placebo controlled trial of prednisolone in children intubated for croup. Lancet 1992; 340:745–748.
219. Roger G, Denoyelle F, Triglia JM, et al. Severe laryngomalacia: surgical indications and results in 115 patients. Laryngoscope 1995; 105:1111–1117.
220. Sotomayor JL, Godinez RI, Borden S, et al. Large-airway collapse due to acquired tracheobronchomalacia in infancy. Am J Dis Child 1986; 140:367–371.
221. Wiel E, Vilette B, Darras JA, et al. Laryngotracheal stenosis in children after intubation. Report of 5 cases. Paediatr Anaesth 1997; 7: 415–419.
222. Balazie J, Masera A, Poljak M. Sudden death caused by laryngeal papillomatosis. Acta Oto-Laryngol 1997; 527:111–113.
223. Somers GR, Tabrizi SN, Borg AJ, et al. Juvenile laryngeal papillomatosis in a pediatric population: a clinicopathologic study. Pediatr Pathol Lab Med 1997; 17:53–64.
224. Hatch DJ. New inhalation agents in paediatric anaesthesia. Br J Anaesth 1999; 83:42–49.
225. Asai T, Fujise K, Uchida M. Use of the laryngeal mask in a child with tracheal stenosis. Anesthesiology 1991; 75:903–904.
226. Fisher JA, Ananthanarayan C, Edelist G. Role of the laryngeal mask in airway management (editorial). Can J Anaesth 1992; 39:1–3.
227. Asai T, Morris. The laryngeal mask and patients with collapsible airways (letter). Anaesthesia 1994; 49:169–170.
228. Wilson IG. The laryngeal mask airway in paediatric practice. Br J Anaesth 1993; 70:124.
229. Baraka A. Bronchoscopic removal of inhaled foreign bodies in children. Br J Anaesth 1974; 46:124–126.

230. Carluccio F, Romeo R. Inhalation of foreign bodies: epidemiological data and clinical considerations in the light of a statistical review of 92 cases. Acta Otorhinolaryngol Ital 1997; 17:45–51.

231. Harboyan G, Nassif R. Tracheobronchial foreign bodies – a review of 14 years' experience. J Laryngol Otol 1970; 84:404–412.

232. Bhatia PL. Problems in the management of aspirated foreign bodies W Afr J Med 1991; 10:156–167.

233. General Dental Council. General anaesthesia in dentistry. Maintaining standards. Guidance to dentists on professional and personal conduct. 1998.

234. Royal College of Anaesthetists. Standards and guidelines for general anaesthesia for dentistry.

235. Standing Dental Advisory Committee. Report of an expert working party. General anaesthesia, sedation and resuscitation in dentistry. 1990.

236. Conscious Decision: a review of the use of general anaesthesia and conscious sedation in primary dental care. Department of Health, London 2000.

237. Payne K, Heydenrych JJ, Martins M, et al. Caudal block for analgesia after paediatric inguinal surgery. S Afr Med J 1987; 72:629–630.

238. Conroy JM, Othersen HB Jr, Dorman BH, et al. A comparison of wound instillation and caudal blocks for analgesia following pediatric inguinal herniorrhaphy. Pediatr Surg 1993; 4:565–567.

239. Fisher QA, McClomiskey CM, Hill JL, et al. Postoperative voiding interval and duration of analgesia following peripheral or caudal nerve blocks in children. Anesth Analg 1993; 76:173–177.

240. Burns AM, Shelly MP, Dewar AK. Caudal analgesia for pediatric daycase surgery: assessment of motor function prior to discharge. J Clin Anesth 1990; 90:27–30.

241. Klimscha W, Chiari A, Michalek-Sauberer A, et al. The efficacy and safety of a clonidine/bupivacaine combination caudal for pediatric hernia repair. Anesth Analg 1998; 86:54–61.

242. Constant I, Gall O, Gouyet L, et al. Addition of clonidine or fentanyl to local anaesthetic prolongs the duration of surgical analgesia after single shot caudal block in children. Br J Anaesth 1998; 80:294–298.

243. Cook B, Doyle E. The use of additives to local anaesthetic solutions for caudal epidural blockade. Paediatr Anaesth 1996; 6:353–359.

244. Dupeyrat A, Goujard E, Muret J, et al. Transcutaneous CO_2 tension effects of clonidine in paediatric caudal analgesia. Paediatr Anaesth 1998; 8:145–148.

245. Jamali S, Monin S, Began C, et al. Clonidine in pediatric caudal anesthesia. Anesth Analg 1994; 78:663–666.

246. Surana R, Quinn F, Puri P. Is it necessary to perform appendicectomy in the middle of the night in children? Br Med J 1993; 306:1168.

247. Naguib M, Samarkandi AH, Ammor A, et al. Comparison of suxamethonium and different combinations of rocuronium and mivacurium for rapid tracheal intubation in children. Br J Anaesth 1997; 79:450–455.

248. Weir PS. Anaesthesia for appendicectomy in childhood: a survey of practice in Northern Ireland. Ulster Med J 1997; 66:34–37.

249. Sfez M, Le Mapihan Y, Gaillard JL, et al. Analgesia for appendectomy: comparison of fentanyl and alfentanil in children. Acta Anaesthesiol Scand 1990; 30:30–34.

250. Sims C, Johnson CM, Bergesio R, et al. Rectal indomethacin for analgesia after appendicectomy in children. Anaesth Intens Care 1994; 22:272–275.

251. Morton NS, O'Brien K. Analgesic efficacy of paracetamol and diclofenac in children receiving PCA morphine. Br J Anaesth 1999; 82:715–717.

252. Lambert AW, Mayor A. Analgesia requirements for appendicectomy: the difference between adults and children. Ann R Coll Surg Engl 2000; 82:111–112.

253. Colbert S, O'Hanlon DM, Courtney DF, et al. Analgesia following appendicectomy – the value of peritoneal bupivacaine. Can J Anaesth 1998; 45:729–734.

254. Mather SJ. Paediatric anaesthetic emergencies. Br J Hosp Med 1993; 50:377–389.

255. Lejus C, Delile L, Plattner V, et al. Randomised, single blinded trial of laparoscopic versus open appendectomy in children: effects on postoperative analgesia. Anesthesiology 1996; 84:801–806.

256. Sfez M. Laparoscopic surgery in pediatrics: the point of view of the anesthetist. Can Anesthesiol 1993; 41:237–244.

257. Blakely ML, Spurbeck W, Lakshman S, et al. Current state of laparoscopic appendectomy in children. Curr Opin Pediatr 1998; 10:315–317.

258. Tytgat SH, Bakker XR, Butzelaar RM. Laparoscopic evaluation of patients with suspected acute appendicitis. Surg Endosc 1998; 12:918–920.

259. Lamparelli MJ, Hoque HM, Pogson CJ, et al. A prospective evaluation of the combined use of the modified Alvarado score with selective laparoscopy in adult females in the management of suspected appendicitis. Ann R Coll Surg Engl 2000; 82:192–195.

260. Lunn JN. Implications of the National Confidential Enquiry into Perioperative Deaths for paediatric anaesthesia. Paediatr Anaesth 1992; 2:69–72.

261. Jones PF. The general surgeon who cares for children. Br Med J 1986; 2:1156–1158.

262. Cook-Sather SD, Tulloch HV, Liacouras CA, et al. Gastric fluid volume in infants for pyloromyotomy. Can J Anaesth 1997; 44:278–283.

263. Salem MR, Wong AY, Fizzott GF. Efficacy of cricoid pressure in preventing aspiration of gastric contents in paediatric patients. Br J Anaesth 1972; 44:401–404.

264. Goudsouzian NG, Denman W, Schwartz A, et al. Pharmacodynamic and hemodynamic effects of mivacurium in infants anesthetized with halothane and nitrous oxide. Anesthesiology 1993; 79:919–925.

265. Andropoulos DB, Heard MB, Johnson KL, et al. Postanesthetic apnea in full-term infants after pyloromyotomy. Anesthesiology 1994; 80:216–219.

266. Uemura S, Woodward AA, Amerena R, et al. Early repair of inguinal hernia in premature babies. Pediatr Surg Int 1999; 15:36–39.

267. Gallagher TM, Crean PM. Spinal anaesthesia in infants born prematurely. Anaesthesia 1989; 44:434–436.

268. Darlow BA, Dawson KP, Mogridge N. Inguinal hernia and low birthweight. NZ Med J 1987; 100:492–494.

269. Kurth CD, Spitzer AR, Broennle AM, et al. Postoperative apnea in preterm infants. Anesthesiology. 1987; 66:483–488.

270. Welborn LG, Rice LJ, Hannallah RS, et al. Postoperative apnea in former preterm infants: prospective comparison of spinal and general anesthesia. Anesthesiology 1990; 72:838–842.

271. Malviya S, Swarz J, Lerman J. Are all preterm infants younger than 60 weeks postconceptual age at risk for postanesthetic apnea? Anesthesiology 1993; 78:1076–1081.

272. Cote CJ, Zaslavsky A, Downes JJ, et al. Postoperative apnea in former preterm infants after inguinal herniorrhaphy. A combined analysis. Anesthesiology 1995; 82:809–822.

273. Gollin G, Bell C, Dubose R, et al. Predictors of postoperative respiratory complications in premature infants after inguinal herniorrhaphy. J Pediatr Surg 1993; 28:244–247.

274. Sims CJ, Johnson CM. Postoperative apnoea in infants. Anaesth Intens Care 1994; 22:40–45.

275. Welborn LG, Greenspun JC. Anesthesia and apnea. Perioperative considerations in the former preterm infant. Pediatr Clin North Am 1994; 41:181–198.

276. Welborn LG, Hannallah RS, Fink R, et al. High dose caffeine suppresses postoperative apnea in preterm infants. Anesthesiology 1989; 71:347–349.

277. Henderson-Smart DJ, Steer P. Methylxanthine treatment for apnea in preterm infants. Cochrane Database Syst Rev 2000; 2:CD000140.

278. Steer PA, Henderson-Smart DJ. Caffeine versus theophylline for apnea in preterm infants. Cochrane Database Syst Rev 2000; 2:CD000273.

279. Tobias JD, Flannagan J, Brock J, et al. Neonatal regional anesthesia: alternative to general anesthesia for urologic surgery. Urology 1993; 41:362–365.

280. Welborn LG, Hannallah RS, Higgins T, et al. Postoperative apnoea in former preterm infants: does anaemia increase the risk? Can J Anaesth 1990; 37:S92.

281. Webster AC, McKishnie JD, Kenyon CF, et al. Spinal anaesthesia for inguinal hernia repair in high-risk neonates. Can J Anaesth 1991; 38:281–286.

282. Flandin-Blety C, Barrier G. Accidents following extradural analgesia in children. The results of a retrospective study. Paediatr Anaesth 1995; 5:41–46.

283. Watcha MF, Thach BT, Gunter JB. Postoperative apnea after caudal anesthesia in an ex-premature infant. Anesthesiology 1989; 71:613–615.

284. Wolf AR, Stoddart P. Neonatal medicine. Awake spinal anaesthesia in ex-premature infants. Lancet 1995; 346 (suppl):13.

285. Williams JM, Tuckey JP, Stoddart PA, et al. Inguinal herniotomy in preterm infants: sevoflurane vs. spinal anaesthesia. 1998

286. Gibson DL, Sheps SB, Hong S, et al. Retinopathy of prematurity-induced blindness: Birth weight-specific survival and the new epidemic. Pediatrics 1990; 86:405.

287. Lin DM, Furst SR, Rodarte A. A double-blind comparison of metoclopramide and droperidol for prevention of emesis following strabismus surgery. Anesthesiology 1992; 76:357–361.

288. Abramowitz MD, Oh TE, Epstein BS, et al. The antiemetic effect of droperidol following outpatient strabismus surgery in children. Anesthesiology 1983; 59:579–583.

289. Hardy JF, Charest J, Girouard G, et al. Nausea and vomiting after strabismus surgery in preschool children. Can Anaesth Soc J 1986; 33:57–62.

290. Yentis SM, Bissonnette B. Ineffectiveness of acupuncture and droperidol in preventing vomiting following strabismus repair in children. Can J Anaesth 1992; 39:151–154.

291. Larsson S, Asgeirsson B, Magnusson J. Propofol–fentanyl anesthesia compared to thiopental–halothane with special reference to recovery and vomiting after pediatric strabismus surgery. Acta Anesthesiol Scand 1992; 36:182–186.

292. Snellen FT, Vanacker B, van Aken H. Propofol–nitrous oxide versus thiopental sodium–isoflurane–nitrous oxide for strabismus surgery in children. J Clin Anesth 1993; 5:37–41.

293. Watcha MF, Simeon RM, White PF, et al. Effect of propofol on the incidence of postoperative vomiting after strabismus surgery in pediatric outpatients. Anesthesiology 1991; 75:204–209.
294. Reimer EJ, Montgomery CJ, Bevan JC, et al. Propofol anaesthesia reduces early postoperative emesis after paediatric strabismus surgery. Can J Anaesth 1993; 40:927–933.
295. Splinter WM, Rhine EJ, Roberts DJ. Vomiting after strabismus surgery in children: ondansetron vs propofol. Can J Anaesth 1997; 44:825–829.
296. Broadman LM, Ceruzzi W, Patane PS, et al. Metoclopramide reduces the incidence of vomiting following strabismus surgery in children. Anesthesiology 1990; 72:245–248.
297. Rose JB, Martin TM, Corddry DH, et al. Ondansetron reduces the incidence and severity of poststrabismus repair vomiting in children. Anesth Analg 1994; 79:486–489.
298. Ummenhofer W, Frei FJ, Urwyler A, et al. Effects of ondansetron in the prevention of postoperative nausea and vomiting in children. Anesthesiology 1994; 81:804–810.
299. Munro HM, Riegger LQ. Reynolds PI, et al. Comparison of the analgesic and emetic properties of ketorolac and morphine for paediatric outpatient strabismus surgery. Br J Anaesth 1994; 72:624–628.
300. Mendel HG, Guarnieri KM, Sundt LM, et al. The effects of ketorolac and fentanyl on postoperative vomiting and analgesic requirements in children undergoing strabismus surgery. Anesth Analg 1995; 80:1129–1133.
301. Blanc VF, Hardy J–F, Milot J, et al. The oculocardiac reflex: a graphic and statistical analysis in infants and children. Can Anaesth Soc J 1983; 30:360–369.
302. Watson DM. Topical amethocaine in strabismus surgery. Anaesthesia 1991; 46:368–370.
303. Morton NS, Benham SW, Lawson RA, et al. Diclofenac vs oxybuprocaine eyedrops for analgesia in paediatric strabismus surgery. Paediatr Anaesth 1997; 7:221–226.
304. Swedlow DB, Lewis LE. Measurement of cerebral blood flow in children. Anesthesiology 1980; 53:S160.
305. Pople IK, Muhlbauer, Sanford RA, et al. Results and complications of intracranial pressure monitoring in 303 children. Pediatr Neurosurg 1995; 23:64–67.
306. Minns RA, Engelman HM, Stirling H. Cerebrospinal fluid pressure in pyogenic meningitis. Arch Dis Child 1989; 64:814–820.
307. Newfield P. Pediatric anesthesia. Minerva Anesthesiol 1989; 55:137–143.
308. Kennedy C, Sokoloff L. An adaptation of the nitrous oxide method to the study of cerebral circulation in children: normal values for cerebral blood flow and cerebral metabolic rate in childhood. J Clin Invest 1957; 36:1130–1136.
309. Shapiro HM. Intracranial hypertension. Therapeutic and anesthetic considerations. Anesthesiology 1975; 43:445.
310. Lassen NA, Christensen NA. Physiology of cerebral blood flow. Br J Anaesth 1976; 46:719.
311. Turner JM, McDowell DG. The measurement of intracranial pressure. Br J Anaesth 1976; 48:735.
312. Oh TE. Intensive care manual, 7th edn. Oxford: Butterworth; 1985:406–407.
313. Wyatt JS, Cope M, Delpy DT, et al. Quantification of cerebral oxygenation and haemodynamics in sick newborn infants by near red spectrophotometry. Lancet 1986; 2:1063–1066.
314. Goiten KJ, Amit Y. Percutaneous placement of subdural catheters for measurement of intracranial pressure in small children. Crit Care Med 1982; 10:46–48.
315. Stein SC, Schut L. Hydrocephalus in meningomyelocoele. Child's Brain 1979; 5
316. Markovitz BP, Duhaime AC, Sutton L, et al. Effects of alfentanil on intracranial pressure in children undergoing ventriculoperitoneal shunt revision. Anesthesiology 1992; 76:71–76.
317. Shupak RC, Harp JR, Stevenson-Smith W, et al. High dose fentanyl for neuroanesthesia. Anesthesiology 1983; 5:579.
318. Jung R, Shah N, Reinsel R, et al. Cerebrospinal fluid pressure in patients with brain tumors: impact of fentanyl verses alfentanil during nitrous oxide oxygen anesthesia. Anesth Analg 1990; 71:241.
319. Milde LN, Milde JH, Gallagher WJ. Effects of sufentanil on cerebral circulation on dogs. Anesth Analg 1990; 70:138.
320. Shapiro HM, Galindo A, Wyte SR, et al. Rapid intraoperative reduction of intracranial pressure with thiopentone. Br J Anaesth 1973; 47:1057.
321. Vandesteene A, Trempont V, Engelman E, et al. Effect of propofol on cerebral blood flow and metabolism in man. Anaesthesia 1988; 43 (suppl):42.
322. Miletich DJ, Ivankovich AD, Albrecht RF, et al. Absence of autoregulation of cerebral blood flow during halothane and enflurane anesthesia. Anesth Analg 1976; 55:100.
323. Eger II E. Isoflurane: a review Anesthesiology 1981; 55:559.
324. Adams RW, Cucchiara RF, Gronert GA, et al. Isoflurane and cerebrospinal fluid pressure in neurosurgical patients. Anesthesiology 1981; 54:57.
325. Scheller MS, Tateishi A, Drummond JC, et al. The effects of sevoflurane on cerebral blood flow. Anesthesiology 1988; 68:548.
326. Clarke DL, Rosner BS. Neurophysiologic effects of general anesthetics. Anesthesiology 1973; 38:

327. Lutz LJ, Milde JH, Milde LN. The cerebral, functional, metabolic and hemodynamic effects of desflurane in dogs. Anesthesiology 1990; 73:125.

328. Bedford RF, Winn HR, Tyson G, et al. Lidocaine prevents increased ICP after endotracheal intubation. In: Schulman K et al, ed. Intracranial pressure, 4th edn. New York: Springer Verlag: 1980.

329. Abou-madi MN, Keszler H, Yacoub JM. Cardiovascular reactions to laryngoscopy and intubation following small and large doses of lidocaine. Can Anaesth Soc J 1977; 24:12.

330. Bedford RF, Persing JA, Poberskin L, et al. Lidocaine or thiopental for rapid control of intracranial hypertension. Anesth Analg 1980; 59:435.

331. Durward QJ, Amacher AL, Maestro RF, et al. Cerebral and cardiovascular responses to changes in head position in patients with intracranial hypertension. J Neurosurg 1983; 53:938.

332. Campkin TV, Flinn RM. Isoflurane and cerebrospinal fluid pressure – a study in neurosurgical patients undergoing intracranial shunt procedures. Anaesthesia 1989; 44:50–54.

333. Bissonnette B, Leon JE. Cerebrovascular stability during isoflurane anaesthesia in children. Can J Anaesth 1992; 39:128–134.

334. Leon JE, Bissonnette B. Transcranial Doppler sonography: nitrous oxide and cerebral blood flow velocity in children. Can J Anaesth 1991; 38:974–979.

335. Alfery DD, Shapiro HM, Gagnon RL. Cardiac arrest following rapid drainage of cerebrospinal fluid in a patient with hydrocephalus. Anesthesiology 1980; 52:443.

336. Mackersie A. Paediatric surgery. In: Walters F, Ingram GS, Jenkinson JL, eds. Anaesthesia and intensive care for the neurosurgical patient, 2nd edn. Oxford: Blackwell Scientific Publications; 1994:309.

337. Goodarzi M, Shier N-H, Ogden JA. Physiologic changes during tourniquet use in children. J Pediatr Orthop 1992; 12:510–513.

338. Mubarak SJ, Wilton NCT. Compartment syndromes and epidural analgesia (editorial). J Pediatr Orthop 1997; 17:282–284.

339. Goodwin MWP, Robinson KN. A pragmatic approach to fasting in paediatric trauma? Paediatr Anaesth 2000; 10.

340. Bricker SRW, McLuckie A, Nightingale DA. Gastric aspirates after trauma in children. Anaesthesia 1989; 44:721–724.

341. Marcus RJ, Thompson JP. Anaesthesia for manipulation of forearm fractures in children: a survey of current practice. Paediatr Anaesth 2000; 10:273–277.

342. Nolan J, Chalkiadis GA, Low J, et al. Anaesthesia and pain management in cerebral palsy. Anaesthesia 2000; 55:32–41.

343. Frei FJ, Haemmerle MH, Brunner R, et al. Minimum alveolar concentration of halothane in children with cerebral palsy and severe mental retardation. Anaesthesia 1997; 52:1056–1060.

344. Dierdorf SF, McNiece WL, Rao CC, et al. Effect of succinylcholine on plasma potassium in children with cerebral palsy. Anesthesiology 1985; 62:88–90.

345. Moorthy SS, Krishna G, Dierdorf SF. Resistance to vecuronium in patients with cerebral palsy. Anesth Analg 1991; 73:275–277.

346. Carr LT, Cosgrove AP, Gringras P, et al. Position paper on the use of botulinum toxin in cerebral palsy. Arch Dis Child 1998; 79:271–273.

347. Porri F, Lemiere C, Birnbaum J, et al. Association between latex sensitization and repeated latex exposure in children. Anesthesiology 1997; 87:599–602.

348. Viscomi CM, Abajian JC, Wald SL, et al. Spinal anaesthesia for repair of meningomyelocele in neonates. Anesth Analg 1995; 81:492–495.

349. Oren J, Kelly DH, Todres ID. Respiratory complications in patients with myelodysplasia and Arnold–Chiari malformation. Arch Dis Child 1986; 140:221–224.

350. Wells TR, Jacobs RA, et al. Incidence of short trachea in patients with myelomeningocele. Pediatr Neurol 1990; 6:109.

351. Hoffman EP, Brown RH, Kunkel LM. Dystrophin: the protein product of the Duchenne muscular dystrophy locus. Cell 1987; 51:919–928.

352. Morris P. Duchenne muscular dystrophy: a challenge for the anaesthetist (editorial). Paediatr Anaesth 1997; 7:1–4.

353. Rosenberg H, Gronert G. Intractable cardiac arrest in children given succinylcholine (letter). Anesthesiology 1992; 77:1054.

354. Sullivan M, Thompson WK, Hill GD. Succinylcholine-induced cardiac arrest in children with undiagnosed myopathy. Can J Anaesth 1994; 41:497–501.

355. Brownell AKW. Malignant hyperthermia: relationship to other diseases. Br J Anaesth 1988; 60:303–308.

356. Chalkiadis GA, Branch KG. Cardiac arrest after isoflurane anaesthesia in a patient with Duchenne's muscular dystrophy. Anaesthesia 1990; 45:22–25.

357. Mitchell MM, Ali HH, Savarese JJ. Myotonia and neuromuscular blocking agents. Anesthesiology 1978; 49:44–48.

358. Kaufman L. Dystrophia myotonica and succinylcholine. Anaesthesia 2000; 55:929.
359. Wedel DJ. Malignant hyperthermia and neuromuscular disease. Neuromuscular Disorders 1992; 2:157–164.
360. Halsall PJ, Ellis FR. Malignant hyperthermia. Curr Anaesth Crit Care 1996; 7:158–166.
361. Mader N, Gilly H, Bittner RE. Dystrophin deficient mdx muscle is not prone to MH susceptibility: an in vitro study. Br J Anaesth 1997; 79:125–127.
362. Clinical Standards Advisory Group. Services for children with cleft lip and palate. London: Clinical Standards Advisory Group; 1998.
363. Hatch DJ. Airway management in cleft lip and palate surgery (editorial). Br J Anaesth 1996; 76:755–756.
364. Gunawardana RH. Difficult laryngoscopy in cleft lip and palate surgery. Br J Anaesth 1996; 76:757–759.
365. Hatch DJ. Magill's endotracheal catheter device for use during repair of cleft lip and palate. Paediatr Anaesth 1995; 5:199–201.
366. Latto IP. Management of difficult intubation. In: Latto IP, Rosen M, eds. Difficulties in tracheal intubation. London: WB Saunders; 1985:99–103.
367. Knill RL. Difficult laryngoscopy made easy with a "burp". Can J Anaesth 1993; 40:279–282.
368. Wrigley S, Black AE, Sidhu V. A fibreoptic laryngoscope for paediatric anaesthesia. Anaesthesia 1995; 50:709–712.
369. Schwartz D, Singh J. Retrograde wire-guided direct laryngoscopy in a 1-month old infant. Anesthesiology 1992; 77:607–608.
370. Sutera PT, Gordon GJ. Digitally assisted tracheal intubation in a neonate with Pierre Robin syndrome. Anesthesiology 1993; 78:983–985.
371. Krucylak CP, Schreiner MS. Orotracheal intubation of an infant with hemifacial microsomia using a modified lighted stylet. Anaesthesiology 1992; 77:826–827.
372. Inada T, Fujise K, Tachibana K, et al. Orotracheal intubation through the laryngeal mask airway in paediatric patients with Treacher Collins syndrome. Paediatr Anaesth 1995; 5:129–132.
373. Bösenberg AT, Kimble FW. Infraorbital nerve block in neonates for cleft lip repair: anatomical study and clinical application. Br J Anaesth 1995; 74:506–508.
374. Bradbury ET, Hewison J, Timmons MJ. Psychological and social outcome of prominent ear correction in children. Br J Anaesth 1992; 47:97–100.
375. Burtles R. Analgesia for "bat-ear" surgery. Ann R Coll Surg 1989; 71:332.
376. Ridings P, Gault D, Khan L. Reduction in postoperative vomiting after surgical correction of prominent ears. Br J Anaesth 1994; 72:592–593.
377. Sossai R, Johr M, Kistler W, et al. Postoperative vomiting in children. A persisting unsolved problem. Eur J Pediatr Surg 1993; 3:206–208.
378. Lefever EB, Potter PS, Seeley NR. Propofol sedation for pediatric MRI. Anesth Analg 1993; 76:919–920.
379. Coventry DM, Martin CS, Burke AM. Sedation for paediatric computerized tomography: a double–blind assessment of rectal midazolam. Eur J Anaesthesiol 1991; 8:29–32.
380. Varner PD, Ebert JP, McKay RD, et al. Methohexital sedation of children undergoing CT scan. Anesth Analg 1985; 64:643–645.
381. Frankville DD, Spear RM, Dyck JB. The dose of propofol required to prevent children from moving during magnetic resonance imaging. Anesthesiology 1993; 79:953–958.
382. Engelman DR, Lockhardt CH. Comparison between temperature effects of ketamine and halothane anesthesia in children. Anesth Analg 1972; 51:98–101.
383. Annis P, Landa J, Lichtiger M. Effects of atropine on velocity of tracheal mucus in anesthetized patients. Anesthesiology 1976; 44:74–77.
384. Opie JC, Chaye H, Steward DJ. Intravenous atopine rapidly reduces lower oesophageal sphincter pressure in infants and children. Anesthesiology 1987; 67:989–990

CHAPTER 7

Assessing and managing pain

Jane M Peutrell

INTRODUCTION

In the 1980s several authors reported that pain control in children was often inadequate and a significant number were in severe pain on the operative and first postoperative days.[1] Medical and nursing staff were more reluctant to prescribe and give potent analgesics to children compared with adults[2–4] and doses were often inappropriate or too infrequent.[1, 3] Medical staff usually prescribed drugs 'PRN' which the nurses interpreted as 'as little as possible'.[1] The situation may have improved over the subsequent decade with the greater awareness of health-care staff and the general public, but still, in the 1990s, 17–65% of children having inpatient surgery in children's hospitals complained of severe postoperative pain.[5–8] In studies of children discharged home after day surgery, 11% had a disturbed night because of pain[9] and 17% suffered pain at the site of operation.[10]

The authors of the report *Pain after Surgery* recommended establishing services to manage postoperative pain.[11] Introducing a pain service for adults improves the quality of pain control[12, 13] and this is supported by audit in children.[5] The Royal College of Anaesthetists[14] recently included 'a service for the relief of acute pain' as a standard for the purchase of anaesthetic services for children.

In this chapter I will discuss the organisation and role of the acute pain service for children in the district hospital; the methods for assessing pain at different ages; and the use of appropriate monitoring protocols. I will then describe some of the techniques for postoperative analgesia in children.

SECTION 1: The acute pain service

ORGANISATION

Many district hospitals have acute pain teams for inpatients led by a consultant anaesthetist with one or more nurses, of whom one is often a clinical nurse specialist. The clinician often has an interest in anaesthesia for adults. Children have many important differences compared with adults (e.g. age-related pharmacology; haemodynamic stability in younger children during regional anaesthesia; cognitive and emotional immaturity affecting responses to noxious stimuli) and clinicians treating their pain must be familiar with their specific problems.[15] It is, therefore, crucial that the lead consultant for paediatric anaesthesia assumes primary responsibility for the children's acute pain service because of his or her special knowledge and training.

A district hospital is unlikely to have an acute pain nurse dedicated to children. However, it is possible to provide a good service if well organised. Any pain nurse with responsibilities for children must have adequate training and experience in the specific aspects of their pain control and should work in close liaison with paediatric nurses. If the acute pain service employs two or more nurses, it is useful for one to develop an interest in paediatrics. A good arrangement may be to identify a trained and enthusiastic children's nurse on each paediatric ward who is interested in pain (a link nurse) to work in liaison with the acute pain nurse.[5] Each can then provide specific expertise to the joint management of children with pain. The acute pain nurse is principal coordinator but both will collaborate with other nurses, junior doctors, surgeons, anaesthetists, pharmacists, parents and children.

ROLE

The authors of the recent *Guidance for the Provision of Paediatric Services*, published by the Royal College of Anaesthetists, recommend that a member of the acute pain service should visit each paediatric surgical ward and review all children after major surgery daily. They also advocate scoring pain for all children having painful surgery.[16]

The acute pain team should also ensure that all children are free of pain when discharged from the recovery area and that good analgesia is provided safely on routine surgical wards. This is achieved by:

1. educating nursing staff (in recovery and on the wards) and junior doctors in various aspects of pain management, e.g. the recognition of pain in babies and children of different ages, use of appropriate pain assessment tools, analgesic techniques and their side-effects and hazards, appropriate drugs, doses and dosing intervals;[15]

2. establishing clear guidelines for the treatment of pain, appropriate monitoring, management of side-effects and criteria for contacting the pain team;
3. clinically reviewing children using more complex analgesic techniques (e.g. epidural infusions or patient-controlled analgesia (PCA)) and giving advice, if required, for the management of others with pain;
4. training (or supervising the training of) children (and their parents) using more complex analgesic systems (e.g. PCA) or pain assessment tools;
5. establishing standards of clinical care (Box 7.1a);
6. auditing quality and reviewing clinical practice;
7. introducing new techniques appropriately and safely.

In addition, practitioners in some institutions will have sufficient clinical cases to support research and development projects.

In general, standardising guidelines and clinical practices throughout the hospital is thought to improve safety.[15] Goddard and Pickup found the introduction of a four-point plan of action (Box 7.1b) significantly improved the quality of postoperative analgesia in children.[5]

EQUIPMENT

It is advisable to standardise infusion pumps throughout the hospital but those chosen must be capable of delivering small rates of infusion safely. Antisiphon valves should be used with all continuous intravenous (IV) infusions of opioids (including PCA). Unless opioids are infused through a dedicated cannula, an antireflux valve should be attached if another infusion is to run concomitantly.

DAY SURGERY

A significant number of children experience pain at home after day surgery.[9, 10, 17] Circumcision is particularly painful.[9, 17] Surprisingly, 18% of parents do not give analgesics to their children when in pain at home.[18]

The anaesthetist with special responsibilities for children should, therefore, establish with day-surgery colleagues guidelines for preventing pain and minimising symptoms. These include:

1. optimising intraoperative analgesics, particularly regional blocks, but avoiding opioids because of high incidence of nausea or vomiting;[19]

Box 7.1 Proposed clinical standards and plan to improve the management of postoperative pain in children[5]

(a) Clinical standards established for the management of postoperative pain at the Sheffield Children's Hospital

1. All children have analgesia prescribed before they leave theatre
2. Analgesia is given when pain is rated as 'bad' or 'most severe pain' (provided it is safe to do so)
3. No child should have a pain score of 'most severe pain' on the ward postoperatively
4. 95% of children will not have a pain score rated as 'bad' or worse for two consecutive hourly assessments

(b) Four-point plan to improve postoperative analgesia

1. Encourage use of non-steroidal analgesic drugs in children older than 2 years
2. Make recommendations for the prescription of a limited number of analgesic drugs (appropriate dose, maximum daily dose, minimal dosing interval, restrictions) and ensure the information is widely available to nurses and medical staff throughout the hospital
3. Ensure the pain control chart is incorporated into routine postoperative observations
4. Educate staff, particularly nurses and junior doctors

2. giving coanalgesics (e.g. paracetamol, non-steroidal anti-inflammatory drugs (NSAIDs)) as premedicants or suppositories during anaesthesia in an attempt to ensure therapeutic plasma concentrations when local anaesthetics have worn off;

3. giving clear instructions to parents to give regular analgesics for 24–48 h rather than waiting for pain to develop;[20]

4. ensuring an adequate supply of analgesics in appropriate doses to take home, including topical anaesthetics if indicated (e.g. after circumcision[21]);

5. ensuring clear lines of communication if the parents have problems after discharge (e.g. telephone contact to hospital practitioner or review from community nursing staff attached to the day-surgery unit).[10]

SECTION 2: Assessment of pain and monitoring protocols

ASSESSMENT

Babies and children have well-developed physiological and behavioural responses to pain. Many are not specific and pain can be difficult to distinguish from other distressing stimuli (e.g. hunger or separation from parents). Assessments of pain should be made in context

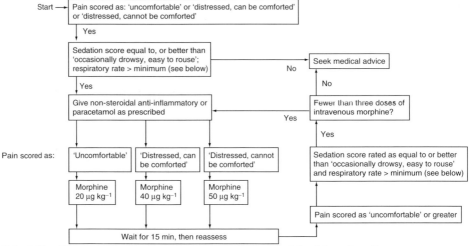

Note: 1. If the child is younger than 3 months, seek medical advice. If 3–6 months, halve all doses of morphine.

2. A qualified nurse will remain with the child for 10 min, and a responsible adult for an additional 30 min after each dose of morphine.

3. A member of the paediatric medical staff must be present on the children's floor of the hospital.

4. Resuscitation equipment and appropriate drugs (e.g. naloxone) must be available on each ward.

5. If child requires more than three doses, patient-controlled analgesia or a morphine infusion may be useful. Please contact the acute pain team.

6. If there are signs of respiratory depression, give oxygen by mask and intravenous naloxone 4 µg kg⁻¹.

Minimum respiratory rates:

Age	Respiratory rate (breaths/min)
< 3 months	25
3–24 months	20
2–8 years	15
> 8 years	12

Fig. 7.1 A protocol for the administration of intravenous morphine by nurses (Kestin, personal communication).

using several measures (e.g. physiological and observed behavioural scores plus reports by the child, if possible) and sources (e.g. parents and health-care workers) to improve accuracy and specificity.

A child's response to a noxious stimulus is influenced by age, cognitive and emotional development, personality, sociocultural background and systemic illness. Carers must be trained to recognise the various indicators of pain in children and babies of different ages (e.g. changes in activity, behaviour and physiological variables) and assess its severity using validated scoring systems. They should make assessments as part of a routine schedule of clinical observations (in the recovery area of theatre and on the general ward) to reduce distress, minimise disturbance and ensure that the severity of pain is assessed and recorded regularly.[22] Pain, once recognised, should be treated according to agreed clinical guidelines (e.g. Fig. 7.1) and the effects of treatment assessed (the assessment–intervention–reassessment cycle[23]).

Three categories of scoring system (or tool) are used to assess pain severity. A numeric score is assigned to aspects of behaviour, changes in physiological variables or the self-reported severity of pain.

Some systems are composite measurements, e.g. the Observer Pain Scale,[24] which uses physiological variables and behaviours (Table 7.1). Strictly, pain scales are ordinal data: there is a graded relationship between severity of pain and the assigned scores but this relationship is probably not arithmetic.

Any tool used to assess pain should be appropriate to the child's age and cognitive development and validated for the clinical context (i.e. postoperative as opposed to chronic pain). A working party from the Royal College of Nursing Institute recently made recommendations for assessing acute pain in children of different ages and its evaluation of some of the available tools is given in Table 7.2. Additional systems are available for premature babies and neonates.[22]

Physiological changes

Pain affects many physiological variables, e.g. heart and respiratory rates, palmar sweating, blood and intracranial pressures, oxygen saturation, cortisol and endorphin concentrations.[25] Physiological changes are important components of assessment in babies and small children

Table 7.1 Objective Pain Scale[24]

Observation	Criteria	Score
Blood pressure	± 10% preoperative	0
	> 20% preoperative	1
	> 30% preoperative	2
Crying?	Yes	0
	Yes, but responds to comforting	1
	Yes, but does not respond to comforting	2
Movement	None	0
	Restless	1
	Thrashing	2
Agitation	Child asleep or calm	0
	Mild	1
	Hysterical	2
Verbal evaluation	Child asleep or states 'no pain'	0
	Mild pain (cannot localise)	1
	Moderate pain (localises verbally or by pointing)	2

Table 7.2 Summary of tools for assessing acute pain in children[22]
(a) Behavioural and physiological signs of pain and distress for use in babies (0–1 month)

Tool and references	Validated	Indicators	Advantages/disadvantages
Objective **P**ain **S**cale (OPS)[24, 37]	Against a linear analogue, CHEOPS and faces scales	Blood pressure, crying, movement, agitation, verbal evaluation/body language	*Advantages* • Easy to use • Five categories • Reliable between observers • Tracks pain over time and scores are reduced with analgesia *Disadvantages* • Blood pressure measurements may upset baby/child • Cannot be used in intubated, paralysed patients • Three out of five categories are similar
Neonatal Facial Coding System[29]	Yes	Bulging brow, eyes squeezed tightly shut, deepening of nasolabial furrow, open lips, mouth stretched, tongue taut	*Notes* • Anatomically based system for assessing facial expression
Crying, **R**equires O$_2$ for saturation above 95%, **I**ncreased vital signs, **E**xpression and **S**leeplessness (CRIES)[26]	Yes	Cry, oxygen saturation, heart rate/ blood pressure, expression, sleeplessness	*Advantages* • Easy to remember and use • Valid and reliable down to 32 weeks' gestation • Reliable between observers • Tracks pain and the effects of analgesia *Disadvantages* • Oxygenation can be affected by factors other than pain • Blood pressure measurement may upset baby

Table 7.2 continued overleaf

Table 7.2 continued from previous page

Tool and reference	Validated	Indicators	Advantages/disadvantages
COMFORT[308]	Yes	Alertness, calmness/agitation, respiratory response, movement, blood pressure, heart rate, muscle tone, facial tension	*Disadvantages* ● Complicated ● Eight categories and many subcategories ● Cannot be used in intubated, paralysed patients
Children's **H**ospital of **E**astern **O**ntario **P**ain **S**cale (CHEOPS)[27, 309]	Yes	Alertness, respiratory response, heart rate, calmness/agitation, physical movement, muscle tone, facial tension	*Disadvantages* ● Complicated behavioural scale ● May not track postoperative pain well in 3–7-year-olds as pain behaviour is inhibited ● 10 categories, of which four are similar ● Confusing (high score = low pain) ● Cannot be used in intubated or paralysed patients

(b) Behavioural and physiological signs of pain and distress for use in infants and toddlers (1 month–3 years)

Tool and reference	Validated	Indicators	Advantages/disadvantages
OPS	See above		
COMFORT	See above		
CHEOPS	See above		
Toddler/**P**reschooler **P**ostoperative **P**ain **S**core (TPPPS)[310]	Yes	Verbal – complaint/cry, groan/moan/grunt, scream, open mouth, brow bulge, restless Motor behaviour – rub/touch, squint	*Advantages* ● Suitable for age 1–5 years ● Tracks pain relief and effects of analgesia ● Correlates with nurse and parental pain assessments *Disadvantage* ● Seven categories

Table 7.2 continued overleaf

203

Table 7.2 continued from previous page

Tool and reference	Validated	Indicators	Advantages/Disadvantages
Nurse observations[311]			*Advantages* ● Easy to incorporate into routine observations ● Experienced nurse is usually accurate *Disadvantages* ● Observer bias ● Lack of training leads to inaccuracy
Parental observations[311, 312]			*Advantage* ● Parental observations are often helpful and accurate

(c) Behavioural and physiological signs of pain and distress and self-report for use in children (3–7 years)

Tool and reference	Validated	Indicators	Notes
OPS	See above		
COMFORT	See above		
CHEOPS	See above		
TIPPS	See above		
Faces[27a, 33, 313]	Yes	Sets of cartoon faces in various stages of pain Number of faces ranges from four to six	Simple and quick ● Younger children tend to choose extremes ● Best with four choices of face ● Some children confuse scale with measurement of happiness

Table 7.2 continued overleaf

Table 7.2 continued from previous page

Tool and reference	Validated	Indicators	Notes
Colour Scales[314, 315]	Yes	Child chooses pens or crayons and colours the outline of a child's body	• Quickly engages child's interest • Fun • Colours allow expression of other aspects of pain • Child describes exact site of pain
Poker Chip Tool[316]	Yes	Four red chips and one white (no pain). Chips represent 'pieces of pain'	• Useful for children 4–13 years
Oucher[31, 39, 314, 317, 318]	Yes	Photographs of children in six stages of distress aligned to a vertical, marked scale rating the degree of pain	• Can use either or both scales to fit child's comprehension/preference • Three multiethnic versions available • Self-report
Horizontal Linear Analogue[314]	Yes	No information available	
Vertical Analogue Scale (VAS)[319]	Yes	Verbal or horizontal line with verbal, facial or numerical anchors on a continuum of pain intensity	• Reliable and versatile • Children must understand concept of proportionality • Intervals may not be equal from a child's perspective
Coloured Analogue Scale (CAS)[320]	Yes	Use sliding indicator on triangular-shaped scale varying in shape and colour	• Assesses pain intensity • Age 5 years + • Very easy to use

Table 7.2 continued overleaf

205

Table 7.2 continued from previous page

Tool and reference	Validated	Indicators	Notes
Adjectival Self-Report[36]	Yes		• Easy to use • Four categories sensitive enough to track pain and effect of analgesia • Uses language a child can understand
Face, Legs, Activity, Cry, Consolability (FLACC)[321]	Yes		• Behavioural scale • Postoperative pain assessment tool

(d) Self-report tools for use in children (7 years +)

Tool and reference	Validated	Indicators	Notes
CAS	See above		
Horizontal Linear Analogue	See above		
Adjectival Self-Report	See above		
Adolescent Pediatric Pain Tool (APPT)[322,323,323a]	Yes	Assesses three dimensions: location, intensity, quality	• Multidimensional tool • Includes word graphic rating scale, VAS, graded graphic numerical and colour scale
Ladder Scale[314]	Not in children	Higher intensities of pain represented by higher rungs on ladder	• Used by wide range of ages

unable to self-report but these changes are not specific for pain and correlate poorly with severity. Most are influenced by many other factors, including behavioural state, postconceptional age and systemic illness. Sweating, for example, does not develop until 36–37 weeks' gestation. Physiological measures should be used in conjunction with other assessments such as behaviour, as, for example, in the CRIES (Crying, Requires O_2 for saturation above 95%, Increased vital signs, Expression and Sleeplessness) neonatal postoperative pain score (Table 7.3).[26]

Observer's assessment of behaviour

Several scales have been developed from observation of behaviour commonly evoked by noxious stimuli such as changes in facial expression or body position, crying and verbalisation. Examples include the Children's Hospital of Eastern Ontario Pain Score (CHEOPS) (Table 7.4);[27] Neonatal Facial Coding System[28, 29] and some components of the Observational Pain Scale (OPS) (Table 7.1).[24]

Behavioural assessments are useful but have limitations:

1. The scales measure distress and only indirectly assess pain and it can be difficult to differentiate from other causes of distress. It may be helpful to determine whether a child is in pain by assessing the effects of interventions such as cuddling or giving sucrose. For example, OPS assesses the effect of comfort on a child who is crying (Table 7.1).[24]
2. Overt distress does not correlate with intensity of pain.[30]
3. Components of some scales may measure sedation rather than analgesia.
4. Complex scoring systems are time-consuming and may be impractical, e.g. CHEOPS (Table 7.4).

Children's assessment of their own pain (self-report)

Most children older than 3 years of age can describe the severity and location of pain if given tools appropriate for their cognitive and developmental levels. Several ordinal scales have been developed, e.g. the Oucher Scale (six photographs of children's faces expressing increasing distress lying alongside a vertical numerical scale),[31] the Faces Scale, in which line drawings are shown of four to nine faces representing increasing intensity between 'no pain' and 'worst pain possible' (Fig. 7.1)[5, 32, 33] or the Poker Chip Tool, with which children quantify the magnitude of pain by selecting one to four poker chips.[34] These scales work best for younger children if the system is simple and the choices limited to three to five. A scale with a smiling face at one end may be less appropriate than one with a neutral expression because children may confuse the representation of 'no pain' with 'happiness'.[35] Children consistently rate pain higher using a scale with a smiling face indicating 'no pain' compared with one with a neutral expression.

Table 7.3 CRIES (Crying, Requires O_2 for saturation above 95%, Increased vital signs, Expression and Sleeplessness) neonatal postoperative pain score[26]

Score	0	1	2
Crying	No	High-pitched	Inconsolable
F_IO_2 to maintain $SpaO_2 > 95\%$	No	< 30%	> 30%
Increased vital signs	Heart rate and blood pressure ≤ preoperative values	Heart rate and blood pressure < 20% preoperative values	Heart rate and blood pressure > 20% preoperative values
Facial expression	No grimace	Grimace	Grimace and grunt
Wakefulness	Asleep	Wakes at frequent intervals	Awake constantly

Table 7.4 Children's Hospital of Eastern Ontario Pain Scale (CHEOPS)[27]

Item	Behaviour	Score	Definition
Cry	None	I	Child is not crying
	Moaning	2	Moaning or quiet vocalising, silent cry
	Crying	2	Cry is gentle or whimpering
	Screaming	3	Full-lunged cry, sobbing (can be scored with or without complaint)
Facial	Smiling	0	Score only if definite positive facial expression
	Composed	I	Neutral facial expression
	Grimacing	2	Score only if definite negative facial expression
Verbal	Positive	0	Child makes any positive statement or talks about other things without complaint
	None	I	Child is not talking
	Other complaints	I	Child complains, but not about pain, e.g. 'I want my mummy!'
	Complaints about pain	2	Child complains about pain
	Complaints about pain and other things	2	Child complains about pain and other things, e.g. 'It hurts, I want my mummy!'
Torso	Neutral	I	Body (not limbs) is at rest; torso inactive
	Shifting	2	Body in motion in a shifting or serpentine fashion
	Tense	2	Body arched or rigid
	Shivering	2	Body shuddering or shaking involuntarily
	Upright	2	Child in a vertical or upright position
	Restrained	2	Body restrained
Touch	Not touching	I	Child is not grabbing or touching the wound
	Reaching	2	Child reaching for, but not grabbing the wound
	Touching	2	Child gently touching wound or wound area
	Grabbing	2	Child grabbing vigorously at wound
	Restrained	2	Child's arms restrained
Legs	Neutral	I	Legs can be in any position but are relaxed; includes gentle swimming or serpentine-like movements
	Squirming/kicking	2	Definitive uneasy or restless movements in the legs and/or striking out with foot or feet
	Drawn up/tensed	2	Legs tensed and/or pulled up tightly to body and kept there
	Standing	2	Standing, crouching or kneeling
	Restrained	2	Child's legs are held down

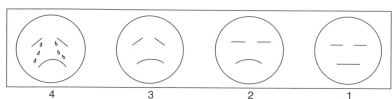

| 4 | 3 | 2 | 1 |

Fig. 7.2 The faces scale for self-report of acute pain in children. 'No pain' is represnted by face I and 'worst pain' by face 4.

Morton describes an ordinal scale using four descriptions of severity of pain in simple language ('no pain'; 'not really sore'; 'quite sore'; 'very sore') for children as young as 4 years of age.[36]

Linear analogue scales, e.g. a horizontal line with a smiling face at one end and a sad face at the other,[37] and other variants[32, 38] are more abstract concepts requiring greater cognitive development. Visual analogue scales held vertically are understood by children at a younger age than horizontal scales.[39] Generally, children older than 5 years can use visual analogue scales reliably to rate pain.[30]

Self-reporting is the most accurate measure of intensity of pain and should override assessments of parents and health-care workers.[22] However, carers must teach children to use the tools and ensure they understand the concepts.

The role of parents

Parents should be encouraged to contribute to pain assessment, particularly in babies and younger children or others unwilling or unable to self-report.[22] In a study,[40] parents determined their child's need for postoperative analgesics using an objective pain scale.[24] Parents, however, consistently overestimate pain compared with their child's self-report using the same tool[41] and their assessments are higher than nurses.[17]

Children with special needs

The recognition and assessment of pain in children with cognitive delay or communication problems, e.g. cerebral palsy, are difficult.[42] Their behaviour is often inconsistent, difficult to interpret because of physical problems, and may mask expressions of pain (e.g. moaning).[43] I am unaware of a validated assessment tool for postoperative pain in these children and health-care workers rely considerably on evaluations made by parents.

MONITORING PROTOCOLS

Several authors recommend hourly assessments of sedation, pain and breathing rates in children given opioids, particularly by continuous infusion.[36, 44] In addition, Morton recommends continuous measurement of transcutaneous oxygen saturation whilst breathing air to improve detection of ventilatory depression (Table 7.5).[36]

From the alveolar gas equation, a small rise in the $PACO_2$ whilst breathing air significantly decreases the oxygen tension (e.g. $PACO_2$ of 8.8 kPa results in a PAO_2 of 10 kPa corresponding to a haemoglobin saturation of approximately 94%).

Schemes developed for use with opioids can be adapted for monitoring during epidural analgesia by additionally recording blood pressure, heart rate and density of motor block regularly. Children having epidural infusions are commonly nursed on standard postoperative wards. In the majority of institutions surveyed in North America, oxygen saturation is monitored continuously and breathing rates recorded hourly. Sedation, pain and measurements of other vital signs tend to be recorded 1- or 4-hourly.[45]

Low oxygen saturation may result from factors other than ventilatory depression, e.g. inadequate analgesia, nausea or vomiting, urinary retention or surgical factors.[36] Although unpredictable respiratory depression is a major concern in neonates having opioids, it is uncommon in infants and children.[44]

Any ward caring for children receiving opioids or epidural analgesia must be adequately equipped with resuscitation equipment and emergency drugs and the nursing staff trained in basic life support. It is useful to include a prescription of naloxone appropriate for the child's weight alongside that for opioids.

Table 7.5 Recommended scheme for monitoring children using patient-controlled analgesia.[36] This can be modified for use during continuous infusions of opioids or epidural analgesia

Time	SpaO₂¹	Respiratory rate	Sedation score Eyes open: 0 = Spontaneously 1 = To speech 2 = To shake **3 = Unrousable (call doctor)**	Pain score 0 = No pain A = Asleep 1 = Not really sore 2 = Quite sore **3 = Very sore (crying – call doctor)**	Nausea score 0 = None 1 = Nausea only 2 = Vomiting ×1 in last hour **3 = Vomiting >×1 in last hour (call doctor)**	Total dose of opioid since reset	Number of presses of button and % good presses **< 60% (call doctor)**	Volume of opioid solution remaining in syringe

¹Breathing air.

SECTION 3: Techniques of postoperative analgesia

Most techniques described for pain control in adults can be adapted for children[11] using appropriate doses of drugs and equipment. In general, we should give analgesia in anticipation of pain and thereafter continuously or at regular intervals for the estimated duration of pain or discomfort and not expect simple analgesics alone to control severe pain.

Different techniques are often synergistic, improving analgesia and reducing the doses of drugs required for each. Common combinations include a regional block plus suppositories of paracetamol and an NSAID or adding clonidine or ketamine to solutions of local anaesthetics for caudal block. Clinicians are increasingly convinced that this multimodal or balanced analgesia is superior to using single drugs or techniques and does not increase side-effects (especially when the components have different sites or mechanisms of action or are synergistic).[15] Suggested schemes for mild, intermediate or severe pain are shown in Table 7.6.

Some techniques for postoperative analgesia are useful for other causes of acute pain, e.g. PCA for the pain of mucositis associated with chemotherapy, sickle-cell crises or haemolytic–uraemic syndrome.

Table 7.6 Suggested scheme for pain control after minor, intermediate, or major surgery. Doses are given later in the text

Minor surgery

e.g. removal of superficial skin lumps; myringotomy; retraction of foreskin

- Loading doses of NSAIDs and paracetamol as oral premedication or suppositories given intraoperatively
- Local anaesthesia if indicated (e.g. infiltration of minor wounds; topical lidocaine (lignocaine) jelly for retraction of foreskin or division of perineal adhesions)
- Oral paracetamol every 6 h for 24 h

Intermediate surgery

e.g. circumcision; herniotomy; otoplasty; tonsillectomy; minor talipes correction

- Loading doses of NSAIDs and paracetamol as oral premedication or suppositories given intraoperatively
- Local block (e.g. caudal; iliac crest block; greater auricular nerve block) if possible; if not, give appropriate dose of longer-acting opioids (e.g. codeine phosphate IM or morphine sulphate IM/IV) during anaesthesia
- Consider adding clonidine or ketamine to local anaesthetic solutions for caudal analgesia, especially for inpatients
- Topical local anaesthetics postoperatively, if indicated (e.g. after circumcision)
- Oral paracetamol every 6 h, and NSAIDs (if indicated) regularly or 'as required' for 24–48 h

Major surgery

e.g. laparotomy; femoral osteotomy; thoracotomy

- Loading doses of NSAIDs and paracetamol as oral premedication or suppositories given intraoperatively (omit NSAIDs if major blood loss is anticipated)
- Regional block (e.g. epidural; fascia iliaca block) or adequate dose of intravenous opioid intraoperatively
- Opioid (e.g. morphine infusion, PCA or NCA) or regional analgesia (continuous infusion or 'top-ups')
- Oral or rectal paracetamol every 6 h and regular NSAIDs (unless contraindicated) for 48–72 h

NSAID, non-steroidal anti-inflammatory drug; IM, intramuscularly; IV, intravenously; PCA or NCA, patient-controlled analgesia or nurse-controlled analgesia.

SYSTEMIC ANALGESICS

Simple analgesics

Simple analgesics are used alone for mild to moderate pain or to supplement other drugs for severe pain. They are usually given orally (O) or rectally (PR). The anaesthetist should discuss suppositories with a parent and the child (if old enough to understand) before administration.[46]

Paracetamol

Paracetamol has analgesic and antipyretic but no anti-inflammatory properties. Plasma concentrations of 10–20 mg l^{-1} (0.07–0.130 mmol l^{-1}) are antipyretic.[47, 48] Although analgesic effectiveness correlates with plasma concentration, the therapeutic range for analgesia is unknown and the values for antipyresis are often taken as a guide for analgesia. However, Anderson and colleagues[49] did find plasma concentrations of 25 mg l^{-1} provided adequate analgesia in 60% of children after tonsillectomy and demonstrated a ceiling effect.

Traditional doses (i.e. 10–15 mg kg^{-1} O/R) of paracetamol are ineffective.[50–52] Regular paracetamol, either 60 mg kg^{-1} day^{-1} O or 90 mg kg^{-1} day^{-1} PR, provides inadequate pain relief after adenoidectomy or adenotonsillectomy,[18] whereas 40 mg kg^{-1} as a single dose before surgery (O or PR) is effective for tonsillectomy in two-thirds of children.[49] Anderson & Holford[53] have stressed the importance of using an adequate amount of drug and giving a loading dose to obtain a therapeutic concentration for a greater proportion of time. From a computer simulation, using known pharmacological data, they proposed a loading dose of 70 mg kg^{-1} with maintenance of 50 mg kg^{-1} every 8 h. However, these data should be interpreted cautiously because pharmacokinetic parameters are very variable between patients. Plasma concentrations of paracetamol also tend to increase with repeated doses because of a time-dependent decrease in elimination, particularly in younger children and babies, probably because of substrate depletion or saturation of sulphate conjugation.[54] The margin of safety with frequent therapeutic doses is thus much lower than generally appreciated, and hepatotoxicity has been reported in children given 60–420 mg kg^{-1} day^{-1} over several days.[54, 55] The therapeutic ratio is probably further reduced in those with febrile viral illnesses.[55–58] Associated fasting, dehydration and fever may make children particularly susceptible to hepatic damage by depleting glutathione stores.

The maximum dose of paracetamol by any route, therefore, should probably not exceed 90 mg kg^{-1} day^{-1} to avoid toxicity, despite some children having inadequate plasma concentrations with these doses. For postoperative analgesia beyond 24 h, we also limit the dose to 60 mg kg^{-1} day^{-1}, given for a maximum of 5 days.

Parents must also be aware of potential hazards and maximum doses. Paracetamol is commonly considered a 'safe' drug and parents may inadvertently increase the dose dangerously if their child's symptoms persist, with the risk of hepatorenal failure and death.[59] Use of inappropriate preparations and miscalculations by parents are the major causes of overdose in children younger than 10 years of age.[58]

Paracetamol alone is inadequate for severe pain. Adding other agents (e.g. NSAIDs) rather than increasing the dose may be safer and more efficacious. Recommendations for using paracetamol in children are given in Table 7.7.

ROUTES OF ADMINISTRATION

Oral delivery is associated with higher peak plasma concentrations and, except in babies (see below), greater bioavailability compared with PR administration.[50] Paracetamol can be given as an elixir 0.7 ml kg^{-1} as premedication 90 min before induction with no effect on the volume of gastric contents.[60] An oral dose of 24–30 mg kg^{-1} every 8 h produces plasma concentrations therapeutic for antipyresis.[61]

Table 7.7 Recommendations for the use of paracetamol after surgery in children

	Loading dose	Maintenance dose
Children		
Oral[61]		24–30 mg kg^{-1} every 8 h
	20 mg kg^{-1}	15 mg kg^{-1} every 4 h
Rectal[64, 65a]	40 mg kg^{-1}	20 mg kg^{-1} every 6 h
Infants		
Oral/rectal[324a]	Total of 60 mg kg^{-1} day^{-1} by any route	
Neonates		
Oral[324]	30 mg kg^{-1}	20 mg kg^{-1} every 8 h
Rectal[324]	40 mg kg^{-1}	30 mg kg^{-1} every 12 h
Premature babies		
Rectal[70]	20 mg kg^{-1}	20 mg kg^{-1} every 8–12 h

Maximum by any route:
- in children: 90 mg kg^{-1} day^{-1} for 24 h, then 60 mg kg^{-1} day^{-1}
- in babies: 60 mg kg^{-1} day^{-1}

The bioavailability of PR paracetamol and peak plasma concentrations depend on formulation,[62] colonic blood flow, volume of rectal contents and defecation. Relative bioavailability compared with oral administration ranges from 0.24 to 0.98[63] and absorption is slower. Peak concentrations occur at 2–3 h.[49, 50, 64] Suppositories must be given in an adequate dose and timed appropriately to ensure therapeutic concentrations when needed. Paracetamol PR 35 or 40 mg kg^{-1} produces therapeutic plasma concentrations in 90% of children within 1–2 h,[65, 66] but concentrations are subtherapeutic after 15–20 mg kg^{-1}.[50, 62, 64, 67]

PARACETAMOL IN BABIES

The uptake of PR paracetamol is more rapid and complete in babies than in children or adults and bioavailability is similar to oral administration.[50, 68] In premature babies, peak plasma concentrations after PR administration correlate inversely with gestational age. Paracetamol 20 mg kg^{-1} PR produces therapeutic plasma concentrations in babies of 28–32 weeks' postconceptional age, but not in more mature preterm babies.[69,70] For full-term neonates, Anderson and colleagues[68] suggest a loading dose PR of 40 mg kg^{-1} and 30 mg kg^{-1} every 12 h. Uptake of oral paracetamol is also more complete in neonates compared with older children and 16 mg kg^{-1} is usually therapeutic.[50] However, Anderson and colleagues[68] used pharmacokinetics variables obtained in neonates, and proposed an oral loading dose of 30 mg kg^{-1} followed by 20 mg kg^{-1} every 8 h.

Babies have reduced glucoronidation partly compensated for by a greater capacity for sulphation compared with older children or adults and conjugation with sulphate is the major pathway of excretion.[70, 71] Although Miller and colleagues[71] found no important age-related differences in the overall rate of elimination of paracetamol for healthy neonates compared with older children or adults, other have reported a prolonged half-life.[68, 72] Elimination is markedly reduced in very preterm babies and half-life varies inversely with gestational age[70] and dosing intervals must therefore be increased.

Recommendations for using paracetamol in babies are given in Table 7.7.

PROPARACETAMOL

Proparacetamol is a water-soluble prodrug rapidly hydrolysed by plasma cholinesterases to paracetamol when given IV. It has been evaluated in children for postoperative pain[73] and used in neonates[72] but is not available in the UK. One gram of proparacetamol produces 0.5 g of paracetamol.

Non-steroidal anti-inflammatory drugs

NSAIDs reversibly inhibit peripheral synthesis of prostaglandins and may modulate prostaglandin synthetase activity in the brain, potentiating the antinociceptive action of opioids.[74] Although usually insufficient for pain after major surgery, they are often adequate for minor or intermediate surgery and are the drugs of choice after many day-case operations. Aspirin is no longer recommended in children and adolescents under 16 years of age because of the association with Reye's syndrome.

Although regional blocks (caudal or penile) produce better pain control than NSAIDs immediately after minor surgery, some authors have found no difference thereafter.[75, 76] However, most practitioners generally consider that pain control is better if local anaesthetic techniques and NSAIDs are used concurrently.[77, 78]

In adequate dose, NSAIDs produce analgesia comparable to opioids after minor or intermediate surgery (e.g. tonsillectomy, correction of strabismus, internal fixation of fractures).[51, 79–81] After major surgery in children, NSAIDs reduce opioid requirements by a third or more.[82–86]

NSAIDs do not depress breathing or cause sedation. Most authors report less vomiting compared with IV opioids,[51, 81, 87, 88] although others found an increased incidence despite less opioid consumption when given to children using PCA.[85]

Major bleeding is a serious potential complication because NSAIDs inhibit aggregation of platelets by reducing synthesis of thromboxane A_2. Some authors have found more perioperative bleeding in children given NSAIDs,[89] particularly ketorolac,[90–92] but the relative risk is unknown. NSAIDs should not be given to children with a coagulopathy, those taking anticoagulants or before operations with a high risk of haemorrhage. Other contraindications include impaired renal function, hypovolaemia, hypotension, angiotensin-converting

---

Box 7.2 Conclusions from the working party of the Royal College of Anaesthetists on the use of non-steroidal anti-inflammatory drugs (NSAIDS) for postoperative pain relief in children[94]

Conclusions based on strongest evidence available

- NSAIDs produce good pain relief after minor to intermediate surgery
- NSAIDs reduce the demand for, and thus the complications associated with, opioids
- Increased bleeding after tonsillectomy has been demonstrated
- The rectal route is effective

Recommendations based on consensus opinion of experts

- Child-friendly formulations should be used whenever possible (e.g. oral syrups, lingual melts, topical eye drops, intravenous formulations) and intramuscular injections should be avoided in a conscious child
- For rectal administration in a conscious child, the consent of parent and child should be obtained
- NSAIDs can be very beneficial in the management of children and this should be borne in mind in assessing risk
- Care is required with NSAIDs in infants < 12 months because of immaturity of renal function
- NSAIDs should be avoided in children with proven asthma (i.e. regular maintenance therapy, previous hospital admissions because of asthma, particularly if admitted to the intensive care unit), especially if associated with nasal polyps, severe eczema or atopy

enzyme inhibitors or hypersensitivity to NSAIDs. Proven asthma is a relative contraindication. 'Aspirin-sensitivity' is extremely rare in childhood and the results of a recent study of the effects of NSAIDs in children using inhaled steroids and bronchodilators for mild to severe asthma were very reassuring (no clinically significant bronchospasm up to 30 min after taking 1–1.5 mg kg^{-1} of oral effervescent diclofenac).[93] Many practitioners are now willing to prescribe NSAIDs to asthmatic children as long as they are not currently taking anti-asthmatic treatment.

A working party from the Royal College of Anaesthetists considered the use of NSAIDs after surgery.[94] Their conclusions for children are given in Box 7.2.

Recommended doses of NSAIDs evaluated in children are given in Table 7.8.

TOPICAL NSAIDS

Topical diclofenac 0.1% instilled on to the cornea before and after strabismus surgery produces better analgesia than oxybuprocaine 0.4% for the first postoperative hour and comparable analgesia thereafter.[95] However, topical ketorolac 0.5% is no better than placebo.[96]

An advantage of NSAIDs over local anaesthetics is that sensation to the cornea is preserved, theoretically reducing the risk of trauma.

Table 7.8 Recommended doses of non-steroidal anti-inflammatory drugs (NSAIDs) in children

	Dose	Notes for use in the UK
Ibuprofen[83, 85]	40 mg kg^{-1} day^{-1} in 3–4 divided doses O/R	• Licensed for postoperative pain • Not recommended in babies < 7 kg • Available as tablets, syrup, soluble or modified-release forms
Ketorolac[81, 325]	1 mg kg^{-1} O (premed) 0.75–0.9 mg kg^{-1} IV (at induction)	• Licensed for postoperative pain • O, IM and IV preparations available but not licensed for children • Associated with increased bleeding after tonsillectomy
*Diclofenac[75–77, 79, 80, 85]	1 mg kg^{-1} R (premed) or IM (at induction) 2–2.5 mg kg^{-1} R (at induction) 1 mg kg^{-1} every 12 h O/R (postop)	• Licensed for postoperative pain • Not licensed in children < 12 months • IM injection not recommended because of pain at site of injection • IV preparation available but not licensed in children
Temoxicam[88]	0.75 mg kg^{-1} IM (at induction)	• Licensed for postoperative pain in children • Long elimination half-life • O, IM or IV preparations available • No pain at site of injection

O, oral; R, rectal; IV, intravenous; IM, intramuscular; premed, as premedication.
*Maximum dose in 24 hours of 3mg kg^{-1}

Systemic opioids

Morphine

Morphine is the commonest opioid for analgesia in children. It is also a useful sedative to smooth emergence from anaesthesia[19] and reduce agitation after major surgery.[97] There are few reports of alternative opioids for pain relief in children.

Morphine is given intermittently or continuously, by a variety of routes, and can be titrated to requirements by the child or carers. Recommended doses for different age groups calculated from known pharmacokinetic variables are given in Table 7.9.

INTERMITTENT ADMINISTRATION

Intermittent administration of drugs produces marked fluctuation in plasma concentration. For opioids, this 'peak-and-trough' pattern may produce inadequate analgesia alternating with excessive sedation. However, intermittent administration of morphine by nursing staff may be helpful after intermediate surgery (combined with local blocks or coanalgesics) (see Fig. 7.1) or for additional sedation in some children who are agitated despite adequate sensory blocks from regional techniques. Alternative methods (e.g. a continuous infusion of morphine or PCA) should be considered if a child needs more than three bolus doses over a relatively short time.

In the 1980s opioids were most commonly given to children IM.[1] With the recognition of children's fears of needles, this technique has become increasingly uncommon. If local nursing practices allow, IV injection is probably the best route for giving morphine intermittently. The injection is painless and analgesia is obtained quickly. To ensure safety, IV morphine must be given according to a strict protocol, including assessments of sedation, breathing rates and severity of pain and adequate observation of the child, as shown in Figure 7.1. Additionally, $SpaO_2$ whilst breathing air should be monitored continuously as a sensitive indicator of ventilatory depression. Alternative routes of administration without needles include injection through indwelling subcutaneous (SC)[98] or IM cannulae sited during general anaesthesia or after topical anaesthesia of the skin. It is our practice to insert a SC cannula over the deltoid muscle for 'rescue analgesia' in children having epidural analgesia with 'top-ups' of local anaesthetics.

Table 7.9 Recommended dosages for morphine administration at different ages. Doses are calculated from known pharmacokinetic variables[270]

Route	Preterm neonates	Term neonates	Infants and children
Oral	-	-	0.3 mg kg^{-1} every 6 h 0.2 mg kg^{-1} every 4 h
Rectal	-	-	0.3 mg kg^{-1} every 6 h 0.2 mg kg^{-1} every 4 h
IV bolus	8 µg kg^{-1} every 4 h 4 µg kg^{-1} every 2 h	30 µg kg^{-1} every 4 h 15 µg kg^{-1} every 2 h	80 µg kg^{-1} every 4 h 40 µg kg^{-1} every 2 h
IV infusion	2 µg kg^{-1} h^{-1}	7 µg kg^{-1} h^{-1}	20 µg kg^{-1} h
IV PCA	-	-	20 µg kg^{-1} bolus
IV PCA plus BI	-	-	20 µg kg^{-1} bolus plus 4 µg kg^{-1} h^{-1}
Epidural	Not recommended	Not recommended	30 µg kg^{-1} every 8 h

IV, intravenous; PCA, patient-contolled analgesia; BI, background infusion.

PR administration is also painless and used in some hospitals for children unable to take medicines by mouth. However, bioavailablity varies enormously depending upon the formulation and extent of first-pass metabolism[99] and clinical effects may be unpredictable. A 7-month-old baby died from ventilatory depression after morphine 440 µg kg^{-1} had been given PR approximately every 4 h.[100] Children given morphine by any route must, therefore, be monitored adequately and frequently reassessed.

CONTINUOUS INFUSION

Continuous delivery of drug ensures a more stable plasma concentration than intermittent administration. Morphine can be infused SC[101] or IV[8, 102–104] and is associated with better pain control than intermittent IM injection,[102, 104] probably because a greater dose is delivered. Recommendations for doses for infusion of morphine in children are given in Table 7.9.

SC administration is contraindicated in sick children with impaired peripheral perfusion (e.g. hypovolaemia or hypothermia) because of the risk of sequestration. With restoration of the circulating volume or rewarming, the morphine may be taken up dramatically, producing ventilatory depression or apnoea.[105]

PATIENT-CONTROLLED ANALGESIA AND VARIANTS

Plasma concentrations associated with adequate analgesia differ widely between patients:[106] a standard rate of opioid delivery may produce excessive sedation in some patients but inadequate pain control in others. PCA allows patients to titrate the drug delivery to their own requirements. Morphine use varies > 15-fold after major orthopaedic operations in children.[85] PCA may confer psychological benefit by giving them control over their own pain and provide analgesia in anticipation of painful procedures (e.g. repositioning, removal of drains or physiotherapy). It can also be used as a measure of the efficacy of other techniques.[85] Morphine PCA produces better analgesia compared with IM injection[107] or continuous infusion in older children (but not those < 9 years),[108] probably because they use more drug when allowed control over delivery.

Bedside and disposable devices have been used in children as young as 4 or 5 years of age, usually with IV delivery of morphine.[6,106–117] A child's ability to understand the technique and operate the control button are important limitations. A pain nurse should see the child and his or her parents before surgery to teach the technique, and assess the child's abilities to understand the concept and use the equipment. The nurse should reinforce this teaching after surgery because some children are reluctant to administer analgesia despite severe pain.[6] An inherent safety feature of PCA is that a child who is oversedated is unlikely to operate the control button. To avoid morphine overdose,[110] parents or nurses should not operate the system except in specific circumstances (e.g. a child who is physically unable to press the control button) and then only in response to a clear request from the child. The desirable features of a PCA machine for children are given in Table 7.10.

In some studies in children, a background infusion of morphine in association with PCA provided superior analgesia to PCA alone without increasing the incidence of side-effects[107] and improved patterns of sleep, probably because of a continuing delivery during sleep.[113, 114, 117] In contrast, studies using background infusions of morphine 10–20 µg kg^{-1} h^{-1} found increased morphine consumption compared with a continuous infusion, a higher incidence of side-effects (e.g. nausea, sedation and hyperaemia),[117] and no improvement in analgesia.[6, 117] Some of these findings are similar to those in adults.[118] Doyle and colleagues, however, gave morphine 4 µg/kg h^{-1} (a low-dose background infusion) plus PCA and found fewer episodes of hypoxaemia, a better pattern of sleep and a similar incidence of nausea or vomiting compared with PCA alone and this is probably the ideal combination.[114] A background infusion does reduce the inherent safety of the system. To improve safety, Lloyd-Thomas & Howard[44] suggested initially increasing the lockout interval and then reducing it as the background infusion is decreased over the first 24 postoperative hours and omitting the

Table 7.10 Desirable features of a patient-controlled analgesia pump for children[326]

- Suitably sized, easily identified and easily used patient control button, which beeps when activated. Alternatives should be available for children unable to use their hands
- The programmes should be easy to use and flexible enough to cope with a wide range of body weights. Programme features should include: bolus dose as mg or μg (or better still as $\mu g\ kg^{-1}$); lockout interval 1 min and above; optional background infusion programmable in $\mu g\ kg^{-1}\ h^{-1}$
- Accepts either standard sizes of syringe or prefilled cartridges to minimise dilution errors
- Compact, light-weight, durable, mains- or battery-operated
- Lockable key pad and syringe holder
- Clear display of stored data. Memory should store 24 h worth of data
- Standard interface for data retrieval, storage, processing and generation of hard copy
- Alarms for: mains/battery failure; occlusion; overdelivery; empty syringe and programming errors

background infusion in children over 10 years. A background infusion should also be omitted when regional blocks have been used (e.g. during orthopaedic operations) because morphine is given during the period of analgesia obtained from local anaesthetic, increasing consumption of morphine without improving analgesia.[113]

Morphine 20 $\mu g\ kg^{-1}$ is probably the ideal bolus dose. Doyle and colleagues found a bolus of 20 $\mu g\ kg^{-1}$ of morphine was associated with better pain control on movement and fewer episodes of hypoxaemia than 10 $\mu g\ kg^{-1}$ in PCA with both combined with a background infusion of 4 $\mu g\ kg^{-1}\ h^{-1}$.[115]

PCA with SC morphine is associated with analgesia comparable to IV delivery but with reduced morphine consumption, a higher percentage of successful demands and a lower incidence of oxygen desaturation. It is possible that children are aware of the SC injection and this feedback may help them to use the technique more effectively.[116]

Guidelines for the initial settings for morphine PCA (IV or SC) in children are given in Table 7.11. These should be adjusted according to the success of demands and pain scores: a rate of successful demands less than 60%, particularly if associated with high pain scores, suggests the settings for the PCA should be adjusted.[36]

Patients using PCA show considerable variability in consumption and plasma concentrations of morphine. Plasma concentrations correlate with morphine consumption but not pain scores. The variability may result from differences in children's psychology, pain threshold or tolerance, or the way individuals use the PCA.[106]

NURSE-CONTROLLED OR PARENT-CONTROLLED ANALGESIA

Parent-assisted or nurse-controlled analgesia (NCA) in which a parent or nurse operates the control button has been described[119, 120] and is useful for children who are too young or physically unable to press the control button.

These techniques have greater potential for overdose because the child does not control the delivery of drug. However, NCA has a low incidence of complications if used according to strict guidelines (Table 7.12)[44] and is popular with nurses because they are able to titrate analgesics to a child's needs. Recommended initial settings are given in Table 7.11. Weldon and colleagues found NCA less satisfactory than PCA in older children because nurses gave fewer doses of morphine.[120] Parents may find controlling their child's analgesia stressful.[119]

EQUIPMENT FOR DELIVERY OF IV MORPHINE

Morphine given by continuous or a PCA/NCA system must be delivered through an antisiphon valve to prevent the contents of the syringe emptying into the child if there is an air

Table 7.11 Schemes for continuous infusion or PCA morphine in children

Continuous infusions of morphine sulphate

Intravenous[103]	1 mg kg^{-1} made up to 50 ml with 0.9% saline/5% glucose (1 ml = 20 µg kg^{-1})
Infusion rate	0.5–2.0 ml h^{-1} = 10–40 µg kg^{-1} h^{-1}
Subcutaneous[101]	1 mg kg^{-1} made up to 20 ml with 0.9% saline (1.0 ml = 50 µg kg^{-1})
Infusion rate	0.3–0.6 ml h^{-1} = 15–30 µg kg^{-1} h^{-1}

Patient-controlled analgesia using morphine*

Intravenous[115]	1 mg kg^{-1} made up to 50 ml with 0.9% saline/5% glucose (1 ml = 20 µg kg^{-1})
Lockout	5 min
Bolus dose	1 ml = 20 µg kg^{-1}
Background infusion	0.1–0.4 ml kg^{-1} h^{-1} = 2–8 µg kg^{-1} h^{-1}
Subcutaneous[116]	1 mg kg^{-1} made up to 20 ml with 0.9% saline (1 ml = 50 µg kg^{-1})
Lockout	5 min
Bolus dose	0.4 ml = 20 µg kg^{-1}
Background infusion	0.1 ml kg^{-1} h^{-1} = 5 µg kg^{-1} h^{-1}

Nurse-controlled analgesia using morphine*

Intravenous[44]	1 mg kg^{-1} made up to 50 ml with 0.9% saline/5% glucose (1 ml = 20 µg kg^{-1})
Lockout	30–60 min
Bolus dose	0.5–1.0 ml = 10–20 µg kg^{-1}
Background infusion	0.5–1.0 ml kg^{-1} h^{-1} = 10–20 µg kg^{-1} h^{-1}
Maximum in 4 h	400 µg kg^{-1}

* Maximum bolus of 1mg

leak (e.g. a cracked syringe or inadequately tightened connections). Alternatively, the syringe driver can be kept at, or below, the level of the patient so venous pressure will prevent discharge of the syringe contents. A one-way valve should be used if the morphine is delivered concurrently with a gravity-driven infusion. This is to prevent reflux of drug along the drip tubing if the cannula occludes and the subsequent delivery of a large dose of morphine when the occlusion is cleared. It is also advisable to run a continuous IV infusion concurrently if a PCA is used without a background infusion to prevent the cannula repeatedly occluding.

COMPLICATIONS ASSOCIATED WITH OPIOIDS

The complications associated with opioids are predictable and similar to those occurring in adults.

Table 7.12 Guidelines for nurse- or parent-controlled analgesia[326]

Criteria for activation of the pump

Pain score 'quite sore' or 'very sore'
Patient request

Contraindications to activation of the pump

Pain score 'asleep' or 'not really sore'
Sedation score 'unrousable'
Breathing rate < 10 breaths min^{-1} in a child 5 years or older or < 20 breaths min^{-1} if younger than 5 years
SpaO$_2$ < 90%

Opioids given postoperatively in appropriate doses and with adequate patient observation have a good record of safety.[8] Ventilatory depression or arrest has been reported in children with PR[100] or SC administration[105] and with PCA.[110, 121] Recommendations for monitoring children given opioids are given in Table 7.5. Oxygen desaturation with the patient breathing air is a good indicator of ventilatory depression (see above).[36]

Although a single dose of morphine during groin surgery doubles the incidence of vomiting from 25% to 56%,[19] many side-effects are influenced by additional factors (e.g. type of surgery, anaesthetic technique). Nausea or vomiting is reported in about 40% of children receiving a continuous infusion of morphine[8, 103] and vomiting affects 33% of those using morphine PCA.[110] Urinary retention occurs in 13–26% of children given systemic morphine (by continuous infusion;[8] PCA or IM).[107] Pruritus (usually of the face) affects 13%, and dysphoria 7%, of children given morphine by continuous infusion.[8]

Myoclonus (morphine jerks) is sometimes a real problem, particularly in younger children, and seems to be related to the dose of morphine.[122]

MORPHINE IN BABIES

Neonates during the first week of life have lower clearance and prolonged elimination half-life for morphine compared with older children but there is considerable variability between patients.[123, 124] Half-life and clearance correlate with gestational age.[124] The delivery of morphine to opioid receptors is probably also increased because of greater brain blood flow in babies, increased partitioning between the cerebrospinal fluid and plasma[125] and possibly increased free fraction of drug.[124] Doses should therefore be reduced and dose intervals increased in preterm babies and neonates. Morphine clearance matures rapidly after birth, finally reaching adult levels by about 6 months–2 years of age.[126, 127]

In a study of a small number of babies and children, serum concentrations of morphine > 20 ng ml^{-1} produced significant ventilatory depression in most, but there was no evidence that babies < 7 days were any more sensitive.[128] However, anecdotally, young babies are sensitive to the respiratory-depressant effects of opioids. The dose of morphine in neonates should be reduced and titrated to effect to take account of different pharmacokinetic variables and the considerable variability between patients (see Table 7.9). Babies older than 6 months given continuous infusions of morphine can be managed safely on a general ward if they are monitored adequately (see Table 7.5). Younger babies should be nursed on a high-dependency or intensive care unit.

Codeine and dihydrocodeine

Codeine or dihydrocodeine can be useful for the pain of intermediate surgery. IM codeine phosphate 1.5 mg kg^{-1} produces analgesia comparable to IM morphine 0.15 mg kg^{-1} after adenotonsillectomy but with a significantly lower incidence of vomiting (30% compared with 60%).[129]

IV codeine is associated with catastrophic hypotension and bronchospasm and is contraindicated in children.

Benzodiazepines

Intermittent muscle spasm is a major component of pain in children with cerebral palsy, particularly after major orthopaedic operations. Muscle spasm may also occur in normal children, e.g. with fractured femur. Benzodiazepines, in low dose to relax muscle tone (e.g. oral diazepam 0.1 mg kg^{-1} 6-hourly or IV midazolam 10–30 µg/kg h^{-1}) are helpful.[42, 130, 131] The doses are considerably lower than used for sedation but the effects are additive with opioids and sedation and ventilation must be monitored carefully.

REGIONAL TECHNIQUES

Regional techniques (usually combined with paracetamol and/or NSAIDs) are the mainstay of pain control in children, and, by avoiding the side effects of opioids, are particularly useful in day surgery.

Recent advances include the increasing preference for peripheral rather than neuraxial techniques the use of catheters inserted around peripheral nerves to allow continuous blockade and the addition of clonidine or ketamine to local anaesthetics to prolong the duration of analgesia.

Topical anaesthesia

Topical lidocaine (lignocaine) spray, jelly or ointment has been recommended for analgesia after circumcision in boys[21, 132] but may be less effective than penile block.[133] Topical lidocaine (lignocaine) 2% (up to 10 ml intraoperatively) produces peak plasma concentrations of $< 5\ \mu g\ ml^{-1}$ (toxic concentration in adults $> 10\ \mu g\ ml^{-1}$).[134] Topical anaesthetics are probably most useful for repeated application to treat postoperative pain in conjunction with other techniques, e.g. paracetamol and NSAIDs.

Local anaesthetic eye drops (e.g. tetracaine (amethocaine) 0.5%, oxybuprocaine 0.4%, proxymetacaine 0.5%) can be instilled on to the cornea during surgery to provide analgesia for squint correction. Additional drops of oxybuprocaine 0.4% can be given for postoperative pain control,[95] although proxymetacaine produces much less initial stinging and is probably a better choice in children. Anecdotally, tetracaine (amethocaine) produces a punctate keratopathy, which may be painful once the local-anaesthetic effect has resolved.

Topical anaesthesia theoretically increases the risk of corneal damage, but this is extremely rare.

Instillation or infiltration with local anaesthetic

Instilling or infiltrating a wound with local anaesthetic is simple and safe. Several authors have found analgesia as good as or almost as good as peripheral nerve or caudal blocks.[135–139] Tobias, however, reported better pain control and quicker recovery in children given caudal block, rather than wound infiltration, for repair of umbilical hernia.[140]

Peripheral nerve and central blockade

Timing of blocks

The timing of a regional block has little or no influence on analgesia after minor surgery,[141, 142] but one established before incision reduces intraoperative requirements for volatile agents, enabling earlier discharge from the recovery ward.[140] This may be useful in babies, particularly ex-prematures, in whom reduced requirements for general anaesthesia may decrease postoperative morbidity.

Peripheral nerve blocks

Since the publication of a prospective survey of regional analgesia in children by the French Language Society of Paediatric Anesthesiologists (ADARPEF) in 1996,[159] peripheral nerve and compartment space blocks are becoming increasingly popular. The analgesia obtained generally compares favourably with central blockade[139, 143–147] (often for a lower dose of local anaesthetic), whilst avoiding some common side effects (e.g. bilateral leg weakness and sensory loss) or potential hazards (e.g. 'total spinal'). The authors of the ADARPEF survey reported no complications amongst >9 000 peripheral blocks compared with 1.2/1000 for epidural analgesia.[159] However, it is difficult to assess subtle changes in sensori-motor function in children and the 'true' incidence of localised nerve damage is unknown.

Most approaches described in adults can be adapted for children and contraindications and complications are similar. Less well-known and particularly useful techniques

221

include block of the infraorbital nerve in babies having cleft lip repair;[148] block of the sciatic-nerve at the back of the thigh[149] or its branches within the popliteal fossa[150, 151, 151a] for correction of talipes; and block of the femoral, lateral cutaneous and obturator nerves in the psoas compartment (fascia iliaca block) for skin grafts or operations of the hip.[152]

Most peripheral blocks are single-injection techniques, but catheters can be inserted into the psoas compartment[156] around the brachial plexus,[153] into the femoral[154] or rectus[155] sheaths, or paravertebral spaces[157] and used for continuous infusion or repeated injections of local anaesthetics.

TECHNIQUE

The technique for peripheral nerve block differs from that in adults. In the UK, regional blocks are usually combined with light general anaesthesia in children and sited after induction.

Nerves with a motor component are best identified with a nerve stimulator in children because anatomy varies with age, the technique of paraesthesia cannot be used, and the volume of local anaesthetic can be reduced if delivered adjacent to a nerve. The use of a nerve stimulator is associated with a very high rate of successful block in children.[160, 161] Insulated needles are more accurate because maximum current density lies at the tip of the needle and the current required to produce a twitch is lowest with the tip adjacent to the nerve. In contrast, the greatest current density in a non-insulated needle occurs along the shaft, so a maximum 'twitch' will be obtained when the needle tip is beyond or through the nerve. My practice is to locate the nerves with a current of 0.5 mA. If a response is produced at less than 0.3 mA, I withdraw the needle a little in the intuitive belief that the needle tip may lie within the nerve. This is different to what is commonly recommended for adults because concurrent general anaesthesia also depresses nerve conduction, so more current is required than in a conscious patient despite the needle lying the same distance from the nerve. There is, however, no research evidence that the use of a nerve stimulator decreases the incidence of nerve damage.

A short bevelled needle is appropriate for techniques using loss of resistance because fascial planes are thinner in children and these needles give a sensitive appreciation of changes in tissue resistance and make 'fascial clicks' more distinctive. For blocks of the ilioinguinal/iliohypogastric nerves or lateral cutaneous nerve of the thigh, we find a 25-mm, 22G spinal needle ideal.

Anaesthetised children cannot complain of pain during injection of local anaesthetic to alert the anaesthetist to potential nerve damage. If there is significant resistance to injection, the anaesthetist should reposition the needle because the tip may lie within a nerve or nerve sheath. Techniques of block not relying on precise localisation of nerve are attractive. For example, in the fascia iliaca block, (developed specifically for children from the study of cadavers)[152] local anaesthetic is injected deep to the fascia iliaca in the groin and spreads through a potential space containing components of the lumbar plexus (femoral, lateral cutaneous nerves of the thigh, genitofemoral and obturator nerves). As local anaesthetic is injected remote from nerves, there is little risk of neuropraxia.

Central blockade – epidural and subarachnoid analgesia

In contrast to adults, children younger than 6–8 years usually have little change in heart rate or blood pressure in association with central blockade with local anaesthetics.[162, 163]

SINGLE-INJECTION CAUDAL ANALGESIA

Caudal analgesia with bupivacaine is the commonest regional technique in children. In most studies, block with local anaesthetic produces similar analgesia to other regional techniques, e.g. block of the dorsal nerve of the penis[143–144] or ilioinguinal nerve[145–147, 164] or wound infiltration.[136, 138, 139] However, it has several disadvantages limiting its use to minor surgery of the lower abdomen and legs. The duration of analgesia from bupivacaine is relatively short (approximately 4–6 h); the volume required to block thoracic dermatomes is large; and sensorimotor block of both legs may delay discharge from the day-surgery unit. Recent developments to prolong analgesia include inserting a catheter and injecting or infusing local anaesthetic postoperatively or adding other drugs to the local anaesthetic solution, such as clonidine or ketamine (see below).

Failure rates range from 1 to 11%[165–168] and landmarks are difficult in 11%.[165] The rate of success depends on age and weight. Failure is commoner in children > 7 years of age (15% compared with 1.4% for younger children)[165, 166] or weighing > 35 kg.[169] This is probably because posterior fusion of the sacrum increases with age and the sacral hiatus becomes smaller. Several attempts are required in 25% of children[166] and this is influenced by the anaesthetist's experience.[165]

TRANSSACRAL APPROACH

Busoni & Sarti[170] described the transsacral approach to the caudal space (between S2 and S3) using an epidural needle and a 'loss of resistance' technique. It is useful in children in whom the sacral hiatus cannot be identified or is obliterated. Although the risk of dural puncture is theoretically higher, it did not occur in the 74 children originally reported.

EPIDURAL CATHETER TECHNIQUES

Single injection of local anaesthetic into the lumbar epidural space[171] has largely been superseded by catheter techniques with the development over the last decade of equipment suitable for children. The aim is to position the catheter tip at a segmental level appropriate to surgery.

Advantages. Epidural analgesia using local anaesthetic solutions provides analgesia comparable with IV morphine[97] and may improve outcome in babies and children at greater risk of postoperative morbidity, although most of the evidence is retrospective or anecdotal. Meignier and colleagues[172] successfully used epidural analgesia in children with respiratory disability having major abdominal operations. There was no deterioration in blood gases, physiotherapy was well tolerated, and no child needed postoperative ventilation. Babies given epidural analgesia for pain control for repair of tracheo-oesophageal fistula had a better postoperative outcome compared with historical controls.[173] In a retrospective analysis of fundoplication, significantly fewer children with epidural infusions of opioids +/- bupivacaine became hypoxic or required postoperative ventilation compared with those given IV boluses of morphine. In fundoplication the duration of hospital admission after epidural analgesia is reduced compared with both intermittent[174] or continuous IV morphine.[175] In otherwise fit children having major abdominal surgery, breathing rates and oxygen saturations are also higher compared with those given IV infusions of morphine.[97] Epidural analgesia reduces the stress response to surgery in children more effectively than clinically useful doses of opioids.[97a]

Equipment for continuous caudal epidural. The sacrum is relatively flat in babies compared with older children and a cannula may guide a catheter cranially more successfully than a Tuohy needle. Catheters can also be withdrawn and readvanced without risk of shearing and the stylet acts as an obturator, reducing the risk of implantation dermoid. A 23G catheter will pass through a 20G cannula and a 19G through an 18G. More recently, BBraun™ have introduced specific equipment for inserting a caudal catheter either through an 18G cannula (the 'Oxford set') or a 20G short-bevelled needle.

223

Equipment for lumbar or thoracic epidurals. Two sizes of Tuohy needle are commonly available in the UK for children (Table 7.13). Paediatric Tuohy needles are short, easily manipulated and usually marked at 0.5-cm intervals.

Fewer dural punctures occur with smaller, compared with larger-gauge, needles in young children.[176] However, fine catheters are more difficult to thread[176] and are associated with significant problems and serious complications. Wilson and colleagues[177] reported frequent technical difficulties with 23G catheters (e.g. kinking or occlusion of the catheter; catheter-connector disconnections) leading to premature loss of postoperative infusions. Many fewer problems occur with 19G catheters.[177, 178] More seriously, van Niekerk and colleagues[179] were unable to aspirate blood or cerebrospinal fluid through two 23G catheters whose tips inadvertently lay intravascularly or within the subarachnoid space. They recommend determining the position of the tip of the catheter radiologically before injecting local anaesthetic.

TECHNIQUE

Perpendicular, midline[162, 176, 181, 183, 184] and paramedian[172] approaches to the lumbar or thoracic epidural space are described in children.

The epidural space is usually identified with a 'loss of resistance' technique using air,[162, 170, 171, 176] saline[163, 170, 172, 176] or carbon dioxide.[176] Air, however, is not ideal. It has been associated with venous air embolism and cardiovascular collapse;[185, 186] produces patchy anaesthesia in 4% of children;[187] and was implicated in the aetiology of catastrophic neurological damage in five babies.[188] Some authors recommended using saline alone or with air (interposing saline between the air and needle) to prevent these complications,[189] although this increases the incidence of dural puncture[176] and dilutes local anaesthetic. Carbon dioxide is an alternative that is easily absorbed and not associated with painful gaps.[176]

Approach for caudal epidural catheters. Catheters can be threaded to the thoracic or lumbar level[97, 179, 190–193] and positioned to within one or two segments of the predicted level in 85–95% of babies or children < 3 years of age.[179, 190–192] The technique may be less reliable in older children,[190, 194] probably because epidural fat becomes denser and lumbar lordosis develops with age. A stylet may improve success,[192] although the potential for neurological damage with these stiffer catheters has not been evaluated. Techniques for identifying the position of the tip include epidurography[179] and, more recently, ultrasound scanning or assessment of motor response to a stimulating catheter.[180]

Compared with thoracic or lumbar approaches, the caudal route is probably a more familiar technique with significantly fewer risks of dural puncture or spinal cord injury. However, the potential for faecal contamination of catheters has made the technique less acceptable. Although Strafford and colleagues found no clinical evidence of infection in a retrospective review of 54 caudal catheters used postoperatively,[195] bacterial colonisation is significantly greater with catheters inserted caudally rather than using a lumbar approach (20% versus 4%).[195a] The technique remains useful in newborn babies, however, because meconium is sterile and unlikely to cause problems. Tunnelling caudal catheters subcutaneously may reduce the risks of faecal contamination.

Table 7.13 Equipment for lumbar or thoracic epidural analgesia in children (Portex™)

Tuohy needle G (length in cm)	Catheter gauge (external diameter in mm)	Position of holes	Number of holes
19 (5)	23 (0.63)	End	1
18 (5)	19 (0.9)	Side	3

Approach for sacral epidural catheters. The sacrum does not begin to ossify until approximately 18 years of age. A sacral approach to the epidural space is useful throughout childhood[170, 176, 183] and is technically easier than lumbar or thoracic approaches.[176] The S2–S3 interspace is the largest and can be identified easily (the S2 vertebra lies at the level of the posterior superior iliac spines)[170] and dural puncture is probably less likely at this level because the dura usually terminates at S2.[170] Catheters can be threaded cranially to thoracic or lumbar levels,[170, 176] or caudally to provide analgesia over sacral dermatomes.[183] The risk of faecal contamination is probably less if caudal catheters are inserted transsacrally rather than through the sacral hiatus.

Approach for lumbar epidural catheters. Catheters are commonly inserted at the lumbar level below the termination of the spinal cord (L3 < 12 months and L2 in older children). The landmarks are indicated by the intercristal line which crosses the vertebral column at L5 in children and L5–S1 in neonates.[196] Several formulae relate age or weight to the depth of the epidural space (Table 7.14). One millimetre per kilogram is a useful guide between the ages of 6 months and 10 years,[197] although there is considerable variability between patients. The depth ranges from 6 to 12 mm in babies < 6 months.[197, 198] For extensive multilevel orthopaedic surgery over a wide range of dermatomes, some authors insert catheters at two segmental levels to ensure adequate analgesia throughout the surgical field.[42]

Approach for thoracic epidural catheters. A thoracic approach to the epidural space is used to position the tip of a catheter reliably at a segmental level appropriate for surgery of the thorax or upper abdomen.[158, 162, 172, 176, 181, 199–202] Although Tobias and colleagues found no clinically significant morbidity associated with thoracic epidural analgesia in a retrospective review of 63 children from 3 months to 18 years,[158] the potential for damage to the spinal cord is probably greater than in adults because distances are small, tissue planes less well defined, and the majority of children are under general anaesthesia when epidurals are inserted. Berde therefore recommends that only practitioners with considerable expertise of the technique in adults and lumbar epidurals in children should attempt a thoracic approach. The technique should be restricted to children with severe illness (such as chronic lung disease or cancer) having major thoracoabdominal surgery[203] in whom the benefits well outweigh the risks.

To reduce the risk of trauma to the spinal cord, catheters can be threaded to thoracic levels from a lumbar interspace.[97] Although useful in neonates,[204] the technique seems unreliable in older children. Blanco and colleagues could advance only 22% of 19G catheters to predicted thoracic levels from an approach at L4–L5 in children < 8 years. The majority of catheters simply coiled within the epidural space near to the point of insertion. The authors' clinical impressions of the ease of insertion did not predict the final

Table 7.14 Distance between skin and epidural space in children			
Investigators	**Approach**	**Level**	**Depth**
Busoni 1990[327]	Midline	L2/3	[2 × age in years] + 10 (mm)
Uemura & Yamashita 1992[328]	Midline	L3/4	[Body weight in kg + 10] × 0.8 (mm)
Hasan et al 1994[198]	Midline	Lumbar	1 + [0.15 × age in years] (cm) 0.8 + [0.05 × body weight in kg] (cm)
Bosenberg & Gouws 1995[197]	Midline	L3/4	Approximately 1 mm kg^{-1} for children 6 months–10 years

225

position of the catheter tips.[184] Age-related changes in anatomy (e.g. the development of the lumbar lordosis from about 12 months of age, increasing density of epidural fat) may partly explain these difficulties. Alternatively, the tip of a catheter threaded through a needle inserted perpendicular in the midline may impinge on the dura, encouraging the catheter to coil rather than advance cranially.[204] In adults, catheters are more successfully threaded using a paramedian approach.[205] Analgesia of thoracic dermatomes can also be obtained by injecting hydrophilic opioids into the lumbar epidural space (see below).

COMPLICATIONS

The authors of a large retrospective study in children over 10 years reported catastrophic neurological damage associated with epidural analgesia in five babies.[188] The aetiology is unclear but age less than 12 weeks, Afro-Caribbean ethnic origin, loss of resistance using air and male sex were risk factors. However, a subsequent prospective study in children (including nearly 18 000 epidurals) found a complication rate of 1.2 per 1000 for epidural block by any approach, with no permanent morbidity or neurological damage. There was significant variability between different age groups. The commonest problems were inadvertent dural puncture or intravascular injection (Table 7.15). Single injections were given to the majority and continuous infusions through catheters were used in fewer than 5% of children.[159]

Table 7.15 Complications of regional anaesthesia in children[159]

Complications	Spinals (n = 506)	Caudal epidural (n = 15 013)	Lumbar epidural (n = 2396)	Sacral epidural (n = 293)	Thoracic epidural (n = 135)
Dural penetration	N/A	4	2	2	0
Uncomplicated	0	0	1	1	0
Postdural headache	0	0	1	1	0
Spinal anaesthesia	N/A	4	0	0	0
Intravascular injection	1	2	3	0	0
No clinical effects	1	0	1	0	0
Convulsions	0	1	1	0	0
Cardiac arrhythmia	0	1	1	0	0
Technical problem	0	2	1	0	0
Delayed installation	0	1	0	0	0
Rectal penetration	0	1	0	0	0
Catheter knotting	N/A	0	1	0	0
Overdose and cardiac arrhythmia	0	1	1	0	0
Transient paraesthesias	0	0	2	0	0
Skin lesion	0	1	0	0	0
Morbidity	1	11	0	2	0
Rate per 1000	2 per 1000	0.7 per 1000	3.7 per 1000	6.8 per 1000	0 per 1000

Dural puncture. The rate of dural puncture for single-injection caudals ranges from 0.1 to 0.3%[165, 166, 169, 206] but in up to half of these, cerebrospinal fluid can not be aspirated and dural puncture is recognised only when the child develops a 'total spinal'.[169]

The rate of dural puncture for lumbar or thoracic approaches is influenced by the type and size of needle and the technique for loss of resistance. The incidence is lower for Tuohy than Potts-Cournand needles; when 20G compared with 17G needles are used in smaller children; and if the epidural space is identified with air instead of saline.[176] The reported rate ranges from 1.5 to 11%.[171, 176, 177] The higher figure included children with marked spinal deformity.[171]

A total spinal may result if a dural puncture is unrecognised and a large volume of local anaesthetic injected. This is a particular risk with fine catheters because cerebrospinal fluid is not aspirated reliably.[179] In a young, anaesthetised child breathing spontaneously, a total spinal is characterised by apnoea and widely dilated pupils, but generally stable cardiovascular variables.[207] Breathing begins to return after about an hour and the ability to move the eyes and arms after about 3 h,[208] with full recovery at about 4 h.[169]

Dural puncture headache is generally considered uncommon in younger children,[209–211] although other authors have not found the incidence to be age-related.[212] Persistent symptoms can be treated with an epidural blood patch using 0.16–0.5 ml kg^{-1} of autologous blood.[213–215]

High block. Unexpected high block associated with a correctly positioned catheter is uncommon. However, Wolf & Walker[216] reported a rising sensorimotor level and extensive sympathetic blockade in a child (characterised by bradycardia, hypoxia and shallow breathing) during a continuous bupivacaine infusion. Unfortunately, the position of the tip of the epidural catheter was not confirmed radiologically.

Vascular penetration. Vascular penetration occurs during 6–13% of caudal blocks.[165, 166, 168, 169] The incidence varies with the anaesthetist's experience[165] and child's weight (commoner in children > 15 kg).[168] Some authors report fewer problems with needles with non-cutting rather than cutting bevels,[166] but this was not confirmed by others.[168] Recognised vascular penetration during lumbar or thoracic epidural block in children occurs in 0.9%.[176]

In the lateral or head-down position epidural veins probably collapse. Often blood cannot be aspirated despite the tip of the needle or catheter lying within a blood vessel.[165, 217, 218] This is a particular problem with catheters of narrow bore (e.g. 23G).[179] There is evidence of intravascular injection of local anaesthetic in just under 1% of caudal blocks,[165, 166] and up to 0.4% of lumbar epidurals.[163] Drugs, particularly local anaesthetic solutions, should be injected slowly to reduce peak plasma concentration, the child should be monitored with an electrocardiagraph to detect the early subtle signs of cardiac toxicity, and the syringe should be repeatedly aspirated for blood throughout injection. Some authors recommend confirming the position of narrow-gauge catheters radiologically before giving analgesic solutions.[179]

Intravascular migration of a 23G catheter with a single orifice has been reported in a child.[219] The problem was recognised when the child had a grand mal seizure immediately after the fourth injection of bupivacaine several hours postoperatively.

Unilateral block. Unilateral block occurs in 2% of caudal[166] and 0.9% of lumbar epidurals.[176] It is probably caused by a dorsomedian septum connecting the dura to the ligamentum flavum limiting spread of analgesic solutions.[220]

Infection. Strafford and colleagues found no evidence of infection associated with epidural infusions in a prospective study of 1450 children after surgery.[195] In a retrospective review of continuous epidural analgesia in 190 children, localised infection around the site of insertion occurred in one child.[221]

Catheter occlusion. Fine-bore catheters (e.g. 23G) have a high resistance to flow and syringe drivers may need a high driving pressure (i.e. up to 600 mmHg). Occlusion during infusion is common, particularly with catheters of narrow gauge (12% of 23G catheters occlude versus 2% of 21G).[177]

Leakage around the site of catheter insertion. Leakage of local anaesthetic around the site of catheter insertion is commoner in small children and is probably due to mismatch between the diameters of the smaller needles and catheters. The rate of infusion can be increased to compensate.[177]

DRUGS

Local anaesthetics. Local anaesthetics must achieve an appropriate segmental level to be effective. For caudal injection the relationship between volume given and height of spread seems to be linear for larger babies and children. The volume required can be calculated using mathematical formulae based on age[222] or weight[223] of the child (Table 7.16) or nomograms.[224] A common and much simpler empirical scheme is given in Table 7.17.[225] Small babies, however, require relatively larger volumes than older children[226] and the spread of local anaesthetic becomes more unpredictable in those > 7 years of age.

For epidural injection at a higher level, spread is always greater cranially than caudally and at thoracic compared with lumbar levels, probably because the epidural space becomes narrower proximally. Radiopaque dye (0.75 ml kg^{-1}) injected through a 20G thoracic or lumbar epidural catheter spreads between 8 and 16 segments.[162]

Bupivacaine. Bupivacaine 0.25% is commonly used for caudal analgesia but is associated with an unacceptable duration of leg weakness.[227] Using more dilute solutions reduces the problem and some authors found that bupivacaine 0.125% produced similar analgesia to bupivacaine 0.25%,[228] but this was not confirmed by others.[229] A dose-finding study determined that a concentration of 0.175% gave the best combination of effectiveness (least requirement for intraoperative volatile anaesthetics and good-quality postoperative pain

Table 7.16 Mathematical schemes to determine the volume of local anaesthetic for caudal analgesia

Lidocaine (lignocaine)[223]
0.056 ml/kg × number of spinal units to be blocked

Lidocaine (lignocaine)[222]
0.06 + (0.007 × age in years) × number of segments to be blocked

Bupivacaine[222]
0.08 + (0.008 × age in years) × number of segments to be blocked

Table 7.17 Volumes of local anaesthetic for caudal analgesia in children using 0.25% plain bupivacaine for volumes ≤ 20 ml and 0.19% for volumes > 20 ml[225]

Area of surgery	Dose (ml kg^{-1})
Lumbosacral	0.5
Thoracolumbar	1.0
Midthoracic	1.25

relief) with rapid recovery and discharge from hospital.[230] In children who are adequately hydrated, caudal block does not delay micturition.[231]

The concentrations and volumes of bupivacaine for thoracic or lumbar epidural analgesia are empirical and calculated to avoid toxicity (Table 7.18).

Bupivacaine is absorbed rapidly from the epidural space. Peak plasma concentrations in children after injection into the caudal or lumbar epidural space of plain solutions of bupivacaine 2–3 ml kg^{-1} occur at 20–40 min and are well below the concentrations associated with convulsions.[163, 164, 182, 232] Plasma concentrations after caudal injection are significantly lower than after ilioinguinal/iliohypogastric nerve blocks.[164]

Peak serum concentrations in babies associated with a single injection of plain bupivacaine 2.5 ml kg^{-1} are also below the convulsive threshold[233] but plasma concentrations often rise during a continuous infusion,[97, 202, 234] despite an increased volume of distribution. After a 4-h infusion, total plasma concentrations are significantly higher in babies younger than 4 months of age compared with children aged 9 months to 6 years.[193] Babies may also be more susceptible to toxicity because firstly, lower concentrations of binding proteins

Table 7.18 Dose of bupivacaine for extradural analgesia in children

	Age	Operative site	Epidural site	Initial dose	Subsequent dose or infusion
Desparmet et al 1987[200]	11 months–15 years	Leg, lower abdomen	Lumbar	0.25%, 0.5 ml kg^{-1}	0.25% 0.08 ml kg^{-1} h^{-1}
[1]Murat et al 1987[329]	7–12 years	Leg	Lumbar	0.5% 1 ml per 10 cm height	
Murat et al 1988[163]	20–135 months	Leg, lower abdomen or penis	Lumbar	0.25%[2] < 20 kg – 0.75 ml kg^{-1} > 20 kg – 1 ml per 10 cm height	
Wilson et al 1993[177]	Newborn–16 years	Abdominal Abdominal or throracic	Lumbar Thoracic	0.25% 0.75 ml kg^{-1} 0.25% 0.5 ml kg^{-1}	0.125% bupivacaine with diamorphine (50 µg ml^{-1}) at 0.1–0.5 ml kg^{-1} h^{-1}
Wolf et al 1993[97]	3–46 months	Abdominal	Lumbar	0.25% 0.05 ml kg^{-1} segment^{-1}	0.25% 0.1–0.4 ml kg^{-1} h^{-1}
Wolfl et a 1993[97a]	0.2–3.9 years	Abdominal	Upper lumbar or thoracic	0.25% up to 1 ml kg^{-1}	0.25% 0.2–0.3 ml kg^{-1} h^{-1} (plus boluses to max. dose of 1.6 mg kg^{-1} in 4 h)

[1]Children with Duchenne's muscular dystrophy.
[2]Bupivacaine with adrenaline (epinephrine).

(notably α_1-acid glycoprotein) produce a higher free fraction of drug;[233] and secondly, increased intra-abdominal pressure (such as occurs in major abdominal surgery) reduces hepatic blood flow and may impair metabolism of local anaesthetics.[234] Proteins binding is influenced by pH: a decrease in pH increases the free fraction of bupivacaine.

Berde reviewed the published pharmacokinetic data for bupivacaine. He recommended a maximum loading dose of 2–2.5 mg kg^{-1} and concluded that an infusion of 0.25 mg kg^{-1} h^{-1} for neonates and 0.4 mg kg^{-1} h^{-1} for older children would be associated with plasma concentrations below 2–2.5 µg ml^{-1}.[235, 236] In the light of more recent information,[97, 193, 202, 234] we also limit the infusion of bupivacaine in babies younger than 6 months to 0.25 mg kg^{-1} h^{-1}. Convulsions have been reported in children at plasma concentrations greater than 2 µg ml^{-1}.[235] Premonitory signs of impending toxicity are not very specific in children and easily misinterpreted. Other analgesic techniques (e.g. IV or epidural opioids) should be added or used instead if pain relief is inadequate despite maximum doses of epidural local anaesthetics.

Central nervous system or cardiac toxicity results from the systemic absorption of an excessive dose of local anaesthetic[237, 238] or inadvertent intravascular injection.[217, 239] Blood is not reliably aspirated through intravascular catheters or needles of narrow bore, and sometimes appears only by aspirating repeatedly throughout the injection.[218] Adrenaline (epinephrine) 5 µg ml^{-1} is sometimes added to help indicate intravascular injection, but is an unreliable marker:[159, 167] the heart rate may slow in some children[218, 240] and rises by less than 10 beats min^{-1} in 29% of children anaesthetised with halothane. The reliability of a test dose of epinephrine (adrenaline) improves if atropine is given beforehand.[167] However, changes in the electrocardiograph trace (e.g. ST elevation, increases in T-wave amplitude and changes in the heart rate) do occur with IV injection of bupivacaine and epinephrine (adrenaline).[218, 240] Whether the changes are due to bupivacaine, epinephrine (adrenaline) or the combination is unknown. Pre-mixed preparations contain neurotoxic preservatives, so epinephrine (adrenaline) if used, must be added freshly, introducing possible error.

To decrease toxicity, local anaesthetics should be injected slowly to reduce the maximum plasma concentration of any given intravenously and the patient should be monitored with an electrocardiograph to detect early changes.[241] When using more than one local anaesthetic solution one should assume the toxicities of each are roughly additive. Substituting the levo-enantiomer for racemic bupivacaine further improves safety whilst providing a similar quality of analgesia.

Ropivacaine. Ropivacaine is a the S(+)-enantiomer of a new homologue of bupivacaine. It is long-acting with possibly less motor than sensory block, and has reduced potential for systemic toxicity. Plasma concentrations with epidural administration in children are comparable with those associated with the same dose of bupivacaine, but peak concentrations occur later (1–2 h).[242–244] The recommended epidural loading dose is up to 3 mg kg^{-1}, with subsequent infusion rates of 0.4 mg kg^{-1} h^{-1}.

Several authors have compared ropivacaine 1 mg kg^{-1} 0.20%, 0.25% or 0.375% with similar doses of bupivacaine for caudal analgesia in children and found similar or improved analgesia but usually with less weakness of the legs.[242, 246–248] In contrast, Khalil and colleagues reported similar sensory and motor effects for the same dose and concentration of drugs (0.25% 1 mg kg^{-1}).[227] The intrinsic vasoconstrictor effects of ropivacaine may preclude concommitant use with adrenaline (epinephrine) or injection around end arteries.

ADDITIVES

Drugs commonly added to local anaesthetic to prolong the duration of epidural analgesia include vasoconstrictors (e.g. adrenaline (epinephrine)), opioid and non-opioid spinal analgesics (e.g. clonidine, ketamine). All solutions injected along the neuroaxis should be free of preservatives because of the risk of neural damage.

Vasoconstrictors. Adrenaline (epinephrine) 1:200 000 (5 μg ml⁻¹) is commonly added to local anaesthetic solutions as a marker of intravascular injection, to reduce systemic absorption (and therefore the risk of toxicity), and to prolong the duration of epidural block. The effect on the duration of analgesia obtained from bupivacaine in children is unclear. Warner and colleagues found significantly prolonged caudal block in children < 5 years of age[249] and Murat and colleagues reported a 47% increase in duration of epidural analgesia in children younger than 2 years.[163] In both studies, the effect was much less pronounced in older children. Other authors, however, found that adrenaline (epinephrine) had no influence on the duration of analgesia with bupivacaine.[231, 250]

Opioids. Epidural opioids can be used alone or combined with local anaesthetics for post-operative pain relief.[171, 177, 181, 191, 199, 251–268] They principally bind to morphine receptors within the substantia gelatinosa of the spinal cord and, depending on the degree of rostral spread within the cerebrospinal fluid, also act on the brain. Epidural opioids produce profound analgesia at systemic concentrations below the therapeutic range[181, 258] but have no effect on vasomotor tone, motor power or other sensory functions. The rationale of using opioids with local anaesthetics is to attempt to improve analgesia but reduce side-effects by decreasing the dose of individual agents. Epidural opioids may produce useful sedation in small children.

Morphine. Morphine is the commonest epidural opioid used in children. It is hydrophilic and spreads rostrally along the neuroaxis: morphine injected caudally can produce analgesia for thoracic[257, 262] or craniofacial surgery.[265]

Caudal morphine 50 μg kg⁻¹ produces a median duration of analgesia of 12 h compared with 5 h for bupivacaine and 45 min for IV morphine, without increasing side-effects.[253] The efficacy of caudal morphine compared with bupivacaine has been confirmed in other studies.[258, 260] Morphine 33 or 67 μg kg⁻¹ injected alone through a caudal catheter lasts longer than 8 h in 75% of children. Increasing the dose to 100 μg kg⁻¹ prolongs analgesia but at the expense of a risk of serious ventilatory depression.[255,269] Krane and colleagues therefore recommend 33 μg kg⁻¹ and subsequently increasing this only if necessary.[269] In a similar study of babies aged 3–12 months, caudal morphine 25 μg kg⁻¹ or 50 μg kg⁻¹ had similar durations of action (mean 7.3 versus 8.7 h) compared with 4 h for IV morphine 50–100 μg kg⁻¹. The incidence of side-effects was similar between all groups. Again the authors of this study recommend giving an initial dose of 25 μg kg⁻¹ and increasing this by 25 μg kg⁻¹ if analgesia lasts less than 4 h.[267]

Lumbar or thoracic epidural morphine 50 μg kg⁻¹ provides analgesia at about 30 min[181] lasting 5–36 h.[171, 176, 181, 191] Higher doses increase the incidence of side-effects but do not extend the duration of analgesia.[252]

There are only a few reports of continuous epidural infusions of morphine. Based on known pharmacokinetic data, Kart recommends giving 30 μg kg⁻¹ every 8 h.[270] Parkinson and colleagues have reported experience of infusions of 4–5 μg kg⁻¹ h⁻¹ in two children having major surgery.[254]

SIDE-EFFECTS

Epidural morphine produces a dose-dependent increase in side-effects.[252] Symptoms such as ventilatory depression, nausea and vomiting, itching and urinary retention affect up to 50% of children given epidural morphine at the sacral level or higher.[176]

Ventilatory depression. Epidural morphine depresses the ventilatory response to carbon dioxide for more than 22 h without affecting respiratory rate.[181] Serious ventilatory depression or arrest has occasionally occurred.[191, 261, 267, 271] Risk factors include age < 12 months, opioids given by other routes and delivery of morphine at a higher segmental level (i.e. through a catheter). The mean onset of ventilatory depression is 3.8 h, shorter than generally observed in adults.[261] Children should be monitored closely for the first 24 h after an injection of lumbar or thoracic epidural morphine and those with particular risk factors, especially those < 12 months of age, should be observed on a high-dependency unit. The relative risks of epidural compared with equianalgesic doses of IV morphine are unknown.

The incidence of ventilatory depression with caudal morphine in children without the recognised risk factors discussed above is not known. Clinically significant respiratory depression was not found in a retrospective review of 500 children > 3 months of age given 30 or 40 µg kg^{-1} of morphine[265] but did occur in a 2.5-year-old more than 3.5 h after injection of morphine 1.5 mg through a catheter inserted 2 cm into the caudal space.[255] Wolf and colleagues suggest discontinuing special monitoring 6 h after a single dose of caudal morphine if the child has no signs of excessive sedation and then continuing general nursing supervision for a further 6 h.[260]

Ventilatory depression can be treated with IV naloxone 5–20 µg kg^{-1} followed, if necessary, with 2–10 µg kg^{-1} h^{-1}.[261]

Itching. Itching associated with caudal morphine 30–70 µg kg^{-1} occurs in 0–13% of children[253, 257, 258, 260–262, 265] and has a similar incidence to IV morphine.[253] It is more common with morphine injected at higher levels (12–75%), when the onset is about 3 h.[176, 181, 256, 267, 272]

Itching is not segmentally distributed[181] and commonly affects the face.[267, 269, 272] It can be treated with IV naloxone with only a slight reduction in the duration of analgesia. Suggested schemes include: 0.5–2 µg kg^{-1} [177, 272] and/or infusions of 1–5 µg kg^{-1} h^{-1}.[176, 272] Other recommendations include diphenhydramine or a small dose of droperidol.[176, 267]

Urinary retention. Urinary retention occurs in 13–39% of children given epidural morphine (25–100 µg kg^{-1}) at the sacral level or higher.[171, 176, 181, 269] The incidence is considerably greater compared with children given local anaesthetic only[171, 176] and is probably dose-related.[252] It may be less common with morphine delivered at a lower segmental level, occurring in 0–30% of children given caudal morphine (30–70 µg kg^{-1}).[260–262, 265] The higher rates seem to occur in studies using larger doses. Krane and colleagues found no significant difference compared with morphine given IV.[253]

Urinary retention can be treated by bladder compression in small children or IV naloxone.

Nausea or vomiting. Nausea and/or vomiting occurs in about 40% of children given epidural morphine 50 µg kg^{-1} above the caudal level.[171, 176, 181] This is a much higher rate than for local anaesthetics alone[171, 176] but the incidence with caudal morphine 50 µg kg^{-1} is not statistically different from that associated with IV morphine or caudal bupivacaine.[251, 253, 258, 260]

Treatment includes naloxone, droperidol (as above) or IV metoclopramide 100–150 µg kg^{-1}.[177]

OTHER OPIOIDS

Lipid-soluble opioids have a more localised action when injected into the epidural space with less rostral spread and potentially reduced risk of complications such as ventilatory depression or itching.

Diamorphine. Caudal diamorphine 30 µg kg^{-1} added to bupivacaine improves immediate pain control and modestly increases the median time to first dose of postoperative analgesia compared with bupivacaine alone (10.5 versus 8.6 h).[266]

Combining bupivacaine 0.125% with diamorphine 50, 83 or 166 µg ml⁻¹ for lumbar or thoracic epidural infusion (0.1 ml/kg h⁻¹) after major surgery seems to make children easier to nurse, possibly because of improved quality of analgesia or central sedation.[177] However, ventilatory depression or excessive sedation has occurred with the two higher doses and a maximum concentration of 50 µg ml⁻¹ is now recommended.

Fentanyl. Fentanyl has a short duration of action and adding 1 µg kg⁻¹ to local anaesthetics does not improve the quality or duration of caudal analgesia[259, 273] and should be infused to be effective. Epidural fentanyl 2 µg kg⁻¹ alone followed by a continuous infusion of 5 µg kg⁻¹ day⁻¹ produces similar analgesia to a single dose of morphine 75 µg kg⁻¹ but with considerably less nausea or vomiting (20% versus 53%) or itching (0% versus 33%).[263] Pietropaoli and colleagues routinely infuse fentanyl (mean rate of 0.9 µg kg⁻¹ h⁻¹) with bupivacaine for epidural analgesia after major surgery in children.[194]

Pethidine. Adding pethidine 0.5 ml kg⁻¹ prolongs the duration of caudal analgesia compared with bupivacaine only but is associated with an unacceptable incidence of vomiting (60% versus 12%).[274]

Clonidine. Clonidine is an α_2-adrenergic agonist at pre- and postsynaptic receptors. Analgesia is thought to result from activity within the dorsal horn of the spinal cord and the effects correlate with cerebrospinal fluid but not blood concentrations.[275] Clonidine is not neurotoxic and is available as a preservative-free solution (150 µg ml⁻¹), although this is not licensed in the UK for anaesthetic or epidural use.

Clonidine 1 or 2 µg kg⁻¹ significantly prolongs the duration of postoperative analgesia obtained from caudal local anaesthetics in children older than 12 months without increasing the incidence of serious side-effects such as ventilatory depression, hypoxia, tachycardia or hypotension, urinary retention[40, 250, 276–278] or elevating the carbon dioxide tension.[279] The time to first analgesia for a caudal mixture of clonidine (1 or 2 µg ml⁻¹) and bupivacaine ranges from 3.6 to 16.5 h compared with 3.2–7.7 h for bupivacaine alone.[40, 250, 276, 277] This is approximately a doubling in duration, although differences between the designs of the studies (e.g. premedication, anaesthetic technique, surgical operation, assessment of pain, criteria for giving postoperative analgesia) may explain the wide range of individual results. The analgesic effects of 1 µg kg⁻¹ are comparable to adding morphine 30 µg kg⁻¹.[280] Increasing the dose from 1 to 2 µg kg⁻¹ does not improve the efficacy of analgesia,[277] and although 5 µg kg⁻¹ with bupivacaine produces very prolonged analgesia (20.9 h), it is associated with modest reductions in blood pressure and heart rate for the first three postoperative hours.[281]

Adding clonidine also allows the use of more dilute solutions of local anaesthetic, reducing the density of any motor block. For example, clonidine (2 µg kg⁻¹) with ropivacaine 0.1% provides better analgesia than ropivacaine 0.2% after lower abdominal surgery in children.[278]

Clonidine has also been infused epidurally in children. Nolan et al[42] recommend combining bupivacaine 0.125% with clonidine 2.5 µg ml⁻¹ for lumbar epidural infusion (0.2–0.3 ml h⁻¹) in children with cerebral palsy having multilevel orthopaedic surgery.

Most authors have found that children given epidural clonidine are more sedated postoperatively,[276, 277, 279, 281, 282] although this is not supported by others.[40, 278] It is unclear whether any increased sedation is actually sedation, improved analgesia or a combination of both. The findings are also confounded by the use of sedative[276, 277, 281, 282] or opioid[276] premedication in many studies, which may interact with clonidine, potentiating the sedative effects. Cook and colleagues used no premedication and reported no increase in sedation.[40] However, plasma concentrations associated with epidural clonidine 2 µg kg⁻¹ produce plasma concentrations in some children that are known to be associated with sedation in adults (i.e. > 0.6 ng ml⁻¹).[245a]

Experience with epidural clonidine is limited in babies. Breschan and colleagues reported recurrent apnoea, oxygen desaturation and bradycardia in a 2-week-old term baby given caudal clonidine 2 μg kg^{-1} and ropivacaine for analgesia for groin surgery under light general anaesthesia.[283]

Some authors now use caudal clonidine for children having day surgery.[40, 277]

Ketamine. Ketamine is principally an antagonist at N-methyl-D-aspartate (NMDA) receptors, which are found throughout the central nervous system (particularly in the dorsal horn). It also has some opioid receptor and local anaesthetic activity (its chemical structure is similar to bupivacaine) and is synergistic with bupivacaine in the epidural space. At clinically effective doses it does not induce side-effects such as confusion or delirium.

Racemic ketamine 10 mg ml^{-1} is available without preservatives but this is not licensed for epidural administration. Suitable preparations are available in the UK but can be imported as Curamed from Pharma GmbH (Postfach 410229, 76202 Karisruhe, Germany). Nerve damage has not been shown in animals given preservative-free solutions and no sequelae are reported in adults.[284]

Because of its spinal analgesic effects, some authors suggest using caudal ketamine instead of local anaesthetics to avoid the morbidity associated with inadvertent intravascular injection.[285] However, ketamine is more commonly given caudally with local anaesthetic solutions to prolong the duration of analgesia without increasing side-effects or producing behavioural changes.[40, 286, 287] Ketamine 0.5 mg kg^{-1} prolongs the analgesia obtained from caudal bupivacaine more effectively than clonidine 2 μg kg^{-1} (approximately ×3 for ketamine, ×2 for clonidine).[40] Increasing the dose to 1 mg kg^{-1} further prolongs the duration of analgesia but is associated with a higher incidence of behavioural side-effects (e.g. strange affect, vacant stares). Semple and colleagues concluded that 0.5 mg kg^{-1} was the optimal dose.[288]

Caudal ketamine 0.5 mg kg^{-1} with bupivacaine 0.25% produces three times the duration of analgesia after orchidopexy than iliac crest block combined with wound infiltration (median 10 h versus 2.9 h) with no difference in sedation or times to micturition and spontaneous movement of the legs.[289]

Several authors add ketamine to bupivacaine for caudal analgesia in children having day surgery.[40, 289, 290] Johnston and colleagues found that ketamine prolongs the analgesic effect of 0.25% bupivacaine more than 0.125% (median 9.5 versus 8 h) but with a longer duration of motor block. The authors concluded that bupivacaine 0.125% with ketamine was more suitable for outpatient surgery.[290]

Recently S(+)-ketamine, one of the two enantiomers of racemic ketamine, has been evaluated.[285] It was thought to have three times the analgesic potency of the racemate, fewer neuropsychiatric side-effects, and is available as a preservative-free formulation. However, in a study of children having herniotomy, Marhofer and colleagues reported that S(+)-ketamine 1.0 mg kg^{-1} was equipotent with bupivacaine 0.25% with adrenaline (epinephrine) (0.75 ml kg^{-1}), and both were superior to ketamine 0.5 mg kg^{-1}.[285] These findings contrast with those of an earlier study of racemic caudal ketamine, in which Naguib and colleagues found that 0.5 mg kg^{-1} provided analgesia comparable with bupivacaine 0.25% (1 ml/kg).[286] I am unaware of a direct comparison in children between the S-enantiomer and the racemate.

Midazolam. Midazolam is an agonist of the benzodiazepine receptor attached to the (γ-aminobutyric acid (GABA) receptor. Within the spinal cord GABA-benzodiazepine receptors are concentrated in the dorsal horn where they modulate nociception.

Epidural analgesia using midazolam has been described in children. Caudal midazolam 50 μg kg^{-1} produces analgesia comparable with bupivacaine 2.5 mg kg^{-1} after inguinal herniotomy but with no motor weakness or behavioural changes[291] and prolongs the duration of analgesia when added to local anaesthetic solutions more effectively than morphine

50 µg kg^{-1}.[292] However, Goresky, in an editorial, raised serious concerns about the potential central nervous system toxicity of midazolam, particularly after inadvertent injection into the subarachnoid space. He recommended further studies in animals and adults to establish the safety and risk–benefit of epidural midazolam.[293]

EPIDURAL PCA

The major disadvantages of intermittent injection of analgesics and the advantages of PCA have been discussed elsewhere (see above). Investigators have also used epidural PCA with opioids alone (fentanyl or morphine),[201, 294] or combined with local anaesthetics[295] in an attempt to allow children older than 5 or 6 years to titrate their own delivery of analgesics. Analgesia in most children was satisfactory, although numbness was a problem in some of those using local anaesthetic solutions. None of the groups reported respiratory depression, although the lockout time for morphine was much shorter than the expected onset of action.[181] Side-effects were similar to those found with epidural opioids given intermittently. The doses and PCA settings used are given in Table 7.19.

I am unaware of comparative studies with other analgesic techniques.

SUBARACHNOID ANALGESIA

Subarachnoid anaesthesia using local anaesthetics was described in children nearly a century ago but the technique became unpopular as general anaesthesia became safer. The technique is advocated by some as the sole anaesthetic for minor lower abdominal surgery in ex-premature babies.[296–301] Compared with older general anaesthetic agents (e.g. thiopentone, halothane), the incidence of postoperative apnoea is significantly reduced.[300] However, it merits compared with light general anaesthesia using newer agents (e.g. sevoflurane or desflurane) combined with a regional block are unclear. In a small study, Williams and colleagues found an excess of clinically silent episodes of bradycardia or apnoea in ex-premature babies anaesthetised with sevoflurane. However, spinal anaesthesia was potentially stressful for the baby and failed in 4/14.[295a]

Several authors have injected morphine 3.75–30 µg kg^{-1} into the lumbar intrathecal space to provide prolonged analgesia after abdominal,[302, 303] cardiac[303, 304] or major spinal surgery.[305, 306] Intrathecal morphine spreads extensively along the neuroaxis and, when injected, the lumbar level provides analgesia for operations on the head and neck.[302]

Intrathecal morphine profoundly depresses the ventilatory response to carbon dioxide and this recovers only partially by 18 h.[307] Clinical evidence of ventilatory depression is common.[304] Krechel and colleagues routinely infuse naloxone postoperatively in all children given intrathecal opioids.[303] Because of the serious risks of ventilatory depression, intrathecal opioids should be reserved for children having major surgery given intensive care postoperatively and are unlikely to be used in the district hospital.

Table 7.19 Epidural PCA in children using (a) morphine[294] or (b) fentanyl[201]

Morphine	
Background infusion	5 µg kg^{-1} h^{-1}
Bolus dose	1.25 µg kg^{-1}
Lockout	15 min
Fentanyl	
Mean background infusion	0.57 µg kg^{-1} h^{-1}
Mean bolus dose	0.50 µg kg^{-1}
Lockout	15 min

REFERENCES

1. Mather L, Mackie J. The incidence of postoperative pain in children. Pain 1982; 15:271–282.
2. Perry S, Heidrich G. Management of pain during debridement: a survey of US burn units. Pain 1982; 13:267–280.
3. Beyer JE, DeGood DE, Ashley LC, et al. Patterns of postoperative analgesic use with adults and children following cardiac surgery. Pain 1983; 17:71–81.
4. Schecter NL, Allen DA, Hanson K. Status of pediatric pain control: a comparison of hospital analgesic usage in children and adults. Pediatrics 1986; 77:11–15.
5. Goddard JM, Pickup SE. Postoperative pain in children: combining audit and a clinical nurse specialist to improve management. Anaesthesia 1996; 51:588–590.
6. Peters JWB, Bandell Hoekstra IENG, Huijer Abu-Saad H, et al. Patient controlled analgesia in children and adolescents: a randomized controlled trial. Paediatr Anaesth 1999; 9:235–241.
7. Romsing J, Walther-Larsen S. Postoperative pain in children: a survey of parents' expectations and perceptions of their children's experiences. Paediatr Anaesth 1996; 6:215–218.
8. Esmail Z, Montgomery C, Court C, et al. Efficacy and complications of morphine infusions in postoperative paediatric patients. Paediatr Anaesth 1999; 9:321–327.
9. Tan SG, May HA, Cunliffe M et al. An audit of pain and vomiting in paediatric day case surgery. Paediatr Anaesth 1994; 4:105–109.
10. Grenier B, Dubreuil M, Siao D, et al. Paediatric day case anaesthesia: estimate of its quality at home. Paediatr Anaesth 1998; 8:485–489.
11. Commission on the Provision of Surgical Services. Pain after surgery. London: Royal College of Surgeons of England and Royal College of Anaesthetists; 1990.
12. Gould TH, Crosby DL, Harmer M, et al. Policy for controlling pain after surgery: effect of sequential change in management. Br Med J 1992; 305:1187–1193.
13. Tighe SQM, Bie JA, Nelson RA, et al. The acute pain service: effective or expensive care? Anaesthesia 1998; 53:382–403.
14. Royal College of Anaesthetists. Guidance for the provision of paediatric anaesthetic services. London: Royal College of Anaesthetists Bulletin 2001; 8:355–359.
15. American Society of Anesthesiologists Task Force on Pain Management, Acute Pain Section. Practice guidelines for acute pain management in the perioperative setting: a report. Anesthesiology 1995; 82:1071–1081.
16. Royal College of Anaesthetists. Guidance for the provision of anaesthetic services. London: Royal College of Anaesthetists; 2001.
17. Knight JC. Post-operative pain in children after day case surgery. Paediatr Anaesth 1994; 4:45–51.
18. Romsing J, Hertel S, Harder A, et al. Examination of acetaminophen for outpatient management of postoperative pain in children. Paediatr Anaesth 1998; 8:235–239.
19. Weinstein MS, Nicolson SC, Schreiner MS. A single dose of morphine sulfate increases the incidence of vomiting after outpatient inguinal surgery in children. Anesthesiology 1994; 81:572–577.
20. Berry FA. Preemptive analgesia for postop pain. Paediatr Anaesth 1998; 8:187–188.
21. Tree-Trakarn T, Pirayavaraporn S. Postoperative pain relief for circumcision in children: comparison among morphine, nerve block, and topical analgesia. Anesthesiology 1985; 62:519–522.
22. Royal College of Nursing Institute. The recognition and assessment of acute pain in children: recommendations. London: Royal College of Nursing Institute; 1999.
23. Morton NS. Pain assessment in children. Paediatr Anaesth 1997; 7:267–272.
24. Hannallah RS, Broadman LM, Belman AB, et al. Comparison of caudal and ilioinguinal/iliohypogastric nerve blocks for control of post-orchiopexy pain in pediatric ambulatory surgery. Anesthesiology 1987; 66:832–834.
25. Sweet SD, McGrath PJ. Physiological measures of pain. In: Measurement of pain in infants and children. International Association for the Study of Pain; Seattle, 1996:59–82.
26. Krechel SW, Bilder J. CRIES: a new neonatal postoperative pain measurement score. Initial testing of validity and reliability. Paediatr Anaesth 1995; 5:53–61.
27. McGrath PJ, Johnson G, Goodman JT, et al. CHEOPS: a behaviour scale for rating postoperative pain in children. Adv Pain Res Ther 1985; 9:395–402.
27a. McGrath PJ, Develoer LL, Hearn MJ. Multidimensional pain assessment in children. Adv Pain Res Ther 1985 (b); 9: 387–393.
28. Grunau RVE, Craig KD. Pain expression in neonates: facial expression and cry. Pain 1987; 28:395–410.
29. Grunau RVE, Johnston CC, Craig KD. Neonatal facial and cry responses to invasive and non-invasive procedures. Pain 1990; 42:295–305.
30. McGrath PJ. Pain assessment in children – a practical approach. Adv Pain Res Ther 1990; 15:5–30.
31. Beyer JE. The Oucher: a user's manual and technical report. Evanston D, ed. Judson Press; 1984:1–13.

32. Maunuksela E-L, Olkkola KT, Korpela R. Measurement of pain in children with self-reporting and behavioral assessment. Clin Pharmacol Ther 1987; 42:137–141.
33. Bieri D, Reeve RA, Champion GD, et al. The faces pain scale for the self-assessment of the severity of pain experienced by children: development, initial validation, and preliminary investigation for ratio scale properties. Pain 1990; 41:139–150.
34. Hester NO. The preoperational child's reaction to immunization. Nurs Res 1979; 28:250–255.
35. Champion GD, Goodenough B, von Beyer CL, et al. Measurement of pain by self-report. In: Measurement of pain in infants and children. International Association for the Study of Pain; Seattle, 1996:123–160.
36. Morton NS. Development of a monitoring protocol for the safe use of opioids in children. Paediatr Anaesth 1993; 3:179–184.
37. Broadman LM, Rice LJ, Hannallah RS. Testing the validity of an objective pain scale for infants and children. Anesthesiology 1988; 69:A770.
38. Abu-Saad H. Assessing children's reponses to pain. Pain 1984; 19:163–171.
39. Beyer JE, Aradine CR. Patterns of pain intensity: a methodological investigation of a self-report scale. Clin J Pain 1987; 3:130–141.
40. Cook B, Grubb DJ, Aldridge LA, et al. Comparison of the effects of adrenaline, clonidine and ketamine on the duration of caudal analgesia produced by bupivacaine in children. Br J Anaesth 1995; 75:698–701.
41. Chambers CT, Giesbrecht K, Craig KD, et al. A comparison of faces scales for the measurement of pediatric pain: children's and parents' ratings. Pain 1999; 83:25–35.
42. Nolan J, Chalkiadis GA, Low J, et al. Anaesthesia and pain management in cerebral palsy. Anaesthesia 2000; 55:32–41.
43. McGrath PJ, Rosmus C, Canfield C, et al. Behaviors caregivers use to determine pain in non-verbal, cognitively impaired individuals. Dev Med Child Neurol 1998; 40:340–343.
44. Lloyd-Thomas AR, Howard RF. A pain service for children. Paediatr Anaesth 1994; 4:3–15.
45. Brenn BR, Rose JB. Pediatric pain services: monitoring for epidural analgesia in the non-intensive care unit setting. Anesthesiology 1995; 83:432.
46. Association of Anaesthetists of Great Britain and Ireland, London, 1999. Information and consent for anaesthesia.
47. Rumack BH. Aspirin versus acetaminophen: a comparative view. Pediatrics 1978; 62:943–946.
48. Kelley MT, Walson PD, Edge JH, et al. Pharmacokinetics and pharmacodynamics of ibuprofen isomers and acetaminophen in febrile children. Clin Pharmacol Ther 1992; 52:181–189.
49. Anderson B, Kanagasundarum S, Woollard G. Analgesic efficacy of paracetamol in children using tonsillectomy as a pain model. Anaesth Intens Care 1996; 24:669–673.
50. Hopkins CS, Underhill S, Booker PD. Pharmacokinetics of paracetamol after cardiac surgery. Arch Dis Child 1990; 65:971–976.
51. Watcha MF, Ruiz MR, White PF, et al. Perioperative effects of oral ketorolac and acetaminophen in children undergoing myringotomy. Can J Anaesth 1992; 39:649–654.
52. Tobias JD, Lowe S, Hersey S, et al. Analgesia after bilateral myringotomy and placement of pressure equalization tubes in children: acetaminophen versus acetaminophen with codeine. Anesth Analg 1995; 81:496–500.
53. Anderson BJ, Holford NHG. Rectal paracetamol dosing regimens: determination by computer simulation. Paediatr Anaesth 1997; 7:451–455.
54. Penna A, Buchanan N. Paracetamol poisoning in children and hepatotoxicity. Br J Clin Pharmacol 1991; 32:143–149.
55. Heubi JE, Barbacci MB, Zimmerman HJ. Therapeutic misadventures with acetaminophen: hepatotoxicity after multiple doses in children. J Pediatr1998; 132:22–27.
56. Alonso EM, Sokol RJ, Hart J, et al. Fulminant hepatitis associated with centrilobular hepatic necrosis in young children. J Pediatr 1995; 127:888–894.
57. Morton NS, Arana A. Paracetamol-induced fulminant hepatic failure in a child after 5 days of therapeutic doses. Paediatr Anaesth 1999; 9:463–465.
58. Riviera-Penara T, Gugig R, Davis J, et al. Outcome of acetaminophen overdose in pediatric patients and factors contributing to hepatotoxicity. J Pediatr 1997; 130:300–304.
59. Blake KV, Bailey D, Zientek GM, et al. Death of a child associated with multiple overdoses of acetaminophen. Clin Pharm 1988; 7:391–397.
60. Anderson BJ, Rees SG, Liley A et al. Effect of preoperative paracetamol on gastric volumes and pH in children. Paediatr Anaesth 1999; 9:203–207.
61. Nahata MC, Powel DA. Kinetics of acetaminophen (Ac) following single strength (SS-Ac) vs double strength (DS-Ac) administration to febrile children. Clin Res 1982; 30:634A.
62. Cullen S, Kenny D, Ward OC, Sabra K. Paracetamol suppositories: a comparative study. Arch Dis Child 1989; 64:1504–1505.

63. Montgomery CJ, McCormack JP, Reichart CC et al. Plasma concentrations after high-dose (45 mg/kg) rectal acetiminophen in children. Can J Anaesth 1995; 42:982–986.

64. Birmingham PK; Tobin MJ, Fanta KB, et al. 24 hour pharmacokinetics of rectal acetaminophen in children: an old drug with new recommendations. Anesthesiology 1995; 83:A1127.

65. Anderson BJ, Woollard G, Holford NHG. Pharmacokinetics of rectal paracetamol after major surgery in children. Paediatr Anaesth 1995; 5:237–242.

65a. Shann F. Paracetamol: when, why and how much? J Pediatr Child Health 1993; 29:84–85.

66. Houck CS, Sullivan LJ, Wilder RT, et al. Pharmacokinetics of a higher dose of rectal acetaminophen in children. Anesthesiology 1995; 83:A1126.

67. Gaudreault P, Guay J, Nicol O, et al. Pharmacokinetics and clinical efficacy of intrarectal solution of acetaminophen. Can J Anaesth 1988; 35:149–152.

68. Anderson BJ; Holford NHG; Woollard G. Paracetamol kinetics in neonates. Anaesth Intens Care 1997; 25:721–722.

69. Lin Y-C, Sussman HH, Benitz WE. Plasma concentrations after rectal administration in preterm neonates. Paediatr Anaesth 1997; 7:457–459.

70. van Lingen RA, Deinum JT, Quak JME, et al. Pharmcokinetics and metabolism of rectally administered paracetamol in preterm neonates. Arch Dis Child 1999; 80:F59–F63.

71. Miller RP, Roberts RJ, Fischer LJ. Acetaminophen elimination kinetics in neonates, children, and adults. Clin Pharmacol Ther 1976; 19:284–294.

72. Autret E, Duterte J-P, Breteau M, et al. Pharmacokinetics of paracetamol in the neonate and infant after administration of proparacetamol chlorhydrate. Dev Pharmacol Ther 1993; 20:129–134.

73. Granry JC, Rod B, Monrigal JP, et al. The analgesic efficacy of an injectable prodrug of acetaminophen in children after orthopaedic surgery. Paediatr Anaesth 1997; 7:445–449.

74. Souter AJ, Fredman B, White PF. Controversies in the perioperative use of nonsteroidal antiinflammatory drugs. Anesth Analg 1994; 79:1178–1190.

75. Moores MA, Wandless JG, Fell D. Paediatric postoperative analgesia. A comparison of rectal diclofenac with caudal bupivacaine after inguinal herniotomy. Anaesthesia 1990; 45:156–158.

75a. Baer GA, Rorarius MG, Kolehmainen S, et al. The effect of paracetamol or diclofenac administered before operation on postoperative pain and behaviour after adenoidectomy in small children. Anaesthesia 1992; 47 (12): 1078–1080.

76. McGowan, May H, Molnar Z, et al. A comparison of three methods of analgesia in children having day case circumcision. Paediatr Anaesth 1998; 8:403–407.

77. Mannion D, Armstrong C, O'Leary G, et al. Paediatric post orchidopexy analgesia – effect of diclofenac combined with ilioinguinal/iliohypogastric nerve block. Paediatr Anaesth 1994; 4: 327–330.

78. Gadiyer V, Gallagher TM, Crean PM, et al. The effect of a combination of rectal diclofenac and caudal bupivacaine on postoperative analgesia in children. Anaesthesia 1995; 50: 820–822.

79. Bone ME, Fell D. A comparison of rectal diclofenac with intramuscular papaveretum or placebo for pain relief following tonsillectomy. Anaesthesia 1988; 43:277–280.

80. Watters CH, Patterson CC, Mathews HML, et al. Diclofenac sodium for post-tonsillectomy pain in children. Anaesthesia 1988; 43:641–643.

81. Munro HM, Riegger LQ, Reynolds PR et al. Comparison of the analgesic and emetic properties of ketorolac and morphine for paediatric outpatient strabismus surgery. Br J Anaesth 1994; 72:624–628.

82. Maunuksela E-L, Olkkola KT, Korpela R. Does prophylactic intravenous infusion of indomethecin improve the management of postoperative pain in children? Can J Anaesth 1988; 35:123–127.

83. Maunuksela E-L, Ryhanen P, Janhunen L. Efficacy of rectal ibuprofen in controlling postoperative pain in children. Can J Anaesth 1992; 39:226–230.

84. Kokki H, Hendolin H, Maunuksela E-L et al. Ibuprofen in the treatment of postoperative pain in small children. A randomized double-blind-placebo controlled parallel study group. Acta Anaesthesiol Scand 1994; 38:467–472.

85. Teiria H, Meretoja OA. PCA in paediatric orthopaedic patients: influence of a NSAID on morphine requirement. Paediatr Anaesth 1994; 4:87–91.

86. Sims C, Johnson CM, Bergesio R, et al. Rectal indomethacin for analgesia after appendicectomy in children. Anaesth Intens Care 1994; 22:272–275.

87. Mendel HG, Guarnieri KM, Sundt LM, et al. The effects of ketorolac and fentanyl on postoperative vomiting and analgesic requirements in children undergoing strabismus surgery. Anesth Analg 1995; 80:1129–1133.

88. Sutherland CJ, Montgomery JE, Kestin IG. A comparison of intramuscular tenoxicam with intramuscular morphine for pain relief following tonsillectomy in children. Paediatr Anaesth 1998; 8:321–324.

89. Thiagarajan J, Bates S, Hitchcock M, et al. Blood loss following tonsillectomy in children. A blind comparison of diclofenac and papaveretum. Anaesthesia 1993; 47:132–135.

90. Rusy LM, Houck CS, Sullivan LJ, et al.. A double-blind evaluation of ketorolac tromethamine versus acetaminophen in pediatric tonsillectomy: analgesia and bleeding. Anesth Analg 1995; 80:226–229.

91. Gallagher JE, Blauth J, Fornadley JA. Perioperative ketorolac tromethamine and postoperative hemorrhage in cases of tonsillectomy and adenoidectomy. Laryngoscope 1995; 105:606–609.

92. Gunter JB, Varughese AM, Harrington JF, et al. Recovery and complications after tonsillectomy in children: a comparison of ketorolac and morphine. Anesth Analg 1995; 81:1136–1141.

93. Short JA, Barr CA, Palmer CD, et al. Use of diclofenac in children with asthma. Anaesthesia 2000; 55:334–337.

94. Royal College of Anaesthetists. Guidelines for the use of non-steroidal anti-inflamatory drugs in the perioperative period. London: Royal College of Anaesthetists; 1998.

95. Morton NS, Benham SW, Lawson RA, et al. Diclofenac vs oxybuprocaine eyedrops for analgesia in paediatric strabismus surgery. Paediatr Anaesth 1997; 7:221–226.

96. Bridge HS, Montgomery CJ, Kennedy RA, et al. Analgesic efficacy of ketorolac 0.5% ophthalmic solution (Accular) in paediatric strabismus surgery. Paediatr Anaesth 2000; 10:521–526.

97. Wolf AR, Hughes D. Pain relief for infants undergoing abdominal surgery: comparison of infusions of I.V. morphine and extradural bupivacaine. Br J Anaesth 1993; 70:10–16.

97a. Wolf AR, Eyres RL, Laussen PC, et al. Effect of extradural analgesia on stress responses to abdominal surgery in infants. Br J Anaesth 1993; 70:654–660.

98. Lavies NG, Wandless JG. Subcutaneous morphine in children: taking the sting out of postoperative analgesia. Anaesthesia 1989; 44:1000–1001.

99. van Hoogdalem EJ, de Boer AG, Breimer DD. Pharmacokinetics of rectal drug administration, part I. General considerations and clinical applications of centrally acting drugs. Clin Pharmacokin 1991; 21:11–26.

100. Gourlay GK, Boas RA. Fatal outcome with use of rectal morphine for postoperative pain control in an infant. Br Med J 1992; 304:766–777.

101. McNicol LR. Postoperative analgesia in children using continuous s.c. morphine. Anaesthesia 1993; 71:752.

102. Bray RJ. Postoperative analgesia provided by morphine infusion in children. Anaesthesia 1983; 38:1075–1078.

103. Beasley SW, Tibbals J. Efficacy and safety of continuous morphine infusion for postoperative analgesia in the paediatric surgical ward. Aust NZ Surg 1987; 57:233–237.

104. Hendrickson M, Myre L, Johnson DG, et al. Postoperative analgesia in children: a prospective study of intermittent intramuscular injection versus continuous intravenous infusion of morphine. J Pediatr Surg 1990; 25:185–191.

105. Wolf AR, Lawson RA, Fisher S. Ventilatory arrest after a fluid challenge in a neonate receiving s.c. morphine. Br J Anaesth 1995; 75:787–789.

106. Tyler DC, Pomietto M, Womack W. Variation in opioid use during PCA in adolescents. Paediatr Anaesth 1996; 6:33–38.

107. Berde CB, Lehn BM, Yee JD, et al. Patient-controlled analgesia in children and adolescents: a randomized, prospective comparison with intramuscular administration of morphine for postoperative analgesia. J Pediatr 1991; 118:460–466.

108. Bray RJ, Woodhams AM, Vallis CJ, et al. A double-blind comparison of morphine infusion and patient controlled analgesia in children. Paediatr Anaesth 1996; 6:121–127.

109. Rodgers BM, Webb CJ, Stergios D, et al. Patient-controlled analgesia in pediatric surgery. J Pediatr Surg 1988; 23:259–262.

110. Gaukroger PB, Tomkins DP, van der Walt JH. Patient-controlled analgesia in children. Anaesth Intens Care 1989; 17:264–268.

111. Lawrie SC, Forbes DW, Akhtar TM, et al. Patient-controlled analgesia in children. Anaesthesia 1990; 46:1074–1076.

112. Irwin M, Gillespie JA, Morton NS. Evaluation of a disposable patient-controlled analgesia device in children. Br J Anaesth 1992; 68:411–413.

113. Skues MA, Watson DM, O'Meara M, et al. Patient-controlled analgesia in children. A comparison of two infusion techniques. Paediatr Anaesth 1993; 3:223–228.

114. Doyle E, Harper I, Morton NS. Patient-controlled analgesia with low dose background infusions after lower abdominal surgery in children. Br J Anaesth 1993; 71:818–822.

115. Doyle E, Mottart KJ, Marshall C, et al. Comparison of different bolus doses of morphine for patient controlled analgesia in children. Br J Anaesth 1994; 72:160–163.

116. Doyle E, Morton NS, McNicol LR. Comparison of patient-controlled analgesia in children by i.v. and s.c. routes of administration. Br J Anaesth 1994; 72:533–536.

117. Doyle E, Robinson D, Morton NS. Comparison of patient-controlled analgesia with and without a background infusion after lower abdominal surgery in children. Br J Anaesth 1993; 71:670–673.

118. Owen H, Szekely SM, Plummer JL, et al. Variables of patient-controlled analgesia 2. Concurrent infusion. Anaesthesia 1989; 44:11–13.

119. Broadman LM, Rice LJ, Vaughan M, et al. Parent-assisted 'PCA' for postoperative pain control in young children. Anesth Analg 1990; 70:S34.

120. Weldon BC, Connor M, White PF. Nurse-controlled vs patient-controlled analgesia following pediatric scoliosis surgery. Anesthesiology 1991; 75:A935.

121. Stack CG, Massey NJ, Mathew AJ. Bradypnoea during patient-controlled analgesia. Anaesthesia 1990; 45:683–684.

122. de Armendi AJ, Fahey M, Ryan JF. Morphine-induced myoclonic movements in a pediatric pain patient. Anesth Analg 1993; 77:191–192.

123. Koren G, Butt W, Chinyanga H et al. Postoperative morphine infusion in newborn infants: assessment of disposition, characteristics and safety. J Pediatr 1985; 107:963–967.

124. Bhat R, Chari G, Gulati A, et al. Pharmacokinetics of a single dose of morphine in preterm infants during the first week of life. J Pediatr 1990; 117:477–481.

125. Lynn AM, McRorie TI, Slattery JT, et al. Age-dependent morphine partitioning between plasma and cerebrospinal fluid in monkeys. Dev Pharmacol Ther 1991; 17:200–204.

126. Lynn AM, Slattery JT. Morphine pharmacokinetics in early infancy. Anesthesiology 1987; 66:138–139.

127. McRorie TI, Lynn AM, Nespeca MK, et al. The maturation of morphine clearance and metabolism. Am J Dis Child 1992; 146:972–976.

128. Lynn AM, Nepesca MK, Opheim KE, Slattery JT. Respiratory effects of intravenous morphine infuions in neonates, infants, and children after cardiac surgery. Anesth Analg 1993; 77:695–701.

129. Semple D, Russell S, Doyle E, et al. Comparison of morphine sulphate and codeine phosphate in children undergoing adenotonsillectomy. Paediatr Anaesth 1999; 9:135–138.

130. Richtsmeier AJ, Barkin RL, Alexander M. Benzodiazepines for acute pain in children. J Pain Symptom Manage 1992; 7:492–495.

131. Geiduschek JM, Haberkern CM, McLaughlin JF, et al. Pain management for children following selective dorsal rhizotomy. Can J Anaesth 1994; 41:492–496.

132. Tree-Trakarn T, Pirayavaraporn S, Lertakyamanee J. Topical analgesia for relief of post-circumcision pain. Anesthesiology 1987; 67:395–399.

133. Chambers FA, Lee J, Smith J, et al. Post-circumcision analgesia: comparison of topical analgesia with dorsal nerve block using the midline and lateral approaches. Br J Anaesth 1994; 73:437–439.

134. Andersen KH. A new method of analgesia for relief of circumcision pain. Anaesthesia 1989; 44:118–120.

135. Reid MF, Harris R, Phillips PD, et al. Day-case herniotomy in children. A comparison of ilio-inguinal nerve block and wound infiltration for postoperative analgesia. Anaesthesia 1987; 42:658–661.

136. Fell D, Derrington MC, Taylor E, et al. Paediatric postoperative analgesia. A comparison between caudal block and wound infiltration of local anaesthetic. Anaesthesia 1988; 43:107–110.

137. Casey WF, Rice LJ, Hannallah RS, et al. A comparison between bupivacaine instillation versus ilioinguinal/iliohypogastric nerve block for postoperative analgesia following inguinal herniorrhaphy in children. Anesthesiology 1990; 72:637–639.

138. Schindler M, Swann M, Crawford M. A comparison of postoperative analgesia provided by wound infiltration or caudal analgesia. Anaesth Intens Care 1991; 19:46–49.

139. Splinter WM, Bass J, Komocar L. Regional anaesthesia for hernia repair in children: local vs caudal anaesthesia. Report of investigation. Can J Anaesth 1995; 42:197–200.

140. Tobias JD. Postoperative analgesia and intraoperative inhalational anesthetic requirements during umbilical herniorrhaphy in children: postincisional local infiltration versus preincisional caudal epidural block. J Clin Anesth 1996; 8:634–638.

141. Rice LJ, Pudimat MA, Hannallah RS. Timing of caudal block placement in relation to surgery does not affect duration of postoperative analgesia in paediatric ambulatory patients. Can J Anaesth 1990; 37:429–431.

142. Holthusen H, Eichwede F, Stevens M, et al. Pre-emptive analgesia: comparison of preoperative with postoperative caudal block on postoperative pain in children. Br J Anaesth 1994; 73:440–442.

143. Yeoman PM, Cooke R, Hain WR et al. Penile block for circumcision? A comparison with caudal blockade. Anaesthesia 1983; 38: 862–866.

144. Vater M, Wandless J. Caudal or dorsal nerve block? A comparison of two local anaesthetic techniques for postoperative analgesia following day case circumcision. Acta Anaesthesiol Scand 1985; 29:175–179.

145. Markham SJ, Tomlinson J, Hain WR. Ilioinguinal nerve block in children. Anaesthesia 1986; 41:1098–1103.

146. Cross GD, Barrett RF. Comparison of two regional techniques for postoperative analgesia in children following herniotomy and orchidopexy. Anaesthesia 1987; 42:845–849.

147. Scott AD, Phillips A, White JB, et al. Analgesia following inguinal herniotomy or orchidopexy in children: a comparison of caudal and regional blockade. J R Coll Surg Edinburgh 1989; 34:143–145.

148. Bosenberg AT, Kimble FW. Infraorbital nerve blocks in neonates for cleft lip repair: anatomical study and clinical application. Br J Anaesth 1995; 74:506–550.

149. Brown TCK, Fisk GC. Regional and local anaesthesia. In: Anaesthesia for children, 2nd edn. Oxford: Blackwell Scientific Publications; 1992:315–316.
150. Kempthorne PM, Brown TCK. Nerve blocks around the knee in children. Anaesth Intens Care 1984; 12:14–17.
151. Konrad C, Johr M. Block of the sciatic nerve in the popliteal fossa: a system for standardization in children. Anesth Analg 1998; 83:1256–1258.
151a. Tobias JD, Mencio GA. Popliteal fossa block for post operative analgesia after foot surgery in infants and children. J Pediatr Orthop 1999; 19:511–514.
152. Dalens B, Vanneuville G, Tanguy A. Comparison of the fascia iliaca compartment block with the 3-in-1 block in children. Anesth Analg 1989; 69:705–713.
153. Cooper MG, Keneally JP, Kinchington D. Continuous brachial plexus neural blockade in a child with intractable cancer pain. J Pain Symptom Manage 1994; 9:277–281.
154. Tobias JD. Continuous femoral nerve block to provide analgesia following femur fracture in a paediatric ICU population. Anaesth Intens Care 1994; 22:616–618.
155. Cornish P, Anderson B, Chambers C. Continuous rectus sheath block analgesia for an infant with bronchopulmonary dysplasia. Paediatr Anaesth 1993; 3:191–192.
156. Paut O, Sallabery M, Schreiber-Deturmeny E et al. Continuous fascia iliaca compartment block in children: a prospective evaluation of plasma bupivacaine concentrations, pain scores, and side effects. Anesth Analg 2001; 92:1159–1163.
157. Shah R, Sabanathan S, Richardson J et al. Continuous paravertebral block for post thoracotomy analgesia in children. J Cardiovascular Surgery 1997; 38:543–546.
158. Tobias JD, Lowe S, O'Dell N, et al. Thoracic epidural anaesthesia in infants and children. Can J Anaesth 1993; 40:879–882.
159. Giaufre E, Dalens B, Gombart A. Epidemiology and morbidity of regional anesthesia in children: a one-year prospective survey of the French-Language Society of Pediatric Anesthesiologists. Anesth Analg 1996; 83:904–912.
160. Bosenberg AT. Lower limb nerve blocks in children using unsheathed needles and a nerve stimulator. Anaesthesia 1995; 50:206–210.
161. Dalens B, Tanguy A, Vanneuville G. Sciatic nerve blocks in children: comparison of the posterior, anterior, and lateral approaches in 180 pediatric patients. Anesth Analg 1990; 70:131–137.
162. Ecoffey C, Dubousset A-M, Samii K. Lumbar and thoracic epidural anesthesia for urological and upper abdominal surgery in infants and children. Anesthesiology 1986; 65:87–90.
163. Murat I, Delleur MM, Esteve C, et al. Continuous extradural anaesthesia in children. Clinical and haemodynamic implications. Br J Anaesth 1987; 69:1441–1450.
164. Stow PJ, Scott A, Phillips A, et al. Plasma bupivacaine concentrations during caudal analgesia and ilioinguinal–iliohypogastric nerve block in children. Anaesthesia 1988; 43:650–653.
165. Veyckemans F, van Obbergh LJ, Gouverneur JM. Lessons from 1100 pediatric caudal blocks in a teaching hospital. Reg Anesth 1992; 17:119–125.
166. Dalens B, Hasnaoui A. Caudal anesthesia in pediatric surgery: success rate and adverse effects in 750 consecutive patients. Anesth Analg 1989; 68:83–89.
167. Desparmet J, Mateo J, Ecoffey C, et al. Efficacy of an epidural test dose in children anesthetized with halothane. Anesthesiology 1990, 72.249–251.
168. Newman PJ, Bushnell TG, Radford P. The effect of needle size and type in paediatric caudal analgesia. Paediatr Anaesth 1996; 6:459–461.
169. Breschan C, Schalk HV, Schaumberger F, et al. Experience with caudal blocks in children over a period of 3.5 years. Acta Anaesthesiol Scand 1996; 109:174–176.
170. Busoni P, Sarti A. Sacral intervertebral epidural block. Anesthesiology 1987; 67:993–995.
171. Dalens B, Tanguy A, Haberer J-P. Lumbar epidural anesthesia for operative and postoperative pain relief in infants and young children. Anesth Analg 1986; 65:1069–1073.
172. Meignier M, Souron R, Le Neel J-C. Postoperative dorsal epidural analgesia in the child with respiratory disabilities. Anesthesiology 1983; 59:473–475.
173. Bosenberg AT, Hadley GP, Wiersma R. Oesophageal atresia: caudo-thoracic epidural anaesthesia reduces the need for postoperative ventilatory support. Paediatr Surg Int 1992; 7:289–291.
174. McNeely JK, Farber NE, Rusy LM, et al. Epidural analgesia improves outcome following pediatric fundoplication. Reg Anesth 1997; 22:16–23.
175. Wilson GA, Brown JL, Crabbe DG et al. Is epidural analgesia associated with an improved outcome following open Nissen fundoplication? Paed Anesth 2001; 11:65–70.
176. Dalens B, Chrysostome Y. Intervertebral epidural anaesthesia in paediatric surgery: success rate and adverse effects in 650 consecutive procedures. Paediatr Anaesth 1991; 1:107–117.
177. Wilson PTJ, Lloyd-Thomas AR. An audit of extradural infusion analgesia in children using bupivacaine and diamorphine. Anaesthesia 1993; 48:718–723.
178. Sage FJ, Lloyd Thomas AR, Howard RF. Paediatric lumbar epidurals: a comparison of 21-G and 23-G catheters in patients weighing less than 10kg. Paed Anaesth 2000; 10:279–282.

179. van Niekerk J, Bax-Vermeire BMJ, Geurts JWM, et al. Epidurography in premature infants. Anaesthesia 1990; 45:722–725.

180. Tsui BCH, Seal R, Koller J et al. Thoracic epidural analgesia via the caudal approach in pediatric patients undergoing fundoplication using nerve stimulation guidance. Anesth Analg 2001; 93:1152–1155.

181. Attia J, Ecoffey C, Sandouk P, et al. Epidural morphine in children: pharmacokinetics and CO_2 sensitivity. Anesthesiology 1986; 65:590–594.

182. Ecoffey C, Desparmet J, Maury M, et al. Bupivacaine in children: pharmacokinetics following caudal anesthesia. Anesthesiology 1985; 63:447–448.

183. Messeri A, Romiti M, Andreucetti T, et al. Continuous epidural block for pain control in bladder exstrophy: report of a case and description of technique. Paediatr Anaesth 1995; 5:229–232.

184. Blanco D, Llamazares J, Rincon R, et al. Thoracic epidural anesthesia via the lumbar approach in infants and children. Anesthesiology 1996; 84:1312–1316.

185. Guinard J-P, Borboen M. Probable venous air embolism during caudal anesthesia in a child. Anesth Analg 1993; 76:1134–1135.

186. Schwartz N, Eisenkraft JB. Probable venous air embolism during epidural placement in an infant. Anesth Analg 1993; 76:1136–1138.

187. Dalens B, Bazin J E, Haberer J P. Epidural bubbles as a cause of incomplete analgesia during epidural anesthesia. Anesth Analg 1987; 66:679–683.

188. Flandin-Blety C, Barrier G. Accidents following extradural analgesia in children. The results of a retrospective study. Paediatr Anaesth 1995; 5:41–46.

189. Sethna NF, Berde CB. Venous air embolism during identification of the epidural space in children. Anesth Analg 1993; 76:925–927.

190. Bosenberg AT, Bland BAR, Schulte-Steinberg O, et al. Thoracic epidural anesthesia via the caudal route in infants. Anesthesiology 1988; 69:265–269.

191. Rasch DK, Webster DE, Pollard TG, et al. Lumbar and thoracic epidural analgesia via the caudal approach for postoperative pain relief in infants and children. Can J Anaesth 1990; 37:359–362.

192. Gunter JB, Eng C. Thoracic epidural anesthesia via the caudal approach in children. Anesthesiology 1992; 76:935–938.

193. Luz G, Innerhofer P, Bachmann B, et al. Bupivacaine plasma concentrations during continuous epidural anesthesia in infants and children. Anesth Analg 1996; 82:231–234.

194. Pietropaoli JA, Keller MS, Smail DF, et al. Regional anesthesia in pediatric surgery: complications and postoperative comfort level in 174 children. J Pediatr Surg 1993; 28:560–564.

195. Strafford M, Wilder RT, Berde CB. The risk of infection from epidural analgesia in children: a review of 1620 cases. Anesth Analg 1995; 80:234.

195a. McNeely JK, Trentadue NC, Rusy LM, Farber NE. Culture of bacteria from lumbar and caudal epidural catheters used for postoperative analgesia in children. Regional Anesthesia 1997; 22: 428–431.

196. Busoni P, Messeri A. Spinal anesthesia in children: surface anatomy. Anesth Analg 1989; 68:418–419.

197. Bosenberg AT, Gouws E. Skin–epidural distance in children. Anaesthesia 1995; 50:895–897.

198. Hasan MA, Howard RF, Lloyd-Thomas AR. Depth of epidural space in children. Anaesthesia 1994; 49:1085–1087.

199. Shapiro LA, Jedeikin RJ, Shalev D, et al. Epidural morphine analgesia in children. Anesthesiology 1984; 61:210–212.

200. Desparmet J, Meistelman C, Barre J, et al. Continuous epidural infusion of bupivacaine for postoperative pain relief in children. Anesthesiology 1987; 67:108–110.

201. Caudle CL, Freid EB, Bailey AG, et al. Epidural fentanyl infusion with patient-controlled epidural analgesia for postoperative analgesia in children. J Pediatr Surg 1993; 28:554–559.

202. Larsson BA, Olsson GL, Lonnqvist PA. Plasma concentrations of bupivacaine in young infants after continuous epidural infusion. Paediatr Anaesth 1994; 4:159–162.

203. Berde C. Epidural analgesia in children. Can J Anaesth 1994; 41:555–560.

204. Vas L, Naregal P, Sanzgiri S, et al. Some vagaries of neonatal lumbar anaesthesia. Paediatr Anaesth 1999; 9:217–223.

205. Blomberg RG, Jaanivald A, Walther S. Advantages of the paramedian approach for lumbar epidural analgesia with catheter technique. A clinical comparison between midline and paramedian approaches. Anaesthesia 1989; 44:742–746.

206. Broadman LM, Hannallah RS, Norden JM, et al. 'Kiddie caudals': experience with 1154 consecutive cases without complications. Anesth Analg 1987; 66:S18.

207. Lumb AB, Carli F. Respiratory arrest after a caudal injection of bupivacaine. Anaesthesia 1989; 44:324–325.

208. Afshan G, Khan FA. Total spinal anaesthesia following caudal block with bupivacaine and buprenorphine. Paediatr Anaesth 1996; 6:239–242.

209. Bolder PM. Postlumbar puncture headache in pediatric oncology patients. Anesthesiology 1986; 65:696–698.

210. Fernbach DJ. Headache after lumbar puncture. Lancet 1981; 2:529.

211. Wee LH, Lam F, Cranston AJ. The incidence of post dural puncture headache in children. Anaesthesia 1996; 51:1164–1166.
212. Kokki H, Salonvaara M, Herrgard E, et al. Postdural puncture headache is not an age related symptom in children: a prospective, open-randomized, parallel group study comparing a 22-gauge Quincke with a 22-gauge Whitacre needle. Paediatr Anaesth 1999; 9:429–434.
213. Ghia JN, Spielman FJ, Stieber SF. The diagnosis and successful treatment of post-lumbar puncture headache in a pediatric patient. Reg Anesth 1984; 9:102–105.
214. McHale J, O'Donovan FC. Postdural puncture symtoms in a child. Anaesthesia 1997; 52:684–694.
215. Roy L, Vischoff D, Lavoie J. Epidural blood patch in a seven-year-old child. Can J Anaesth 1995; 42:621–624.
216. Wolf AR, Walker SM. Development of a high block in an infant during an epidural bupivacaine infusion. Anaesth Intens Care 1991; 19:583–586.
217. Ved SA, Pinosky M, Nicodemus H. Ventricular tachycardia and brief cardiovascular collapse in two infants after caudal anesthesia using a bupivacaine–epinephrine solution. Anesthesiology 1993; 5:1121–1123.
218. Fisher QA, Shaffner DH, Yaster M. Detection of intravascular injection of regional anaesthetics in children. Can J Anaesth 1997; 44:592–598.
219. Dickson MAS, Doyle E. The intravacular migration of an epidural catheter. Paediatr Anaesth 1999; 9:273–275.
220. Finkel JC. The epidural dorsomedian septum as a possible cause for unilateral epidural anaesthesia in an infant. Paediatr Anaesth 1999; 9:456–459.
221. Wood CE, Goresky GV, Klassen KA, et al. Complications of continuous epidural infusions for postoperative analgesia in children. Can J Anaesth 1994; 41:613–620.
222. Schulte-Steinberg O, Rahlfs VW. Spread of extradural analgesia following caudal injection in children. Br J Anaesth 1977; 49:1027–1033.
223. Takasaki M, Dohi S, Kawabata Y, et al. Dosage of lidocaine for caudal anesthesia in infants and children. Anesthesiology 1977; 47:527–529.
224. Busoni P, Andreuccetti T. The spread of caudal analgesia in children: a mathematical model. Anaesth Intens Care 1986; 14:140–144.
225. Armitage EN. Regional anaesthesia. In: Sumner E, Hatch D, eds. Textbook of paediatric anaesthetic practice. London: Baillière Tindall; 1989:217.
226. Spear RM. Dose–response in infants receiving caudal anaesthesia with bupivacaine. Paediatr Anaesth 1991; 1:47–52.
227. Khalil S, Campos C, Farag AM, et al. Caudal block in children: ropivacaine compared with bupivacaine. Anesthesiology 1999; 91:1279–1284.
228. Wolf AR, Valley RD, Fear DW, et al. Bupivacaine for caudal analgesia in infants and children: the optimal effective concentration. Anesthesiology 1988; 69:102–106.
229. Joshi W, Connelly NR, Dwyer M, et al. A comparison of two concentrations of bupivacaine and adrenaline with and without fentanyl in paeditric inguinal herniorrhaphy. Paediatr Anaesth 1999; 9:317–320.
230. Gunter JB, Dunn CM, Bennie JB, et al. Optimum concentration of bupivacaine for combined caudal–general anaesthesia in children. Anesthesiology 1991; 75:57–61.
231. Fisher QA, McComisky CM, Carmel M, et al. Postoperative voiding interval and duration of analgesia following peripheral or caudal nerve blocks in children. Anesth Analg 1993; 76:173–177.
232. Eyres RL, Bishop W, Oppenheim RC, et al. Plasma bupivacaine concentrations in children during caudal epidural analgesia. Anaesth Intens Care 1983; 11:20–22.
233. Mazoit JX, Souron R, le Neel J-C. Pharmacokinetics of bupivacaine following caudal anesthesia in infants. Anesthesiology 1988; 68:387–391.
234. Larsson BA, Lonnqvist PA, Olsson GL. Plasma concentrations of bupivacaine in neonates after continuous epidural infusion. Anesth Analg 1997; 84:501–505.
235. Berde CB. Convulsions associated with pediatric regional anesthesia. Anesth Analg 1992; 75:164–166.
236. Berde C. Bupivacaine toxicity secondary to continuous caudal epidural infusion in children. Anesth Analg 1993; 77;1305–1306.
237. Agarwal R, Gutlove DP, Lockhart CH. Seizures occurring in paediatric patients receiving continuous infusion of bupivacaine. Anesth Analg 1992; 75:284–286.
238. McClosky JJ, Haun SE, Deshpande JK. Bupivacaine toxicity secondary to continuous caudal epidural infusion in children. Anesth Analg 1992; 75:287–290.
239. Maxwell LG, Martin LD, Yaster M. Bupivacaine-induced cardiac toxicity in neonates: successful treatment with intravenous phenytoin. Anesthesiology 1994; 80:682–686.
240. Freid EB, Bailey AG, Valley RD. Electrocardiographic and hemodynamic changes associated with unintentional intravascular injection of bupivacaine with epinephrine in infants. Anesthesiology 1993; 79:394–398.
241. Berde C. Regional anesthesia in children: what have we learned? Anesth Analg 1996; 83:897–890.

242. Koinig H, Krenn CG, Glaser C, et al. The dose–response of caudal ropivacaine in children. Anesthesiology 1999; 90:1339–1344.

243. Habre W, Bergesio R, Johnson C, et al. Pharmacokinetics of ropivacaine following caudal analgesia in children. Paediatr Anaesth 2000; 10:143–147.

244. Ala–Kokki TI, Partenen A, Karinen J, et al. Pharmacokinetics of 0.2% ropivacaine and 0.2% bupivacaine following caudal blocks in children. Acta Anaesthesiol Scand 2000; 44:1099–1102.

245. Ivani G, Mereto N, Lampugnani E et al. Ropivacaine in paediatric surgery: preliminary results. Paediatr Anaesth 1998; 8:127–129.

245a. Ivani G, Bergendahl HTG, Lampugnani E, Eksborg S et al. Plasma levels of clonidine following epidural bolus injection in children. Acta Anaesthesiologica Scandinavica 1998; 42:306–311.

246. Da Conceicao MJ, Coelho L, Khalil M. Ropivacaine 0.25% compared with bupivacaine 0.25% by the caudal route. Paediatr Anaesth 1999; 9:229–233.

247. Da Conceicao MJ, Coelho L. Caudal anaesthesia with 0.375% ropivacaine or 0.375% bupivacaine in paediatric patients. Br J Anaesth 1998; 80:507–508.

248. Luz G, Innerhofer P, Haussler B, et al. Comparison of ropivacaine 0.1% and 0.2% with bupivacaine 0.2% for single-shot caudal anaesthesia in children. Paediatr Anaesth 2000; 10:499–504.

249. Warner MA, Kunkel SE, Offord KO, et al. The effects of age, epinephrine, and operative site on duration of caudal analgesia in pediatric patients. Anesth Analg 1987; 66:995–998.

250. Jamali S, Monin S, Begon C, et al. Clonidine in pediatric caudal anesthesia. Anesth Analg 1994; 78:663–666.

251. Jensen BH. Caudal block for postoperative pain relief in children after genital operations. A comparison between bupivacaine and morphine. Acta Anaesthesiol Scand 1981; 25:373–375.

252. Glenski JA, Warner MA, Dawson B, et al. Postoperative use of epidurally administered morphine in children and adolescents. Mayo Clin Proc 1984; 59:530–533.

253. Krane EJ, Jacobson LE, Lynn AM, et al. Caudal morphine for postoperative analgesia in children: a comparison with caudal bupivacaine and intravenous morphine. Anesth Analg 1987; 66:647–653.

254. Parkinson SK, Porter CT, Little WL, et al. The use of continuous epidural morphine infusions in small children: a report of two cases. Reg Anesth 1989; 14:152–154.

255. Krane EJ. Delayed respiratory depression in a child after caudal epidural morphine. Anesth Analg 1988; 67:79–82.

256. Amaranath L, Andrish JT, Gurd AR, et al. Efficacy of intermittent epidural morphine following posterior spinal fusion in children and adolescents. Clin Orthop Rel Res 1989; 249:223–226.

257. Rosen KR, Rosen DA. Caudal epidural morphine for control of pain following open heart surgery in children. Anesthesiology 1989; 70:418–421.

258. Wolf AR, Hughes D, Hobbs AJ, et al. Combined morphine–bupivacaine caudals for reconstructive penile surgery in children: systemic absorption of morphine and postoperative analgesia. Anaesth Intens Care 1990; 19:17–21.

259. Jones RDM, Gunawardene WM, Yeung CK. A comparison of lignocaine 2% with adrenaline 1:200 000 and lignocaine 2% with adrenaline 1:200 000 plus fentanyl as agents for caudal anaesthesia in children undergoing circumcision. Anaesth Intens Care 1990; 18:194–199.

260. Wolf AR, Hughes D, Wade A, et al. Postoperative analgesia after paediatric orchidopexy: evaluation of a bupivacaine–morphine mixture. Br J Anaesth 1991; 64:430–435.

261. Valley RD, Bailey AG. Caudal morphine for postoperative analgesia in infants and children: a report of 138 cases. Anesth Analg 1991; 72:120–124.

262. Irving GA, Butt AD, van der Veen B. A comparison of caudal morphine given pre- or post-surgery for postoperative analgesia in children. Paediatr Anaesth 1993; 3: 217–221.

263. Lejus C, Roussiere G, Testa S, et al. Postoperative extradural analgesia in children: comparison of morphine with fentanyl. Br J Anaesth 1994; 72:156–159.

264. Bailey AG, Valley RD, Freid EB, et al. Epidural morphine combined with epidural or intravenous butorphanol for postoperative analgesia in pediatric patients. Anesth Analg 1994; 79:340–344.

265. Mayhew JF, Brodsky RC, Blakey D, et al. Low-dose caudal morphine for postoperative analgesia in infants and children: a report of 500 cases. J Clin Anaesth 1995; 7:640–642.

266. Kelleher AA, Black A, Penman S, et al. Comparison of caudal bupivacaine and diamorphine with caudal bupivacaine alone for repair of hypospadias. Br J Anaesth 1996; 77:586–590.

267. Haberkern CM, Lynn AM, Geiduschek JM, et al. Epidural and intravenous bolus morphine for postoperative analgesia in infants. Can J Anesth 1996; 43:1203–1210.

268. Kundra P, Deepalakshmi K, Ravishankar M. Preemptive caudal bupivacaine and morphine for postoperative analgesia in children. Anesth Analg 1998; 87:52–56.

269. Krane EJ, Tyler DC, Jacobson LE. The dose response of caudal morphine in children. Anesthesiology 1989; 71:48–52.

270. Kart T, Christrup LL, Rasmussen M. Recommended use of morphine in neonates, infants and children based on a literature review: part 2 – clinical use. Paediatr Anaesth 1997; 7:93–101.

271. Vila R, Miguel E, Montferrer N, et al. Respiratory depression following epidural morphine in an infant of three months of age. Paediatr Anaesth 1997; 7:61–64.
272. Rose JB, Francis MC, Kettrick RG. Continuous naloxone infusion in paediatric patients with pruritus associated with epidural morphine. Paediatr Anaesth 1993; 3:255–258.
273. Campbell FA, Yentis SM, Fear DW, et al. Analgesic efficacy and safety of a caudal bupivacaine–fentanyl mixture in children. Can J Anaesth 1992; 39:661–664.
274. Santhosh Kumar TP, Jacob R. A comparison of caudal epidural bupivacaine with adrenaline and bupivacaine with adrenaline and pethidine for operative and postoperative analgesia in infants and children. Anaesthesia and Intensive Care 1993; 21:424–428.
275. Nishina K, Mikawa K, Shiga M, et al. Clonidine in paediatric anaesthesia. Paediatr Anaesth 1999; 9:187–202.
276. Lee JJ, Rubin AP. Comparison of a bupivacaine–clonidine mixture with plain bupivacaine for caudal analgesia in children. Br J Anaesth 1994; 72:258–262.
277. Klimscha W, Chiari A, Michalek-Sauberer A, et al. The efficacy and safety of a clonidine/bupivacaine combination in caudal blockade for pediatric hernia repair. Anesth Analg 1998; 86:54–61.
278. Ivani G, De Negri P, Conio A, et al. Ropivacaine–clonidine combination for caudal blockade in children. Acta Anaesthesiol Scand 2000; 44:446–449.
279. Dupeyrat A, Goujard E, Muret J, et al. Transcutaneous CO_2 tension effects of clonidine in paediatric caudal analgesia. Paediatr Anesth 1998; 8:145–148.
280. Luz G, Innerhofer P, Oswald E, et al. Comparison of clonidine 1 μg.kg^{-1} with morphine 30 μg.kg^{-1} for post-operative caudal analgesia in children. Eur J Anaesthesiol 1999; 16:42–46.
281. Motsch J, Bottiger BW, Bohrer H, et al. Caudal bupivacaine for combined epidural and general anaesthesia in children. Acta Anaesthesiol Scand 1997; 41:877–883.
282. Ivani G, Mattioli G, Rega M, et al. Clonidine–mepivacaine mixture vs plain mepivacaine in paediatric surgery. Paediatr Anaesth 1996; 6:111–114.
283. Breschan C, Krumpholz R, Likar R, et al. Can a dose of 2 μg.kg^{-1} caudal clonidine cause respiratory depression in a neonate. Paediatr Anaesth 1999; 9:81–83.
284. Cook B, Doyle E. The use of additives to local anaesthetic solutions for caudal epidural blockade. Pediatr Anaesth 1996; 6:353–359.
285. Marhofer P, Krenn CG, Plochl W, et al. S(+)-ketamine for caudal block in paediatric anaesthesia. Br J Anaesth 2000; 84:341–345.
286. Naguib M, Sharif AM, Seraj M, et al. Ketamine for caudal analgesia in children: comparison with caudal bupivacaine. Br J Anaesth 1991; 67:559–564.
287. Lee HM, Sanders GM. Caudal ropivacaine and ketamine for postoperative analgesia in children. Anaesthesia 2000; 55:806–810.
288. Semple D, Findlow D, Aldridge LM, et al. The optimal dose for caudal epidural blockade in children. Anaesthesia 1996; 51:1170–1172.
289. Findlow D, Aldridge LM, Doyle E. Comparison of caudal block using bupivacaine and ketamine with ilioinguinal nerve block for orchidopexy in children. Anaesthesia 1997; 52:1090–1113.
290. Johnston P, Findlow D, Aldridge LM, et al. The effect of ketamine on 0.25% and 0.125% bupivacaine for caudal epidural blockade in children. Paediatr Anaesth 1999; 9:31–34.
291. Naguib M, el Gammal M, Elhattab YS, et al. Midazolam for caudal analgesia in children: comparison with caudal bupivacaine. Can J Anaesth 1995; 42:758–764.
292. Gulec S, Buyukkidan B, Oral N, et al. Comparison of caudal bupivacaine, bupivacaine–morphine and bupivacaine–midazolam mixtures for postoperative analgesia in children. Eur J Anaesthesiol 1998; 15:161–165.
293. Goresky GV. The clinical utility of epidural midazolam for inguinal hernia repair in children. Can J Anaesth 1995; 42:755–757.
294. Bellamy CD, McDonnell FJ, Colclough GW et al. Epidural infusion/PCA for pain control in pediatric patients. Anesth Analg 1990; 70:S19.
295. Birmingham PK, Wheeler M, Suresh S, et al. Patient controlled epidural analgesia in children: can they do it? Anesthesiology 1998; 89:A1167.
295a. Williams JM, Stoddart PA, Williams SAR, Wolf AR. Post-operative recovery after inguinal herniotomy in ex-premature infants: comparison between sevoflurane and spinal anaesthesia. Br J Anaesth 2001; 86:366–371.
296. Abajian JC, Mellish RWP, Browne AF, et al. Spinal anesthesia for surgery in the high-risk infant. Anesth Analg 1984; 63:359–362.
297. Harnik EV, Hoy GR, Potolicchio S, et al. Spinal anesthesia in premature infants recovering from respiratory distress syndrome. Anesthesiology 1986; 64:95–99.
298. Mahe V, Ecoffey C. Spinal anesthesia with isobaric bupivacaine in infants. Anesthesiology 1988; 68:601–603.
299. Gallagher TM, Crean PM. Spinal anaesthesia in infants born prematurely. Anaesthesia 1989; 44:434–436.

300. Welborn LG, Rice LJ, Hannallah RS, et al. Postoperative apnea in former preterm infants: prospective comparison of spinal and general anesthesia. Anesthesiology 1990; 72:838–842.

301. Sartorelli KH, Abajian JC, Kreutz JM, et al. Improved outcome utilizing spinal anesthesia in high-risk infants. J Pediatr Surg 1992; 27:1022–1025.

302. Tobias JD, Deshpande JK, Wetzel RC, et al. Postoperative analgesia. Use of intrathecal morphine in children. Clin Pediatr 1990; 29:44–48.

303. Krechel SW, Helikson MA, Kittle D, et al. Intrathecal morphine (ITM) for postoperative pain control in children: a comparison with nalbuphine patient controlled analgesia (PCA). Paediatr Anaesth 1995; 5:177–183.

304. Jones SEF, Beasley JM, MacFarlane DWR, et al. Intrathecal morphine for postoperative pain relief in children. Br J Anaesth 1984; 56:137–140.

305. Dalens B, Tanguy A. Intrathecal morphine for spinal fusion in children. Spine 1988; 13:494–498.

306. Goodarzi M. The advantages of intrathecal opioids for spinal fusion in children. Paediatr Anaesth 1998; 8:131–134.

307. Nichols DG, Yaster M, Lynn AM, et al. Disposition and respiratory effects of intrathecal morphine in children. Anesthesiology 1993; 79:733–738.

308. Ambuel B, Hamlett KW, Marx CM, et al. Assessing distress in pediatric intensive care environments: the COMFORT Scale. J Pediatr Psychol 1992; 17:95–109.

309. Barrier G, Attia J, Mayer MN, et al. Measurement of postoperative pain and narcotic administration in infants using a new clinical scoring system. Intens Care Med 1989; 15:S37–S39.

310. Tarbell SE, Cohen IT, Marsh JL. The Toddler-Preschooler Postoperative Pain Scale: an observational scale for measuring postoperative pain in children aged 1–5. Preliminary report. Pain 1992; 50:273–280.

311. Manne S, Jacobsen PB, Redd W. Assessment of acute paediatric pain: do child self-report, parent ratings and nurse ratings measure the same phenomenon? Pain 1992; 48:45–52.

312. McGrath PJ, Finley GA, Ritchie J. Parent's roles in pain assessment and management. IASP Newsletter 1994; Mar-Apr:3–4.

313. Whaley L, Wong DL. Nursing care of infants and children. St Louis, MO Mosby; 1987.

314. Beyer J, Wells N. The assessment of pain in children. Pediatr Clin North Am 1989; 36:837–854.

315. Eland JM. Minimizing pain associated with prekindergarten intramuscular injections. Issues Comprehensive Paediatr Nurs 1981; 5:361–372.

316. Hester NO, Foster RL, Kristensen K. Measurement of pain in children: generalizability and validity of the Pain Ladder and Poker Chip Tool. In: Tyler DC, Krane EJ (eds).

317. Beyer JE, Aradine CR. Content validity of an instrument to measure young children's perception of the intensity of their pain. J Pediatr Nurs 1986; 1:386–395.

318. Aradine CR, Beyer JE, Tompkins JM. Children's pain perception, before and after analgesia. J Pediatr Nurs 1988; 3:11–23.

319. Scott J, Huskisson EC. Graphic representation of pain. Pain 1989; 2:175–184.

320. McGrath PJ, Seifert CE, Speechley KN, et al. A new analogue scale for assessing children's pain: an initial validation study. Pain 1996; 64:435–443.

321. Merkel S, Voepel-Lewis T, Shayevitz JR, et al. The FLACC: a behavioural scale for scoring post operative pain in young children. Pediatr Nurs 1997; 23:293–297.

322. Tesler MD, Savedra MC, Holzemer WL, et al. The word-graphic rating scale as a measure of children's and adolescents' pain intensity. Res Nurs Health 1991; 14:361–371.

323. Savedra MC, Tesler MD, Holzemer WL, Wilkie DJ, Ward JA. A testing tool to assess postoperative pediatric and adolescent pain. In Tyler DC, Krane EJ (eds). Pediatric pain: advances in pain research therapy, vol. 15. New York: Raven Press; 1990:79–84.

323a. Savedra MC, Holzemar WL, Teler MD, Wilkie DJ. Assessment of postoperative pain in children and adolescents using the adolescent pediatric pain tool. Nursing Research 1993; 42:5–9.

324. Anderson BJ. What we don't know about paracetamol in children. Paediatr Anaesth 1998; 8:451–460.

324a. Wilson JT, Brown DR, Bocchini JA et al. Efficacy, disposition and pharmacodynamics of aspirin, acetaminophen and choline salicylate in young febrile children. Therapeutic Drug Monit 1982; 4:147–180.

325. Watcha MF, Jones MB, Lagueruela RG, et al. Comparison of ketorolac and morphine as adjuvants during pediatric surgery. Anesthesiology 1992; 76:368–372.

326. Gillespie JA, Morton NS. Patient-controlled analgesia for children: a review. Paediatr Anaesth 1992; 2:51–59.

327. Busoni P. Anatomy. In: Saint-Maurice C, Schulte-Steinberg O, eds. Regional anaesthesia in children. Norwalk, CT: Appleton & Lange/Mediglobe; 1990:pp 16–25.

328. Uemura A, Yamashita M. A formula for determining the distance from the skin to the lumbar epidural space in infants and children. Paediatr Anaesth 1992; 2:305–307.

329. Murat I, Esteve C, Montay G, et al. Pharmacokinetics and cardiovascular effects of bupivacaine during epidural anaesthesia in children with Duchenne muscular dystrophy. Anesthesiology 1987; 67:249–252.

FURTHER READING

General

Anand KJS, Stevens BJ, McGrath PJ. Pain in Neonates 2nd edition. Vol 10 of Pain Research and Clinical Management. Amsterdam: Elsevier Science 2000.

McKenzie I et al. Manual of acute pain management in children. Churchill Livingstone 1997

Morton NS (ed). Acute paediatric pain management. London: WB Saunders 1998

Assessment of pain

Findley GA, McGrath PJ (eds). *Measurement of pain in infants and children.* Progress in Pain Research and Management volume 10. IASP Press: Seattle 1996

Morton NS. Pain assessment in children. Paediatr Anaesth 1997; 7: 267–272

Non-steroidal anti-inflammatory drugs and paracetamol

Romsing J, Walther-Larsen S. Peri-operative use of nonsteroidal anti-inflammatory drugs in children: analgesic efficacy and bleeding. Anaesthesia 1997; 52: 673–683

Opioids

Kart T, Christup LL, Rasmussen M. Recommended use of morphine in neonates, infants and children based on a literature review: part 1 – pharmacokinetics. Paediatr Anaesth 1997; 7: 5–11

Regional analgesia – general

Dalens B. Regional anesthesia in infants, children and adolescents. Lippincott, Williams & Wilkins 1995.

Peutrell JM, Mather SJ. A Handbook of Regional Anaesthesia for Babies and Children. Oxford: Oxford University Press 1996

Wulf H, Johr M (eds). Regional Anesthesia in Children. Ballière's Clinical Anesthesiology, volume 14. London: Baillière Tindall 2000.

Regional analgesia – epidural and subarachnoid blocks

Cook B, Doyle E. The use of additives to local anaesthetic solutions for caudal epidural blockade. Paediatr Anaesth 1996; 6:353-359.

Rowney DA, Doyle E. Epidural and subarachnoid blockade in children. Anaesthesia 1998; 53: 980–1001

CHAPTER 8

Examples of good practice

Jane M Peutrell, Kathy Wilkinson,
Anna-Maria Rollin

INTRODUCTION

Throughout this book, authors have discussed the published recommendations for a surgical service for children, suggested ways to implement them and given criteria for referral to a specialist hospital. In this chapter, several clinicians working in district or major acute hospitals describe how they examined the services provided in their own hospitals and then adapted and implemented the various recommendations to meet local needs and improve and develop anaesthetic and surgical services for children.

ORGANISATION
Achieving change and setting standards

Changing established practice is difficult, particularly if change involves staff from many departments. Practitioners may feel very threatened if the drive for change comes from one individual, such as the designated paediatric anaesthetist. A method used in some hospitals is for representatives from all specialties to discuss the service in a multidisciplinary working party or paediatric surgery forum.

> . . . for the benefit of our local population and in the spirit of enlightened self-interest, the Senior Medical Staff Committee established a Paediatric Surgery Committee to identify ways of improving the quality of our surgical services for children to meet

acceptable standards. The committee was multidisciplinary from the outset with representatives from all departments involved with children admitted for surgery. In particular, we included those clinicians likely to have a continuing paediatric practice if we successfully retained children's surgical services in our hospital.

(Epsom General Hospital)

In 1999, a group of interested clinicians from many specialties established the Paediatric Surgery Forum. Our aims are to represent children's needs within the hospital, review our current policies, examine relevant recommendations and publications, and plan the future provision of surgical services for children.

(Norfolk and Norwich Healthcare Trust)

Assessing current workload through audit is often an essential first step to inform decision-making.

In 1993, in response to the report of NCEPOD 1989 [National Confidential Enquiry into Perioperative Deaths], we audited children's surgical services in our hospital. We found we actually dealt with few very young children, and that when the total number was divided amongst the number of anaesthetists and surgeons involved, we realised the clinicians were probably not obtaining sufficient experience to maintain their skills. It was also apparent we were vulnerable and we were concerned one of the colleges would stop paediatric surgery in our hospital if we continued to practise as we had been.

(Epsom General Hospital)

One of the first tasks of the designated paediatric anaesthetist was to look at workload. We used the information system in theatre and stratified the data obtained over 6 months into four age groups (neonates, 1–12 months, 1–4 years, 4–16 years). We examined elective and emergency workload, the experience of the anaesthetist, and the type of surgery.

The results were interesting and reassuring. We anaesthetised 1100 children over the 6 months. All neonates and 90% of babies younger than 12 months were anaesthetised by consultants. The remainder, all having very minor surgery, were managed by senior specialist registrars.

We are fortunate to have an adequate workload to maintain the skills of a number of anaesthetists and have decided to share the workload amongst several colleagues rather than concentrate it on only one or two. We will continue to audit our workload regularly to ensure we have adequate continuing experience; to review the arrangements for emergency surgery; and identify changing patterns of work.

(Frenchay Hospital, Bristol)

The multidisciplinary working party can jointly review the national guidelines in the light of local circumstances and establish and publish policies and codes of practice for its hospital. For example:

The Paediatric Surgery Committee examined the published guidelines and standards, adopted some and adapted others to our local needs to produce a set of principles. These were accepted by the Senior Medical Staff Committee as the hospital standard.

(Epsom General Hospital)

We have agreed guidelines for surgery that are appropriate for our hospital. Essentially, we are happy to manage children older than 1 year, with no significant anaesthetic or medical risks, who are not expected to need intensive or high-dependency care after surgery.

(Barnsley District General Hospital)

We have published a strict code of practice for surgery and anaesthesia in children. This gives guidance for the minimum age of the child, the seniority of the attending doctors, experience and availability of other staff in theatre and on the wards (e.g. registered sick children's nurses (RSCNs)) and the availability of appropriate equipment and facilities. Consultant anaesthetists with regular paediatric experience directly supervise anaesthesia in all children younger than 5 years, and we expect the surgeons involved to have current paediatric skills and not to undertake occasional practice.

(Southend General Hospital)

Our hospital and departmental policy is for a consultant paediatric anaesthetist to be notified of every child younger than 10 years requiring surgery. A consultant is present for anaesthesia in children younger than 3 years. Children aged 3–5 years are cared for either by a consultant or post-fellowship registrar.

(Norfolk and Norwich Healthcare Trust)

We published a policy document that has been widely distributed. Amongst other things, it specifies that all children younger than 5 years of age should be anaesthetised by consultants, and children should only have surgery later than 10 p.m. if life or limb is threatened.

(Musgrove Park, Taunton)

The competence of the surgical service provided for children may vary from time to time because of leave and the consultant cover available out of hours. Whether surgery can be provided safely in the local hospital will also be determined by the complexity of surgery and the medical condition of the child. Local guidelines can be sensitive to this variability of 'competence', as shown, for example in Figure 8.1.

However, local guidelines should not be so proscriptive that they prevent appropriate management of a child with a life-threatening condition.

We included in our 'house rules' the essential proviso that in a life-threatening emergency, a child should be anaesthetised by the most senior appropriately experienced anaesthetist available.

(Epsom General Hospital)

THE ROLE OF THE NOMINATED CONSULTANT FOR PAEDIATRIC ANAESTHESIA

Several bodies recommend that district hospitals admitting children for surgery should have named consultants in anaesthesia and the relevant surgical specialties responsible for leading children's services (see Ch. 1). Many hospitals have adopted this recommendation, although the specific role of the nominated individual depends on local circumstances. In some small hospitals, the lead consultant for anaesthesia provides most of the clinical service, including some cover out of hours:

The department has one 'designated paediatric anaesthetist' who anaesthetises all babies younger than 6 months and who is involved with many of the children less than 3 years of age. The designated paediatric anaesthetist is available 'out of hours' to assist with resuscitation or anaesthesia for children when requested to by colleagues. These arrangements allow the designated anaesthetist to meet 'Lunn's criteria' for adequate clinical practice.

(Dumfries & Galloway Royal Infirmary)

However, this arrangement can be onerous and leave a shortfall in cover when the individual is away. More commonly, the named anaesthetist organises and coordinates the

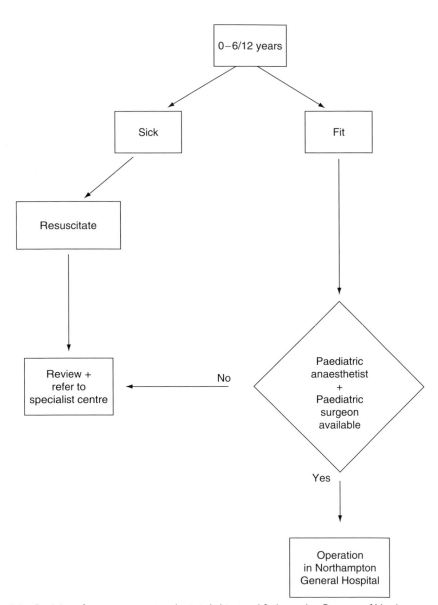

Fig. 8.1a Guidelines for emergency anaesthesia in babies aged 0–6 months. Courtesy of Northampton General Hospital.

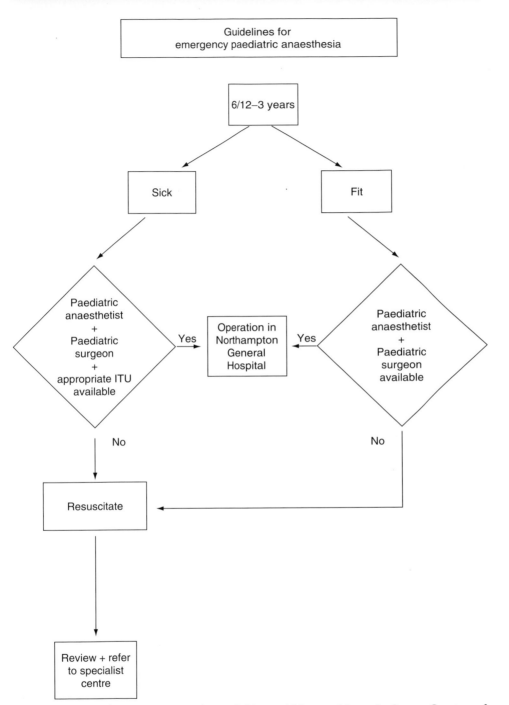

Fig. 8.1b Guidelines for emergency anaesthesia in babies or children aged 6 months–3 years. Courtesy of Northampton General Hospital.

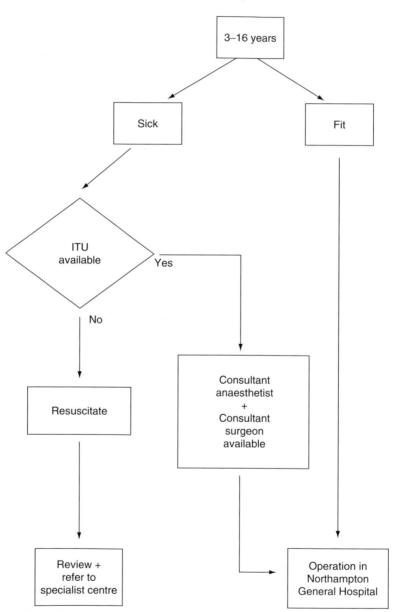

Fig. 8.1c Guidelines for emergency anaesthesia in children aged 3–16 years. Courtesy of Northampton General Hospital.

paediatric service but shares clinical responsibilities with a number of colleagues. For example:

The 'lead clinician for children':

- has authority to speak on behalf of the members of the anaesthetic group to effect change;
- is allowed to attend the divisional meetings of other specialties so that the anaesthetic service can respond (if appropriate) to the needs of other services;
- is recognised by all as responsible for organising the anaesthetic service for children.

(South Tees Acute Hospitals NHS Trust)

The lead anaesthetist also commonly provides clinical and educational support to colleagues:

The designated anaesthetist also acts as a source of support for his or her colleagues. We tried to create an atmosphere in which consultants were able to admit they needed help and would request assistance anaesthetising children.

(Barnsley District General Hospital)

STAFFING
Consultants
General considerations

It is no longer acceptable for babies and children to be cared for by clinicians who have neither adequate training nor sufficient continuing clinical experience. Several professional bodies have made recommendations for the specialist training and minimum clinical case load of those surgeons or anaesthetists managing babies and children (see Ch. 1) and many district hospitals have successfully adopted these. For example:

Anaesthetists caring for children younger than 3 years of age must either have a minimum of one operating list of children each week or anaesthetise at least 12 babies < 6 months, 50 children < 3 years, and 300 children < 10 years. This information should be recorded and regularly reviewed.

(Southend General Hospital)

As part of the review of clinical services, it is essential to identify clinicians fulfilling the criteria for adequate training and determine the number for whom the paediatric case load within the hospital will provide sufficient continuing experience.

An audit showed that we had enough cases to ensure adequate clinical experience for four anaesthetists to maintain their skills managing children. One of these nominated paediatric anaesthetists can be contacted at any time.

(Barnsley District General Hospital)

As a department, we agreed to provide a team of three anaesthetists to anaesthetise all babies younger than 12 months of age. These three also cover the majority of elective lists for children, especially for the more challenging general surgical or orthopaedic operations (including scoliosis surgery).

(Musgrove Park Hospital, Taunton)

However, it can be difficult to persuade colleagues to relinquish what is often a very enjoyable part of their practice.

We (the Paediatric Surgery Committee) then examined details. For example, we adopted the national guidelines for appropriate training and continuing experience (approximately one half-day of paediatric practice per week). These were our greatest stumbling blocks. Clinicians who had practised 'occasional' paediatric surgery or anaesthesia for decades were reluctant to stop. It took considerable pressure from peers (mainly through the Senior Medical Staff Committee) to establish these principles – and we did include a 'grandfather clause' so clinicians close to retirement were not compelled to change their patterns of work.

(Epsom General Hospital)

Clinicians working in a small hospital may also not acquire sufficient experience locally to comply with all aspects of the recommended case load or may feel professionally isolated. To remedy these problems, some practitioners obtain further experience by arranging regular clinical attachments to specialist centres.

The designated paediatric anaesthetist takes up to 1 week (as a block) each year to work in different specialist children's hospitals to increase his experience of managing babies or children having major operations.

(Dumfries & Galloway Royal Infirmary)

Alternatively, and particularly in larger hospitals which are within commuting distance from the referral centre, a 'hub-and-spoke' model has been adopted (see Ch. 1).

Three weeks out of four the 'local' general surgeon with an interest in children runs a paediatric clinic and operates on children. During the fourth week the clinic and operating list are run by a specialist paediatric surgeon from the nearest teaching hospital in conjunction with the 'local' surgeon. General practitioners may refer children to the clinic they deem most suitable and cross-referral between the two specialists is common. This 'hub-and-spoke' model has proved beneficial to patients, their parents, consultants and trainees.

(Epsom General Hospital)

Orthopaedic and ear, nose and throat surgeons have been jointly appointed to our district general and the specialist paediatric hospitals. These surgeons can see children in their outpatients clinic here and, depending on the complexity of the surgery, age of the child or their medical condition, can plan surgery for either the specialist or district hospital.

(Barnsley District General Hospital)

Cover for emergency surgery and resuscitation

It is important to determine, well in advance, exactly what procedures can be done locally and which children should be transferred for treatment by liaising closely with the hospital providing tertiary care.

We have established strong anaesthetic and surgical links with our nearest specialist children's hospital so we can have sensible discussions with colleagues there about the management of children needing emergency operations.

(Barnsley District General Hospital)

Clinicians providing cover out of hours should also meet the accepted standards. In a large hospital, a separate on-call rota may be possible.

We have two lead consultants for paediatric anaesthesia who, along with four other anaesthetists with training in paediatric anaesthesia, provide anaesthetic cover at all times for children and babies. This includes providing support to the paediatric

high-dependency unit and helping colleagues to manage children in casualty or the intensive care unit.
(Derriford Hospital, Plymouth)

A separate rota for paediatric anaesthesia/surgery may not be feasible within smaller hospitals. A less satisfactory arrangement is to offer all emergency work in babies or children to the designated anaesthetist (or surgeon), as described above. However, outside specialist centres, very few babies or small children require surgery that is so urgent it cannot be scheduled within normal hours when the paedatric team is available. If the out-of-hours workload is actually very small, then local informal arrangements may be adequate.

[From a review of the paediatric workload we found] the number of emergencies occurring out of hours approximated to one each week and we have established an informal rota to cover this.
(Frenchay Hospital, Bristol)

With a small department, we don't have a separate rota for emergencies occurring out of hours, but we have an informal 'shadow on-call', that seems to work well.
(Barnsley District General Hospital)

If, at any time, the local hospital is unable to provide a service that meets recommended standards, then all babies and children younger than 3 years of age needing surgery should either be transferred to one which can, or have their surgery delayed (if possible) until the criteria can be met, assuming this can be achieved within an acceptable time. However, staff at the local hospital must be able to resuscitate and stabilise any sick child competently before transfer. As for their surgical services, many respondents have examined and then established or improved their hospital facilities for resuscitating and stabilising sick babies and children.

We have built a resuscitation area adjacent to the intensive care unit, specifically for babies and children. Here we can resuscitate and stabilise children and initiate intensive care in a purpose-built and properly equipped facility before transfer elsewhere.
(Barnsley District General Hospital)

Maintaining the skill of other colleagues

Unfortunately, concentrating all paediatric anaesthetic experience in very few hands can cause problems managing acutely sick babies or children who present to small district general hospitals out of hours, particularly if there is only one children's anaesthetist.

Having only one designated paediatric anaesthetist in a small district hospital raises the problem about what to do when he or she is away. Resuscitation is very frightening for a practitioner who is not allowed (because of the various recommendations) to anaesthetise healthy children electively.
(Dumfries & Galloway Royal Infirmary)

However, it is possible for other clinicians to maintain their abilities to resuscitate and stabilise sick babies and children either by joining colleagues' routine lists or undertaking specific training in resuscitation.

To maintain skills, the designated paediatric anaesthetist commonly joins colleagues to manage babies or children with more complex problems.
(South Tees Acute Hospitals NHS Trust)

Whenever possible, young or ill children are anaesthetised jointly by the designated paediatric anaesthetist and his consultant colleague (see Fig. 8.2) in an attempt to maintain the skills of everybody. If the designated paediatric anaesthetist is unavailable to resuscitate a sick child, a colleague who has completed a PALS [Paediatric Advanced Life Support] or APLS [Advanced Paediatric Life Support] is asked for help.

(Dumfries & Galloway Royal Infirmary)

All consultants and doctors in non-training grades are encouraged to complete an APLS course.

(Barnsley District General Hospital)

Half of the anaesthetic consultants and all the RTOs [resuscitation training officers] have attended PALS or APLS courses. The designated paediatric anaesthetist and RTOs regularly teach paediatric resuscitation to staff in our hospital.

(Dumfries & Galloway Royal Infirmary)

Doctors in training

Trainees in schools of anaesthesia based on the larger, major acute hospitals sometimes obtain all their senior house officer and specialist registrar experience in paediatrics within their base hospital, rather than in a specialist children's hospital. It is important that clinical resources are used efficiently to provide effective training. For example:

Scheduling children on specific lists has enabled us to provide better training, including a paediatric module for registrars.

(Musgrove Park, Taunton)

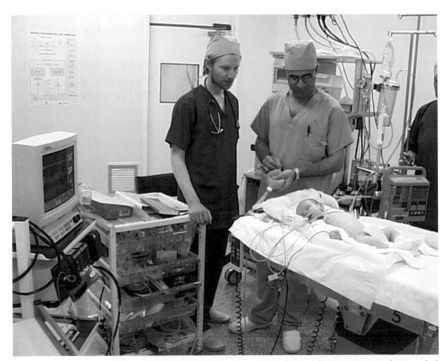

Fig. 8.2 The designated paediatric anaesthetist (left) assists a consultant colleague to anaesthetise a baby. Note the paediatric anaesthetic cart. Courtesy of Dumfries and Galloway Royal Infirmary.

We devised a 3-month module for specialist registrars. Before starting, trainees complete a questionnaire with which we assess their experience. We then tailor the module to the individual trainee's needs. We developed packs for teaching in theatre and a syllabus of core topics. During the attachment, each trainee is expected to complete an appropriate project.
(*Derriford Hospital, Plymouth*)

Many trainees work in several hospitals within a region and it is helpful to them to have consistent clinical guidelines and policies and coordinated training across the region.

We have a consultant nominated as 'paediatric trainer' who attends regular meetings at our regional centre (Great Ormond Street) along with representatives from other anaesthetic departments in the region to formulate regional policies and guidelines for clinical practice. These recommendations facilitate change locally and provide a consistent approach throughout the region.

The group also coordinates training in paediatric anaesthesia. Trainees benefit from having the same policies within all the hospitals in which they work and clinical attachments are coordinated to provide adequate experience in this important aspect of clinical practice.
(*Southend General Hospital*)

Other staff

Anaesthetists and surgeons provide only part of the surgical service, with other staff significantly influencing its quality and standards. All other staff within theatre (such as anaesthetic assistants and recovery nurses) involved in the management of babies and children should have specific training in the paediatric aspects of anaesthesia and recovery (including resuscitation) and adequate clinical experience (see Ch. 1). This is particularly important in the care of the youngest patients.

Anaesthetic assistance for a baby is provided by senior ODPs [operating department practitioners] who are trained PALS providers. The paediatric theatre team is led by an RSCN and four others provide cover for the children's recovery ward.
(*Norfolk and Norwich Healthcare Trust*)

Theatre and recovery nurses, operating department practitioners and ancillary staff with training or a special interest in paediatrics were encouraged to develop their skills, and so form a 'paediatric team'.
(*Epsom General Hospital*)

Although there are no specific qualifications for nurses or ODPs in 'children's theatre', they can develop their skills by a combination of formal courses, particularly in resuscitation (e.g. paediatric life support (PLS), PALS, APLS), clinical attachments to specialist centres and in-house training.

All RSCNs and ODA/Ps working in the day unit are trained in PLS.
(*Barnsley District General Hospital*)

We have established a formal training programme in paediatric resuscitation for senior nurses in intensive care, paediatric wards, accident and emergency departments. We encourage junior nurses and theatre staff to attend one-day PLS courses. We run three PALS courses 'in house' each year.
(*Barnsley District General Hospital*)

The Trust allows a couple of anaesthetic or recovery nurses to accompany the designated paediatric anaesthetist for his 1-week visit each year to different specialist children's hospitals.

(Dumfries & Galloway Royal Infirmary)

We place a high priority on training and education. We run PLS courses regularly and encourage theatre and ward staff to attend. The department has funded some staff to attend relevant external courses, such as APLS courses or the Annual Paediatric Anaesthesia Update in Manchester. This is important for staff education and morale and to disseminate new ideas and information.

(Derriford Hospital, Plymouth)

RUNNING THE CLINICAL SERVICE
Operating department facilities

Staff in many hospitals have attempted to improve the quality – and particularly the safety – of the services for babies and children. Rationalising surgery for children on few sites concentrates resources, enabling the smaller number of staff to obtain sufficient continuing experience.

Until recently, children and babies were operated on in one of four units. Two of these had no nurses or operating department assistants trained in paediatrics and dealt with few children each year. We have now limited surgery to one of two sites: a day-surgery unit with special facilities for children (including a children's waiting area suitably equipped and recently redecorated in primary colours) and main theatres. In this way we are able to concentrate resources and expertise and provide a service of quality.

(Derriford Hospital, Plymouth)

Many official bodies and professional groups advocate having special facilities for children separate from adults (see Ch. 1). Some larger hospitals manage sufficient numbers of children to justify a dedicated theatre which can be fully equipped specifically for paediatric surgery.

Most children have surgery in dedicated paediatric theatres with a 'child-friendly' induction area. The theatre is equipped to a high standard with an efficient, independent heating system, appropriate monitoring and equipment.

(Norfolk and Norwich Healthcare Trust)

Ensuring the emergency theatre is also of an adequate standard for paediatric surgery allows emergency operations in babies or children at any time.

Emergency operations take place in our 24-hour emergency theatre which we have recently upgraded to the standard of the paediatric theatre. This enables us to do emergency operations in children without interrupting elective lists.

(Norfolk and Norwich Healthcare Trust)

Having a dedicated paediatric theatre is not feasible everywhere, and there is often a balance between the requirements of specialist surgeons (e.g. for an ophthalmic microscope) and the need to provide adequate facilities for babies and children. A popular solution is to equip several trolleys or carts that can be taken to wherever children are anaesthetised. This is particularly useful when providing anaesthesia in remote sites, such as in the radiology department.

We have organised standardised trolleys with all the equipment required for babies and children. They also each contain a paediatric formulary and protocols and algorithms for the management of pain, treatment of anaesthetic emergencies (e.g. anaphylaxis) and for the resuscitation of babies and children. Uniform equipment and information is therefore wherever babies and children are anaesthetised.

(Derriford Hospital, Plymouth)

We developed a 'paediatric cart' (see Fig. 8.2) containing everything from masks, tubes and laryngoscopes to peripheral and central venous cannulae to use in the operating theatre, recovery and the resuscitation room in casualty.

(Dumfries & Galloway Royal Infirmary)

A similar cart or trolley can be used to house standardised rescucitation equipment for children.

We have standardised resuscitation equipment for children in special trolleys throughout the Accident and Emergency department, wards and theatres. This equipment is housed in special trolleys, which also contain Broselow tapes and intraosseous needles.

(Dumfries & Galloway Royal Infirmary)

Other facilities within theatre, including reception and recovery, should also be provided specifically for children of *all* ages, including adolescents.

Until recently, children waited in a small reception area in the theatre complex alongside adults. They lay on hospital trolleys, dressed in theatre gowns with only a few books and posters for entertainment. In 1998, we opened a completely separate waiting room for children with adjacent changing facilities situated opposite the entrance to main theatre. The play room is brightly decorated and well stocked with toys, games and other distractions for children and young people aged 1 to 16 years of age (Fig. 8.3). It is staffed by a play specialist. The children remain in their

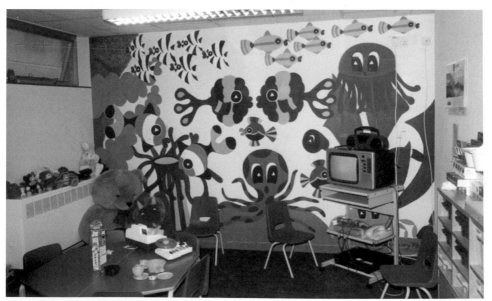

Fig. 8.3 The children's waiting room in the main theatre complex of Derriford Hospital, Plymouth. Courtesy of Derriford Hospital, Plymouth.

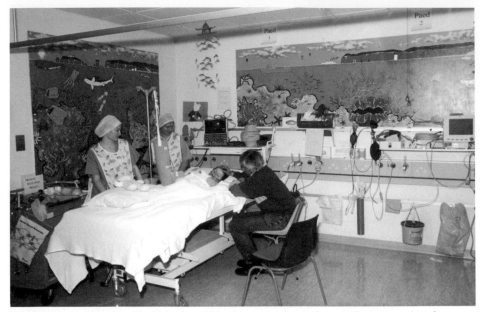

Fig. 8.4 A parent comforts his child in the children's recovery bay in the main theatre complex of Derriford Hospital, Plymouth. Note the paediatric resuscitation trolley (left), and the child-friendly decorations. Courtesy of Derriford Hospital, Plymouth.

own clothes until immediately before surgery and many 'drive' themselves to the atre in a special electric car.

> *(Derriford Hospital, Plymouth)*

Clinical areas, such as the recovery ward, should be fully equipped specifically for children (Fig. 8.4) but can be made 'child-friendly' with appropriate decorations, e.g. the Norfolk and Norwich hippopotamus (Fig. 8.5).

> We transformed a partitioned area of recovery using murals, decorative curtains and mobiles to make it more suitable for children (Fig. 8.4). Recovery staff wear coordinated aprons.
>
> *(Derriford Hospital, Plymouth)*

Some hospitals also provide facilities especially for parents:

> Using charitable funds, we have furbished a private area for parents within the hospital canteen. This is adjacent to the recovery ward to which it is linked by phone.
>
> *(Norfolk and Norwich Healthcare Trust)*

Scheduling of surgery

Despite earlier opposition from some surgical or anaesthetic colleagues, many departments now successfully schedule children for elective surgery on specific paediatrics lists within each specialty.

> I had long argued that we should have dedicated children's lists but had been thwarted by several surgeons who continued to 'dabble' in the more straightforward procedures for children and were resistant to change. However, the situa-

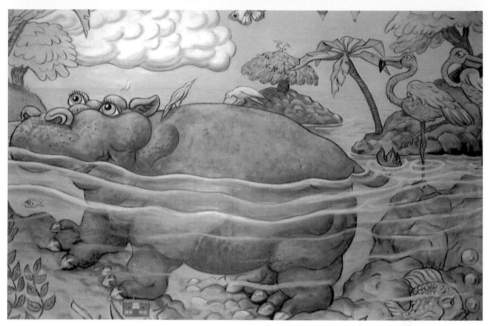

Fig. 8.5 The Norfolk and Norwich hippopotamus. Courtesy of Norfolk and Norwich Healthcare Trust.

tion has improved more recently with appointments of new consultants. The paediatric orthopaedic surgeon established dedicated paediatric lists, and the paediatric general surgeon has greatly developed the general surgical service for children. With the decision by the urologists that only one surgeon would operate on children, we now have a situation where all children having general or urological surgery are anaesthetised by myself (the designated paediatric anaesthetist).
(Musgrove Park, Taunton)

However, it is often more difficult to organise non-elective but urgent work in a similar way. One solution is to have an 'urgent children's list' every week on to which surgeons or other clinicians can book babies or children needing urgent investigations or treatment (e.g. imaging, bone marrow aspirates).

For some children needing certain investigations or procedures, a regular, fixed commitment by an anaesthetist was not appropriate because of inadequate numbers of children within each specialty. A flexible anaesthetic session was established on which cases are booked as required. Cases include semielective procedures (e.g. endoscopies, injection of joints in children with juvenile arthritis, radiological investigations, bone marrow aspiration) or more urgent operations (e.g. inguinal hernia repairs in babies, cryotherapy for retinopathy of prematurity).
(South Tees Acute Hospitals NHS Trust)

Working in teams

Many of our contributors stressed the importance of team working in developing services, improving quality and providing feedback.

The most major surgery here is orthopaedic. The orthopaedic surgeon and I (as the 'designated paediatric anaesthetist') have built this practice slowly as we gained

each other's confidence and the ward and theatre staff became appropriately trained. We only operate on these cases if we are both available.
(Dumfries & Galloway Royal Infirmary)

By working with a small dedicated group of nurses, we all know what each member of the team is capable of, and I (as the designated paediatric anaesthetist) get excellent feedback about quality of blocks or efficacy of analgesia, for example. It has also enabled me to organise and carry out research with their full cooperation.
(Musgrave Park, Taunton)

Postoperative pain relief

Many techniques used in adults can be adapted safely for children.

We have introduced several analgesic techniques that are new to our hospital (for children). These include Entonox, subcutaneous opioid analgesia and PCA [patient-controlled analgesia] with hand-sets specifically designed for children. We have recently written a comprehensive booklet giving advice to staff on managing pain in children.
(Barnsley District General Hospital)

Improving analgesia for one group of children may improve the quality of pain relief for others. For example:

For major orthopaedic surgery, we use lumbar epidurals intraoperatively and PCA or NCA [nurse-controlled analgesia] postoperatively. These developments have improved the care of other children. For example, femoral nerve block for children with fractured femur and PCA or NCA for analgesia after appendicectomy are now routine techniques. We have 'banned' intramuscular opioids. This required considerable effort but it has been very satisfying to observe the improvements over the last few years.
(Dumfries & Galloway Royal Infirmary)

It is unlikely that a hospital, other than specialist children's hospital, will provide a dedicated paediatric pain team, but it is possible to provide a good service if well organised. However, babies and children have many important differences compared with adults that are relevant to the management of their pain and those involved in their care must understand these differences. Many district hospitals have therefore developed a multidisciplinary approach, with individual clinicians and nurses bringing their particular expertise to the overall care of children.

A paediatric pain group was set up consisting of representatives from the paediatric and anaesthetic consultants, the acute pain team, paediatric nurses, pharmacy staff, and from departments usually dealing with adults (e.g. accident and emergency, outpatients, recovery). The aim of this group was to provide consistent and effective pain relief for children by improving communication and organising better training.
(King's Mill Centre, Sutton-in-Ashfield)

We have established a multidisciplinary pain group of paediatricians, anaesthetists, the paediatric pharmacist, staff from the accident and emergency department, and nurses from many areas of the hospital, including dermatology and radiology (two 'forgotten' places for children). The group is led by an extremely committed paediatrician. We meet monthly and coordinate all pain management for children throughout the hospital.
(Barnsley District General Hospital)

A good arrangement for the nursing aspects of care is to identify an RSCN on each paediatric ward who is enthusiastic and interested in pain relief, to work in liaison with the acute pain nurse as a link nurse.

> We have established a network of link nurses with specific responsibilities for managing pain in children and introduced new observation charts on which pain scores are recorded routinely.
> *(South Tees Acute Hospitals NHS Trust)*

> The Acute Pain Nurse Specialist has a network of 'link nurses', one on each ward. They take a lead in education at ward level, trouble-shooting simple problems and providing feedback to the Pain Group. This has proved far more effective than organising formal 'study days' for which attendance can be difficult.
> *(King's Mill Centre, Sutton-in-Ashfield)*

Providing good pain relief to children can be particularly difficult if the junior surgical staff rotate frequently and are more used to adult practice. Many contributors have found that either introducing simple guidelines or providing information booklets, which are widely available for reference, can lead to a huge improvement.

> We had a problem with the prescription of analgesics, partly due to the large number of 'transient' surgical trainees with mainly adult practice. We devised 'The Paediatric Analgesia Ladder', which demonstrates a stepwise approach to analgesia, together with appropriate doses. The 'Ladder' is displayed on a laminated yellow card on the walls of all departments involved with children, providing a useful reference for nursing or medical staff.
> *(King's Mill Centre, Sutton-in-Ashfield)*

> The designated paediatric anaesthetist and other members of the acute pain team have written a local guide to managing, and introduced a credit card-sized tool for assessing, pain in children. The acute pain team includes the children's wards on its rounds.
> *(Dumfries & Galloway Royal Infirmary)*

Information

Adequate written information was one of the recommendations of the Audit Commission in its report *Children First: A Study of Hospital Services* (see Ch. 1). Many hospitals run preadmission programmes (Fig. 8.6) to inform children and their parents about what to expect during admission for surgery. These often include discussion, guided tours, videos and information booklets (Fig. 8.7a-c).

> We run a 'Saturday club' (Fig. 8.8) in the Children's Day Ward for parents and children to attend before planned surgery at which we show a well produced video of a child being admitted to hospital and induced for anaesthesia. There is also a chance to use some of the equipment.
> *(Norfolk and Norwich Healthcare Trust)*

> We have sessions for preoperative preparation and have designed our own story book and video about admission to hospital. We have a theme (Hampton Hog, the Northampton hedgehog) running throughout the preparation sessions and admission to hospital, including pictures of the hedgehog on the walls which the child can follow from the ward to theatre.
> *(Northampton General Hospital NHS Trust)*

Fig. 8.6 The Saturday get-together. Courtesy of the Children's Hospital, Lewisham.

SATURDAY GET TOGETHER

FOR YOU AND YOUR FAMILY

A HOSPITAL ADMISSION IS A STRESSFUL TIME FOR YOU AND YOUR CHILD.

TO HELP YOU OVERCOME THIS WE WOULD LIKE TO INVITE YOU TO A PRE-ADMISSION TALK AND A TOUR OF THE UNIT.

THIS WILL GIVE YOU THE OPPORTUNITY TO ASK ANY QUESTIONS YOU MAY BE CONCERNED ABOUT.

THE VISIT STARTS AT 9.30 A.M. <u>PROMPT</u> AND LASTS APPROXIMATELY 1.1/2 HOURS.

WE MEET ON THE DAY CARE WARD, WHICH IS ON THE SECOND FLOOR OF THE "A" BLOCK.

SOME COMMENTS WE HAVE RECEIVED.

"COMING ON SATURDAY REALLY HELPED US. I COULD ASK THE QUESTIONS THAT I FORGOT ABOUT IN THE OUTPATIENTS DEPARTMENT"

"IT WAS NICE TO SEE WHERE THE WARD WAS AND TO FIND OUT THE ROUTINE OF OP DAY"

WELCOME TO FRANCES WARD

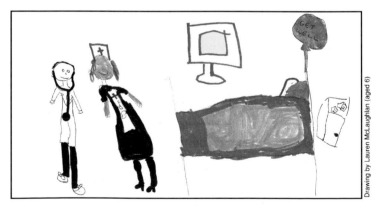

Drawing by Lauren McLaughlan (aged 6)

FAMILY INFORMATION

Fig. 8.7a The Jenny Lind information booklet for children admitted to the Frances Ward, Norfolk and Norwich Healthcare Trust. Courtesy of Norfolk and Norwich Healthcare Trust.

INTRODUCTION

As you will be aware, your child is to be admitted for the day to Frances Ward. Our aim is to create a friendly informal atmosphere and we hope that your short time on the ward will be as pleasant as possible. We are sure there will be many questions that you and your child have about coming into hospital and this leaflet aims to answer these.

If after reading this you still have any queries, do not hesitate to contact the ward between the hours of 7am - 7pm Monday to Friday.
Telephone: 01603 287170

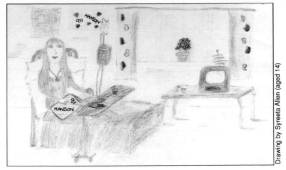

Drawing by Syreeta Allen (aged 14)

Preparation for the day - Preparing your child

It is important that children of all ages are well prepared before coming into hospital. Keep explanations to your child simple but honest.

Reassure your child that you will be with them all the time during their stay, except during their "special sleep" (anaesthetic) if they are being admitted for an operation.

You and your child are encouraged to come to "Saturday Club" a week or so before your admission date. It lasts for approximately 90 minutes on a Saturday morning and is designed to overcome fears and anxieties for all concerned prior to admission. You will find an invitation for your child and family with this leaflet.

Playing hospital games and reading stories will also help younger children to prepare for a hospital visit. Your local library should be able to help you find some suitable books.

Fig. 8.7b The Jenny Lind information booklet for children admitted to the Frances Ward, Norfolk and Norwich Healthcare Trust. Courtesy of Norfolk and Norwich Healthcare Trust.

Eating and drinking before an operation or medical procedure

Morning operations:
No food or milk after midnight / bedtime
A drink of squash or water before 6am

Afternoon operations:
A light breakfast (toast or cereal) before 8am with a drink of juice
Your child will be given a drink of squash or water before 11am
on the ward

IF YOUR CHILD IS UNDER 1 YEAR PLEASE RING THE WARD FOR INSTRUCTIONS REGARDING FEEDING

If your child is to have medical treatment or investigations, please ensure you are clear about any restrictions regarding eating or drinking. If you are unsure please telephone the ward.

What to do if your child becomes unwell

If your child develops a cold or is unwell before their admission date, please telephone the ward for advice. Contact your G.P. as usual if he or she needs medical attention.

Preparing yourselves!

Other Children - if you have other children, you will need to arrange for them to be looked after for the day. This may include arranging for them to be collected from school. If you are feeding a baby you are welcome to bring the baby (and feeds) with you.

Transport - you will need to arrange transport to and from the hospital. It is not suitable to use public transport for your journey home so you will need to have a car, a lift or a taxi.

Fig. 8.7c The Jenny Lind information booklet for children admitted to the Frances Ward, Norfolk and Norwich Healthcare Trust. Courtesy of Norfolk and Norwich Healthcare Trust.

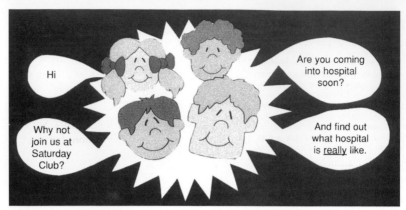

Fig. 8.8 Invitation cards to the Saturday club for children. Courtesy of Norfolk and Norwich Healthcare Trust.

Same-day admissions

Many hospitals are moving towards admitting children having inpatient surgery on the day of operation. This practice requires good communication between the staff involved in the child's care and adequate preoperative assessment and planning.

> Even those children staying in hospital after surgery are usually admitted on the day of their operations. If necessary, the anaesthetist can see a particular child for pre-operative assessment the week before.
> *(Norfolk and Norwich Healthcare Trusts)*

The day-surgery unit

Day surgery has developed enormously over the last decade. To comply with the recommendations for organising day surgery and to improve efficiency, it is better to admit children directly to the day unit, rather than the children's (inpatient) wards. However, this has major implications for the physical structure and facilities within the unit and staffing. Unless children are admitted for the majority of sessions during the week, it is unlikely than the required number of RSCNs will be included in the complement of permanent staff working within the day-surgery unit. A reasonably flexible arrangement is to bring in appropriately qualified nurses from the children's wards to work with the day-surgery staff during children's operating sessions. For this to function efficiently, the paediatric work must be organised properly.

> . . . to comply with the recommended standards to have registered children's nurses on duty, we arranged for a team of nurses to be seconded from the children's (inpatient) wards whenever children are admitted for surgery. To make efficient use of these nurses, we have had to organise the operating lists more effectively. All surgeons wanting to operate on children were allocated specific paediatric lists and were not permitted to admit children at any other time. For the first time, we were able to allocate appropriately trained consultant anaesthetists to these lists.
> *(Musgrove Park, Taunton)*

The facilities within the day unit, as elsewhere, should comply with the published standards for a surgical service for children.

We realised the majority of children in the future would be admitted as day patients. The new day-surgery unit was built with an admission and preoperative holding area specifically for children. This is suitably decorated and equipped with toys, videos and other distractions. Children are anaesthetised in the anaesthetic room of the theatre nearest to this facility, which is decorated and equipped specially for children.

(Barnsley District General Hospital)

Admitting a child to hospital has considerable impact on the whole family. Some units are able to offer considerable flexibility in an attempt to reduce disruption, for example:

We stagger admissions to the day-surgery unit to minimise disruption to the child and family.

(Norfolk and Norwich Healthcare Trust)

Information for parents and children is essential for efficiency and safety. Preadmission programmes and information are often provided specifically for the day-surgery unit, where policies and practice are likely to differ from the inpatient wards. Establishing contact with children and their families well before surgery is likely to improve efficiency by reducing cancellations either because children are inadequately starved or inappropriately admitted (complex medical history, poor social circumstances) or allowing time to arrange admission of a substitute if one develops an intercurrent infection. Written information (especially about preoperative starvation) is particularly important, because parents have a lot to remember.

We send written information to children and their parents before the children are admitted to our day-surgery unit. We include a telephone number to ring if the parents need any more information or advice. We have found this particularly useful in the winter, when we ask parents to ring if their child develops a cold. This has significantly reduced late cancellations and avoids unnecessary trips to hospital.

(Barnsley District General Hospital)

The nurses organise 'preadmission parties' to inform children and their parents about what to expect.

(Musgrove Park, Taunton)

Adequate information for the postoperative care of children at home is vital. Follow-up, either by a home support nurse or telephone interview, provides support to parents, allaying their anxieties and giving feedback to clinicians and nurses involved in their children's care.

[The nurses] also phone the day after surgery to follow the children up and find out about their experiences.

(Musgrove Park, Taunton)

Advice about analgesia is particularly important because many children suffer significant pain after day surgery and parents are sometimes reluctant to give pain relief.

We provide free 'take-away' packs containing combinations of paracetamol, ibuprofen and codeine (depending on age and the anticipated severity of pain). We include clear instructions to try and avoid 'tears at bedtime'.

(Barnsley District General Hospital).

Index

Note: Page references in **bold** and *italics* refer to tables/boxed material and figures respectively.